Restoring the Brain

This thoroughly updated second edition of *Restoring the Brain* is the definitive book on the theory and the practice of infra-low frequency brain training. It provides a comprehensive look at the process of neurofeedback within the emerging field of neuromodulation and essential knowledge of functional neuroanatomy and neural dynamics to successfully restore brain function.

Integrating the latest research, this thoroughly revised edition focuses on current innovations in mechanisms-based training that are scalable and can be deployed at any stage of human development. Included in this edition are new chapters on clinical data and case studies for new applications; using neurofeedback for early childhood developmental disorders; integrating neurofeedback with psychotherapy; the impact of low-frequency neurofeedback on depression; the issue of trauma from war or abuse; and physical damage to the brain.

Practitioners and researchers in psychiatry, medicine, and behavioral health will gain a wealth of knowledge and tools for effectively using neurofeedback to recover and enhance the functional competence of the brain.

Hanno W. Kirk, PhD, LICSW, has been a lecturer/trainer for the past 40 years and is the principal author of *Psychosocial and Behavioral Aspects of Medicine*. After retiring from active college teaching and touring all-day seminars, he has been using neurofeedback since 2006 in his private practice in Lewisburg, WV. He has been a presenter at major national and international conferences on biofeedback and neurofeedback.

T0266844

Restoring the Brain

Neurofeedback as an Integrative Approach to Health

2nd Edition

Hanno W. Kirk

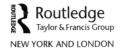

Routledge
Taylor & Francis Group

NEW YORK AND LONDON

Second Edition published 2020
by Routledge
52 Vanderbilt Avenue, New York, NY 10017

and by Routledge
2 Park Square, Milton Park, Abingdon, Oxon, OX14 4RN

Routledge is an imprint of the Taylor & Francis Group, an informa business

Library of Congress Cataloging-in-Publication Data
A catalog record for this title has been requested

ISBN: 9780367225858 (hbk)
ISBN: 9780367225865 (pbk)
ISBN: 9780429275760 (ebk)

Typeset in Gill Sans
by Swales & Willis, Exeter, Devon, UK

Brian Othmer (1968–1991)

This book is dedicated to the memory of Brian Othmer, whose struggles from early childhood with the behavioral consequences of temporal lobe epilepsy led to his and his parents' engagement with EEG neurofeedback, beginning in 1985. In his journal Brian writes of his commitment to making the benefits of neurofeedback more broadly available. With his life cut short due to a nocturnal seizure, that task fell to others. This book is part of Brian's legacy.

Contents

Foreword

It is a great pleasure to write a foreword to *Restoring the Brain: Neurofeedback as an Integrative Approach to Health*. In this successor to the earlier edition, an impressive roster of experts and practitioners provide an update of the developments in the field of neurofeedback. The new volume is a welcome, perhaps even necessary, addition to the growing literature in the vibrant and expanding field of neurofeedback. Its publication is a testament to the success of the original volume and to the growing interest in, and acceptance of, neurofeedback as a mainstream approach to the treatment of a wide range of neurological and psychiatric disorders. The international list of contributors to the volume further attests to the increasingly global embrace of neurofeedback as a viable treatment modality. The book is organized as a logical progression of three broad themes: History and theory; neurofeedback in clinical practice settings; and applications.

The first part, Development, History, and Theory of Neurofeedback, opens with a chapter by Hanno Kirk. Here a strong case is made in support of the thesis that the historically dominant neurochemical perspective is not the only window on brain function, and that the bioelectric perspective offers a different, equally important approach to understanding the complex processes in the brain. Consequently, psychopharmacology should not be regarded as the only therapeutic approach; and that, by implication, protocols aiming to modify the electric activity in large neuronal assemblies and networks offer a complementary or even alternative approach. This is followed by a chapter by Siegfried Othmer, with a cogent and incisive review of the history of neurofeedback from the original discovery of encephalogram by Hans Berger; to the foundational research by M. Barry Sterman; to the ever-expanding array of applications, including seizure disorders, ADHD, and others.

In a chapter by Siegfried Othmer and Sue Othmer, a case is made for the importance of infra-low frequency training (ILF), as well as for reconceptualization of standard models of neurofeedback. The relationship between the regulatory, developmental, and frequency hierarchies is discussed. The final chapter in this section, by David A. Kaiser, focuses on the importance of glial cells, particularly of astrocytes, as well as on the fact that these cells operate in the infra-low frequency range. In light of the ubiquitous presence of glia and its importance in multiple regulatory brain functions, this further strengthens the case for the infra-low frequency training.

The second part, Neurofeedback in Clinical Practice Settings, opens with a chapter by Meike Wiedemann. Here the evolution of clinical practice from the earlier standard protocols to the more individualized infra-low frequency training is discussed, as well as the ways of integrating various (both old and new) neurofeedback approaches into powerful composite treatment plans. In a chapter by Doreen MacMahon, the role of neurofeedback in integrative medical practice, dealing with a wide range of medical conditions, is discussed in relationship to medication efficacy, nutrition and other factors. The promise and efficacy of neurofeedback use in combination with psychotherapy and psychopharmacology is discussed in a chapter by Keerthy Sunder, which also includes two illustrative cases where neurofeedback proved to be effective: in Postpartum Bipolar Disorder and Severe Generalized Anxiety Disorder with Alcohol Dependence. Finally, Stella Legarda discusses the use of neurofeedback in neurology practice. Six distinct brain training protocols are described and the neurological conditions for which neurofeedback treatment has shown to be effective are listed.

In the third part, Specific Applications Areas of Neurofeedback, the use of neurofeedback in a range of specific disorders is discussed. In a chapter by Roxana Sasu, successful use of neurofeedback (particularly of the Othmer Method) is described in children and adolescents with ADHD, Autism Spectrum Disorder, and other conditions, some of which defy clear diagnosis in terms of existing taxonomies and are characterized by a range of cognitive and affective symptoms. A follow-up chapter, by Roxana Sasu and Siegfried Othmer, focuses on ADHD and the use of Continuous Performance tests of sustained attention in the assessment of neurofeedback treatment efficacy. In a chapter by Evvy Shapero and Joshua Prager, a multidisciplinary approach to chronic pain treatment is described. Here neurofeedback is a component of an eclectic treatment protocol which also includes pharmacology, psychotherapy, physical exercise, breathing exercises, and a range of other techniques.

In a chapter by Vera A. Grin-Yatsenko and Yuri Kropotov, the use of Infra-Low Frequency Neurofeedback in healthy and depressed individuals is described. In healthy controls the treatment resulted in the decrease of inner tension and increase on cognitive performance. In depressed patients the treatment resulted in dramatic improvement of mood and decrease in anxiety. In her chapter, Monica Dahl discusses the use of neurofeedback in the treatment of post-traumatic stress disorder (PTSD) and traumatic brain injury (TBI) in war veterans. The effect is both one of clinical symptom reduction and of the enhancement of multiple cognitive abilities and emotional states. Finally, the use of neurofeedback in the treatment of insomnia is described in a chapter by Terrence Moore. Here the basic concepts and underlying physiology of circadian rhythms and sleep–wake cycle, various approaches to the treatment of sleep disorders, and the efficacy of neurofeedback are discussed.

In the concluding chapter, The Future of Neurofeedback, Siegfried Othmer discusses the place of neurofeedback in the broader context of neuromodulatory approaches, whose ascendancy and proliferation we have witnessed during the last few decades. He predicts that as the field of neuromodulation in its various forms matures, a major bifurcation will take place into the methodologies of clear clinical utility and those holding out the promise of optimizing performance in healthy individuals.

On the whole, *Restoring the Brain* is a very impressive, highly competent, and thoughtful review and examination of the current state of neurofeedback, as well as its future. The book is a fitting tribute to the growing maturity and acceptance of neurofeedback in a wide range of clinical and non-clinical applications. The time of this exciting approach has come and the book is an eloquent tribute to it ascendancy.

Elkhonon Goldberg, Ph.D., ABPP
New York, 2019

Preface

For many years, neurofeedback (NF) was considered by many as a topic too soft to be taken seriously by science and medicine. This is still the case in some quarters, but increasingly mainstream science is turning an inquisitive gaze on NF as key objections are being resolved one after another. This fundamental shift did not come about because of what transpired in the neurofeedback field itself but rather from developments within the hard sciences, especially in neuroimaging, with demonstrations that not only key physiological measures, like heart rate, but also levels of brain activity (as measured by the BOLD signal) can be controlled through conscious effort or even sub-consciously. This naturally resulted in scientists from a variety of fields incorporating neurofeedback in their research by means of various neuroimaging techniques. Often this was done under labels such as neuromodulation or closed-loop brain training.

The neuroimaging findings had a profound effect within the neurofeedback field as well, particularly in the area of infra-low frequency (ILF) NF: neuroimaging furnished the missing evidence that key mechanisms related to health and disease are organized within the ILF regime. More importantly, they showed that accessing local variations (e.g. controlling activity of a well-circumscribed brain area) is not only possible but can be a vehicle for influencing global brain function. It then becomes plausible that using measures of global brain activity as the lever for altering brain function is not only possible but likely to be more effective than alternative methods because it operates on the wider system and not just on one (or more) nodes or hubs.

In addition, technical advances allowed new and more effective variants of the method, especially in the area of ILF NF. In summary, the surge of interest in NF has led to revolutionary new insights at levels of basic research, achieving new demonstrations of fundamental capabilities of controlling previously inaccessible aspects of our brain activity. Further, it has yielded practical implementations of new NF applications and theoretical insights about how NF may actually operate. Not all of these new insights have been communicated via scientific papers because the NF practice is primarily – often exclusively – aimed at delivering personalized service to satisfy the needs of each trainee. Such an approach is not readily amenable to the constraints imposed by formal research, in particular the need to repeat in an identical way a specific and unalterable protocol to obtain a statistically significant result for a narrowly defined population. The introduction of new methods, the proliferation of variants, and the individualization of training protocols accentuates the problem, leading to a progressive divergence of clinical practice from its roots in academic research.

The book divides into three main parts. The four chapters of the first part of the book cover not only the basic theory behind recent advances but also the relevant history. In the four chapters of the second part, NF is set in the context of integrative medical practice, the related clinical disciplines psychiatry and neurology. In the third and last part of the book, six chapters cover key applications, with some supported by summary results from thousands of cases. The last chapter of the book dares to venture into projecting the future at a time when technological maturity of the methods will lead to distinct applications, some with clear clinical objectives and others offering access to personalized and self-managed tools for maintaining optimum functioning status.

This second edition of *Restoring the Brain* arrives a mere five years after publication of the first edition. Given the combination of a growing interest and the new findings and data collected here, it comes none too soon. The book is a must for neurofeedback practitioners who wish to be up to date with developments in their field, for professionals entering the field, and for those wishing to investigate the claims. They must become aware of the arguments made by the dedicated scientist-practitioners who have driven the development. They have numerous successful applications of NF behind them that cannot yet be captured in high-impact papers because of their diversity and heterogeneity.

Prof Andreas A. Ioannides
Laboratory for Human Brain Dynamics, Nicosia
Cyprus, 2019

Notes on Editor and Contributors

Editor

Hanno W. Kirk, PhD, LICSW, has been a lecturer/trainer for the past 40 years. After retiring from active college teaching and touring all day seminars, he has been using neurofeedback since 2006 in his private practice in Lewisburg, WV. He has been a presenter at major national and international conferences on biofeedback and neurofeedback and he is principal author of *Psychosocial and Behavioral Aspects of Medicine.*

Contributors

Monica Dahl, EdD, is in private practice using neurofeedback with a special interest in veterans in Key West, FL. She developed a hypnotherapy training manual for the International Medical and Dental Hypnotherapy Association, for which she received Educator of the Year award. From 1985–1995 she taught Mind Power classes for human development and peak performance.

At the request of the US State Department she taught stress reduction for family members of staff at the American Interest Section in Havana, Cuba in 2003. For her doctorate in counseling psychology she used research on the effects of neurofeedback training for PTSD symptom reduction for her dissertation. As a volunteer member of the Homecoming4Veterans program, she provides pro bono neurofeedback training for service men and women.

Vera A. Grin-Yatsenko, PhD, MD, is a research scientist at the Institute of the Human Brain of the Russian Academy of Sciences. Over 25 years she has conducted clinical research and development in EEG, quantitative EEG, neurophysiological mechanisms of EEG-based biofeedback, event-related potentials (ERPs), and objective diagnosis of ADHD. She conducted EEG/qEEG research in depression, anxiety, attention disorders, and schizophrenia. Since 2013 her research has focused on how ILF neurofeedback impacts brain functionality in healthy subjects vs. mentally disordered individuals. She has published over 30 peer-reviewed journal articles, book chapters, abstracts, and papers. Her MD is from St. Petersburg State Pediatric Medical Academy, Russia, and her PhD from the Military Medical Academy, St. Petersburg.

David A. Kaiser, MFA, PhD, has 30 years' experience with EEG and neurotherapy. He was editor of the *Journal of Neurotherapy* for a decade, founder of the

American Neurotherapy Association, and currently trains professionals at Kaiser Academy in functional EEG and evidence-based neurotherapy. His research focuses on EEG neuromarkers of mental health problems, family neurodynamics, and perceptual relativity.

Prof. Juri Kropotov has been head of the research laboratory at Bechtereva Institute of the Human Brain of the Russian Academy of Sciences for 30 years. He developed the theory of action programming and models of realistic neuronal networks, and a methodology for assessing functional neuromarkers of the human brain, published as *Functional Neuromarkers for Psychiatry* (2016). He created an international database of event-related potentials (ERP), described in his book *Quantitative EEG: Event-related Potentials and Neurotherapy* (2009). For his ground-breaking research discoveries, he has been awarded prestigious awards and honorary degrees both in his home country as well as internationally. He is the author of 244 scientific papers, including 13 books published in Russian, German, Polish, and English.

Stella B. Legarda, MD, is a career neurologist-epileptologist who began incorporating clinical neurofeedback as part of her practice in 2010. She co-authored manuscripts published in peer-reviewed medical journals illustrating the value of infra-low frequency brain training in neurology practice. In 2013 Dr. Legarda was the first neurologist to join the specialty group practice Montage Medical Group in Monterey, CA, and over time three more neurologists have joined the revolutionary initiative there to improve neurological care by training brain behavior. Dr. Legarda is certified by the American Board of Clinical Neurophysiology and the American Board of Psychiatry and Neurology with special qualifications in child neurology and epilepsy.

Doreen McMahon, MD, currently practices EEG neurofeedback and integrative medicine at NOVA NeuroIntegrative Medicine in McLean, VA. Having received her neurofeedback training under the supervision of Sue Othmer, BCIAC, and Siegfried Othmer, PhD, she is certified in the Othmer Method of EEG neurofeedback. She is board certified in family medicine and a member of the American Academy of Family Physicians and Virginia Academy of Family Physicians. She is a graduate of the University of Maryland School of Medicine in Baltimore, MD.

P. Terrence Moore, MD, FAASM, received his MD from Tulane University School of Medicine in New Orleans. He is board certified in the specialties of neurology by the American Board of Psychiatry and Neurology and sleep medicine by both the American Board of Sleep Medicine and American Board of Psychiatry and Neurology. He is a fellow of the American Academy of Sleep Medicine, a member of the American Academy of Neurology and the medical director of two AASM accredited sleep centers in the Dallas area. He has trained with Sue Othmer, BCIAC, and Siegfried Othmer, PhD, two international leaders in the field of neurofeedback.

Siegfried Othmer, PhD, has been active in in all aspects of EEG neurofeedback: instrumentation development, professional training, clinical service delivery, clinical research, and publication in both professional and popular media along with his wife Susan. The Othmers have built a large practitioner network that now extends to over 50 countries around the world. Siegfried Othmer is the author of *ADD: The Twenty-Hour Solution* (with co-author Mark Steinberg) and *Brian's Legacy*, the remarkable story of their son who was struggling with epilepsy. Siegfried Othmer received his PhD in physics at Cornell University, Ithaca, NY, in 1970.

Sue Othmer, BCIAC, is clinical director of the EEG Institute in Woodland Hills, CA. She has been working clinically with neurofeedback. Since 1988 she has divided her time between doing clinical work, teaching professional courses on neuro-feedback, and developing new neurofeedback instrumentation and protocols. With scientific rigor she amassed reams of clinical data while developing the infra-low frequency approach to neurofeedback. She is author of *Neurofeedback Clinicians' Protocol Guide*, now in its seventh edition.

Joshua P. Prager, MD, directs a comprehensive interdisciplinary functional reha-bilitation program in Los Angeles dedicated to treatment of intractable pain. It specializes in complex regional pain syndrome, neuromodulation (the implantation of devices to control pain and movement disorders by implantation of devices in the nervous system). He has been on the full-time faculty at both Harvard Medical School and the David Geffen School of Medicine at UCLA. He has lectured inter-nationally and nationally and has won numerous awards from medical societies and patient organizations. Dr Prager is Harvard, Stanford, UCLA trained and holds board certifications in Internal Medicine, Anesthesiology, as well as in Pain Medicine.

Roxana Sasu, MD, RN, is part of the clinical staff and faculty of the EEG Insti-tute. She divides her time between clinical work and teaching professional training courses at the EEG Institute, CA, as well as in Europe. She is also part of the Insti-tute's ongoing research and data collection for improving the efficacy of neurofeed-back. Born in Brasov, Romania, she received her MD from Carol Davila Faculty for General Medicine and Pharmacy, Bucharest, Romania, in 1998. She also has a Mas-ter's in Marketing and Business Communication. In the US she is practicing under a Registered Nursing (RN) license.

Evvy J. Shapero, MA, is affiliated with the California Pain Medicine Center and has been providing neurofeedback for the Comprehensive, Multidisciplinary, Func-tional Rehabilitation Pain Program. As a faculty member at the EEG Institute, CA, she teaches Alpha-Theta to new clinicians. Evvy has a private practice in West LA, working with clients afflicted with chronic pain, anxiety, obsessive compulsive disor-der, ADD/ADHD, PTSD, migraines, sleep disorders, and panic disorder. She is also a certified clinical hypnotherapist. Her MA in Clinical Psychology is from Antioch University, CA.

Evvy is a co-founder of *Glamour Project*, a 501 (c) (3), dedicated to improving the lives of homeless women through kindness, compassion, and photography.

Keerthy Sunder, MD, is an integrative psychiatrist and Chief Medical Officer and Founder of Brain Tune, a Brain Optimization program in California. As a faculty member of the University of California at Riverside School of Medicine, CA, and a board member of the Academy of Integrative Health and Medicine, he is actively involved in training the next generation of clinicians to adopt neuromodulation and gut–brain optimization approaches for wellness across the life span. He is author of *Face your Addictions and Save your Life* and the creator of an online meditation program for health and wellness (www.tunemybrain.com). He is a diplomate of the British Royal College of Obstetricians and Gynecologists, American Board of Psychiatry and Neurology and American Board of Addiction Medicine.

Meike Wiedemann, PhD, is a neurobiologist and associate professor for membrane physiology at the University of Hohenheim, Germany. She led several projects on the effects of microgravity on the central nervous system for the German Space Agency (DLR) and the European Space Agency (ESA). She has a private neurofeedback practice in Stuttgart, Germany. She is head of the EEG Info teaching team for Europe and teaches the German version of ILF-Neurofeedback professional training courses.

Acknowledgments

The venture of creating a technical book with 16 different contributors writing on different aspects of neurofeedback requires close coordination and cooperation between editor and the writers. I was fortunate to have a group of individuals who were open and receptive to accepting guidance and editorial suggestions for changes. A special thank you goes to Siegfried Othmer, who in addition to writing or co-authoring three chapters and the Conclusion, went through all the chapters to check them for technical accuracy as well as congruence between chapters.

This book would not have been possible without the pioneering work of Sue Othmer and the clinicians at the EEG Institute. With infinite patience and assiduous clinical data collection, she ventured into unknown territory as she built upon the traditional EEG-band, fixed protocol, prescriptive model of neurofeedback and pioneered individualized endogenous neuromodulation. In 2006, Sue extended this approach into the infra-low frequency range. The thrust into this domain could not have been accomplished, however, without the technical innovations introduced by Bernhard Wandernoth of bee Medic. This evolutionary development became the prime mover for the first edition. Its revolutionary implications for clinical practice are the impetus for this second edition.

Thanks also goes to Devin Cardona, the graphic artist who took the illustrations submitted by the authors and put them into the format required by the publisher.

A note of appreciation goes to Nina Guttapalle, the Editor for Mental Health at Taylor & Francis who patiently guided me through the pre-production process. Similarly, a commendation goes to Daradi Patar, the Editorial Assistant, who took the manuscript and readied it for typesetting. A shout out also goes to Natalie Thompson who guided the manuscript through the final production process.

Introduction

Hanno W. Kirk

The most promising development in the nascent field of brain–computer interfaces is that of having the brain witness its own function directly. The brain then reacts in real time, to its own lasting benefit, by analogy to ordinary skill learning. Witnessing this process unfold allows it to be shaped to ever greater utility and clinical effectiveness for each person. Over its more than ten-year existence, the evolutionary development of this therapeutic method has taken us to the foundations of the regulatory hierarchy. Since brain function is organized on a frequency basis, this is also the bottom of the frequency hierarchy. The name for this process of endogenous neuromodulation is Infra-Low Frequency (ILF) Neurofeedback.

One of the motivations for producing this second edition is that since 2013, when we wrote the first edition, we have made giant strides in the conduct and understanding of infra-low frequency brain training. At that time we were aware of the efficacy of symptom-based training in the infra-low frequency domain but there was only a fuzzy understanding of why it was producing such consistent positive clinical improvements not only for target symptoms, but also global enhancement of brain functioning. The intensive collection and analysis of clinical data, as well as research by other "brain" scientists on slow cortical potentials (see Chapter 12), mean we now have a clear theoretical basis for how and why ILF brain training works so well. In Chapter 2, Siegfried Othmer recounts the clinical process of how we cautiously and incrementally came to use ever lower frequencies. In Chapter 3 he lays out the theoretical foundation for how and why ILF brain training works. Under the auspices of the clinical research team at the EEG Institute in Woodland Hills, California, as well as from hundreds of neurofeedback practitioners involving thousands of patients, reams of statistical data were collected and analyzed. Some of these data are presented in various chapters in this edition. In Chapter 4, David A. Kaiser adds to the justification of the theoretical explanation in his succinct description of the key role that astroglia play in the brain's regulatory regime and self-maintenance. These cells, which make up 90% of the volume of the brain, oscillate in the ultra-low frequency domain, thus giving scientific support to the theoretical basis for the effectiveness of infra-low frequency brain training.

Another new part of this second edition are chapters by clinicians describing their successful use of ILF Neurofeedback to new applications. In Chapter 8, a neurologist details the use of ILF Neurofeedback in remediating brain instabilities. Chapter 9 looks at how ILF can be used successfully for early developmental and childhood emotional and behavioral problems while Chapter 10 finds new hope in the use of ILF training for ADHD. Remediating chronic pain with ILF and Alpha-Theta training is the topic for Chapter 11. Two prominent Russian researchers then tell of their work using ILF for depression in Chapter 12, and this is followed in Chapter 13 by an unusual classic AB -AB- AB design case study of a veteran with

PTSD and brain trauma, comparing the effects of intermittent standard care at the Veterans Administration with periods of ILF and Alpha-Theta training. Finally, Chapter 14 looks at how ILF training can be used successfully for sleep and insomnia issues.

There are also chapters by medical doctors who relate how they have integrated ILF into their practice specialties, such as family practice (Chapter 6); psychiatry (Chapter 7); neurology (Chapter 8); pain management (Chapter 11); and sleep medicine (Chapter 14).

In the concluding chapter Siegfried Othmer looks at a future where neurofeedback is seen as an economically and temporally efficient way for both preventive as well as rehabilitative integrative care along the life span.

Part I

Development, History, and Theory of Neurofeedback

Chapter 1

Changing the Paradigm from Neurochemical to Neuroelectrical Models

Hanno W. Kirk

Communication patterns in the brain are mediated by chemical and electrical signals. Because of the enormous clinical and commercial potential of psychiatric medications thus far, only the chemical paradigm has received significant interest from the scientific community. The electric patterns in the brain have been almost entirely ignored.

Bessel A. van der Kolk,[1]
Author of the *Body Keeps the Score:*
Brain, Mind, and Body in the Healing of Trauma

1.1 The Early Days of Speculation

Our understanding of how the brain functions has changed dramatically over the centuries. Through much of time the heart was celebrated as the central locus of thought, emotions, and even the soul. The contents of the skull were regarded as an undifferentiated biomass. While an ancient Egyptian papyrus, attributed to a battlefield surgeon, noted that head trauma affected physical function, there was no anatomical knowledge of the brain. In the 1st century BC, Greek philosophers theorized that the brain was where the mind was located, and that it might be the seat of sensations. In the 2nd century AD, the great Roman physician and anatomist Galen used dissection and produced detailed hand-drawn maps of the brain and the spinal cord. Galen believed that soul and mind consisted of *pneumo*, or spirits emanating from the heart, and that the role of the brain was to ennoble these spirits in human beings. Galen's "hydraulic" view of spirits moving around the body like fluids was to dominate thinking into the Renaissance.[2]

The intensely curious Renaissance genius Leonardo da Vinci used anatomical dissection to study all parts of the body, including the brain. He left behind beautifully detailed and accurate anatomical drawings of the brain, including the cavities, or ventricles. Da Vinci's slight departure from the heart-centered spirits view was his belief that perception and cognition resided not in the brain "substance" itself, but in these cavities. Without modern tools, however, he and others could only speculate. A radical departure from this spirit-dominated view of the body came in the 17th century, when Rene Descartes declared that the mind and the body were distinct. This dualistic view has largely dominated Western medical thinking ever since. Even today it seems to inform how the brain is seen as an organ driven by biochemical actions, yet somehow separate from the myriad of mental activities sparked by electrical networks. Brain surgeons and neurologists look at neurological dysfunctions in terms of a physical pathology, but only minimally concern themselves with mental health issues deriving from these conditions.

Psychiatrists, in turn, tend to look at mental dysfunctions with little understanding of how they are impacted by dysregulation of the neural networks in the brain, as well as by biomedical issues in other parts of the body, like the gut. Part of the effort of this book is to move away from this arbitrary dualistic view and instead take an integrative view of mind and body, one that recognizes that seamless interplay between physical and mental health can be used for enhancing overall functioning.

Modern understanding of the nervous system, and later of brain functions, had to await the technological advances in the 19th and 20th centuries. In succession, they were the invention of the microscope; the development of the Golgi staining method for nerve tissue; the development of a refined sensitive galvanometer for measuring the electrical action potentials in the nerves; the invention of micropipettes; and, ultimately, the appearance of the electron microscope in 1950. Each of these breakthroughs allowed for more detailed examination of theories and assumptions that had previously been based on speculation.

In the 1880s, Italian scientist Camillo Golgi invented a silver chromate staining solution that made the study and identification of neural tissue in the spinal cord and in muscular tissue possible for the first time under the microscope. However, because he was limited by the low amplification of microscopes in the 1890s, Golgi drew a critical conclusion that turned out to be incorrect. He believed that the nerve tissue he was identifying with his staining technique was comprised of a seamless network (reticulum) through which nerve impulses could travel in either direction. This became known as the *Reticular Theory*.[3]

At about the same time, Spanish pathologist Santiago Ramon y Cajal, using Golgi's new staining technique, came to a completely different conclusion. He was able to identify and follow individual long axons to their termination. Through this, he demonstrated that the neuron was the principal structural and functional unit of the nervous system. This became known as the *Neuron Doctrine*.[4] This doctrine states that each nerve cell is separate and individual, bounded like all other cells in the body by its plasma membrane. He argued that the junction (or synaptic gap) between neurons was essential in regulating the transmission of signals in the nervous system. From his discovery of the axonal growth cone, he experimentally demonstrated that the relationship between nerve cells was contiguous, rather than continuous as Golgi had supposed.[5] The Neuron Doctrine was initially very controversial and was opposed by Golgi and other histologists, who continued to defend the Reticular Theory past the turn of the 20th century.[6, 7]

However, Cajal's discoveries, including his detailed drawings and lucid prose explanations, had a major influence on the work of British physiologist Charles Sherrington. After meeting Cajal in Spain, Sherrington turned his attention to the connection between the brain and the spinal cord. He observed that signal conduction in the long nerve trunks of the spinal cord was much faster than in the grey matter of the brain. To explain the differential in the speed of conduction, Sherrington hypothesized that neurons had to have gaps between them, to which he gave the term "synapse" in 1897. He argued that the synaptic gap between neurons was essential in the regulation of the transmission of signals in the nervous system.[8] If a synaptic gap existed, then the burning question became what was happening at this gap?

In 1921, the Austrian pharmacologist Otto Loewi, inspired by a dream, conducted experiments on the vagus nerve of frog hearts. He found that during the stimulation of the vagus nerve, a substance was formed. From these experiments, he concluded that *neurohumoral* substances were critical in nerve transmission, but it was difficult to identify this vagus-stimulating neurohumoral substance, which turned out to be acetylcholine (ACH). As Loewi later realized, the difficulty was that "acetylcholine produces only a very short-acting effect [and] is speedily metabolized." This is why other scientists had trouble replicating his findings.[9] The problem of proving the existence and function of these seemingly ephemeral substances, which later became known as neurotransmitters (NTs), turned into a 40-year scientific quest to determine what role these chemical substances played in neurotransmission.

Another group of scientists believed that the transmission of the nerve impulses was accomplished simply by electrical "sparks" flying across the synaptic gaps from one neuron to another. The idea of electrical transmission was seemingly substantiated by the work of German physiologist Emil du Bois-Reymond. After inventing a highly refined and sensitive galvanometer, he was able to observe that nerve impulses were accompanied by electrical discharges. He identified that there could be fluctuations of these discharges from negative to positive, and back again. He found that this corresponded to variation in the action potential as nerve impulses traveled from the brain and through the spinal cord to cause muscle contractions. With only low-amplification microscopes and crude measuring tools, du Bois-Reymond could only speculate on the mystery of how this nerve transmission was accomplished. In a textbook of the time, he wrote:

> Of known natural processes that might pass on excitation, only two are, in my opinion, worth talking about – either there exists at the boundary of the contractile substance – a stimulating secretion ... or the phenomenon is electrical in nature.[10]

Even though du Bois-Reymond considered that chemical change was part of muscle contraction, he did not consider that the transmission between nerve and muscle was chemical. Based on his observations with the galvanometer, du Bois-Reymond tended to place more emphasis on the concept of electrical transmission. Indeed, he became known as the father of the field of electrophysiology.[11]

1.2 The Soups and the Sparks

Du Bois-Reymond's speculation that the process might be either chemical or electrical had defined the debate over the nature of neural transmission that was to continue over the next 60 years. Elliott Valenstein called the debate between the two scientific camps *The War of the Soups and the Sparks* (2005). The chemists and pharmacologists argued for the primacy of neurohumoral secretions in triggering neurotransmission.[12] The physiologists proposed that nerve conduction was achieved primarily by electrical impulses traveling along neural pathways and then into the muscles.

At the beginning of the 20th century, the intensive study of the nervous system by various eminent scientists produced exciting speculation and debate about which side was right. The research on the autonomic nervous system conducted between 1890 and 1920 laid the foundations for later studies on the role of chemicals. Two well-known anatomists, Walter Haskell and John Langley, conducted research at Cambridge University that led to the discovery of the sympathetic and parasympathetic nervous systems. Their studies, and those of Wilhelm Feldberg, led to the positive identification of ACH at the junction of motor neurons and muscle when the muscle contracted. Much of the systematic search for evidence to support chemical transmission of nerve impulses was conducted under the leadership of Henry Dale at the Institute of Medical Research outside London.[13] A spirited debate developed between the "Soups" group, headed by Dale, and the "Sparks" group, whose most prominent proponent was the Australian physiologist John Eccles. Eccles did not believe that the "ACH hypothesis", derived from Feldberg's work with parasympathetic ganglia, applied to the central nervous system. The neurophysiologists, who recorded electrical impulses with a multistage vacuum tube that displayed on fast-responding cathode ray oscilloscopes, were sure that their impressive visual data proved that neurotransmission was electrical. As Valenstein records, there was "also a tendency of the neurophysiologists to look down on the pharmacologists, who spent their time investigating 'spit, sweat, snot and urine'."[14] The principal flaw in the Sparks hypothesis was that neurotransmission did not occur at the speed of electrical transport. To account for this discrepancy, Eccles came up with various explanations that seemed plausible at the time. He cleverly proposed that "wave interference" slowed the transmission. He also attempted to explain the excitation and inhibition phenomenon were caused by "eddy currents" of different polarities. Then, in 1947, he posited a new theory based on a dream. He claimed that interneurons (previously identified with the Golgi staining method) were responsible for producing inhibition at the synapse level.

Four years later it was Eccles who disproved his own theory and confirmed the chemical neurotransmission theory. Two technological advances allowed for this. In 1950, magnification provided by the electron microscope brought into view individual cells and even their constituent parts. The second innovation, coming in 1951, was the micropipette, the glass microelectrode filled with saline solution capable of penetrating the outer membrane of single neurons. This allowed for the precise measurement of the voltage changes that characterized inhibitory and excitatory states. Using these two innovations, Eccles and two colleagues conducted an all-day experiment in August 1951 in his Australian laboratory. The results produced were contrary to his expectations. He was quick to admit that he had been wrong and acknowledged that the "large post-synaptic potential" evoked could not be accounted for by a "trans-synaptic flow of current" but could only be accounted for by "the chemical transmitter mechanism." The riddle of the change in charge

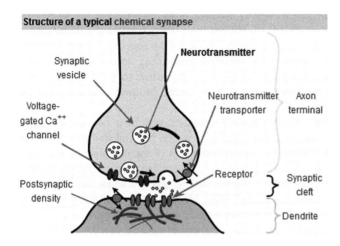

Figure 1.1 Structure of a typical chemical synapse.

had been explained by the discovery of the difference in polarity between the core of the neuron and its outer membrane. With this breakthrough and its publication in a prominent journal in 1952,[15] the War of the Soups and the Sparks had come to an end.[16] The use of the electron microscope and micropipettes spurred almost feverish research in a number of prestigious institutions and made the study of neuron function the new frontier of science. The 1950s was a heady time for these researchers as they came up with one discovery after another. Neuroscience was acknowledged to be a separate field of study with its own publications.[17] The new tools for investigation of the nervous system at the electron microscope level also allowed for exploration of the staggering complexity of the human brain. There are some 100 billion neurons in the brain, composed of 150 different cell types. They vary in size from a robust 100 microns in diameter for the long motor neurons extending down the spinal cord to 4 microns for the interneurons. In addition, there are trillions of glial cells, including astrocytes, which jointly make up 90% of the volume of the cortex.[18] (The critical functions of astrocytes are explained in Chapter 4.) While one area of research focused on the identification and differences in the function of the various neurons, or clusters thereof, another segment focused on the neurochemical mechanisms operating at the synapse level of axons (see Figure 1.1).

1.3 The Neurochemical Paradigm

Once chemical substances had been confirmed as initiating electrical action potentials, the attention of much research turned to the identification and role of NTs in every facet of functioning of the brain and the nervous system. Indeed, once the primacy of NTs had been established, the reigning paradigm for understanding the brain was from the perspective of these neurochemical agents and their action upon physiological function, as well as behavior. With the emphasis on the role of neurochemicals from the 1950s onward, we also see the entry of the then-nascent pharmaceutical industry into the research field. With the enormous profit potential of marketing drugs to correct neurochemical "imbalances" in the brain, the study of how the timing and organization of the brain was related to the patterns of neu-roelectrical currents, measured in waves with specific bandwidths and amplitudes, fell into relative neglect.

There was much excitement as neuroscientists, with their new technological tools, deciphered the detailed mechanisms by which NTs fulfilled their roles at the synapse level. One of the first accomplishments of the new field of neurosci-ence was to identify the chemical substances in the mechanisms of excitation and inhibition at the synapse of individual neurons. The first two to be identified were ACH and gamma-aminobutyric acid (GABA). The excitatory substance is ACH, a complex organic molecule. The inhibitory organic molecule is GABA.

Neurons have a resting membrane potential of approximately −70 millivolts (mV) that results from a relative dearth of sodium ions intracellularly compared to the extracellular matrix. Stimulating input from other axons causes this charge to become more positive (depolarizing) until reaching a critical voltage threshold, trig-gering the generation of an action potential that results in a rapid and temporary reversal of this resting membrane potential from negative to positive. This occurs as sodium ions rush into the cell through sodium channels, leading to the progression of the action potential down the axon. In myelinated (sheathed) neurons, sodium channels are localized at specialized areas known as *nodes of Ranvier*. The action potential generated at one node creates depolarization at the next, so that the signal propagates rapidly from one node to the next in a process known as *saltatory conduction*. When this electrical pulse reaches the axon terminal, an NT (such as acetylcholine) is released via an influx of calcium. NTs bind to specific receptors at the postsynaptic membrane, which then contribute to the generation of the next action potential. This process occurs in both central and peripheral nervous systems, including the neuromuscular junction which couples the nervous system to the motor system. NTs are quickly inactivated, typically through reuptake at the presynaptic terminal or, in the case of ACH, through enzymatic cleavage within the synaptic cleft.[19]

ACH and GABA are only two among scores of chemical messengers that have been described in the nervous system. These messengers may be categorized as neurotransmitters, neuromodulators, and neurohormones, depending on the nature of the substance and its mechanism of action. Some chemicals may act in more than one manner. In general, a neurotransmitter is a specific chemical that is released within the synaptic cleft, causing a change in the potential, i.e. micro volt-age, at the postsynaptic membrane.[20]

Neuromodulators are typically released from neurons and affect groups of other neurons or effector cells that have appropriate receptors. These often act through what are known as second messengers. Neurohormones, on the other hand, are released from neurons into the circulation and affect cells at a distant site. An example of this would be the release of oxytocin from the neurohypophysis to induce labor. It is important to note that many such receptors previously thought to reside only within the nervous system have also been found in the gut, the circulatory system, and the immune system. The chemical messenger model posits that brain function is dependent on proper "levels" of neurochemicals within its circuitry. For example, it has long been thought that low levels of the neurotransmitter serotonin are responsible for symptoms of depression. Further, it has been demonstrated that molecules such as enkephalins and endorphins are important in mediating pain transmission at both physical and psychological levels. Moreover, endorphins may be involved in what is popularly referred to as the "runner's high", because vigorous exercise may stimulate its release. A huge proportion of the pharmaceutical industry is based on manipulation of neurochemistry to alter brain function.

An excitatory NT system worth mentioning in this brief overview is the histamines. Histamines respond to the presence of irritating or pathogenic substances introduced into the body either via ingestion, inhalation, or injury. Their main function appears to be to increase blood supply, especially white blood cells, to the area affected to fight or neutralize the alien substance. The problem is that this is an inflammatory response that is usually experienced as unpleasant (as in congested sinuses or bronchial areas, watery eyes, sneezing, etc.). Here, again, the pharmaceutical industry came to the rescue with a wide range of antihistamines, and non-steroidal anti-inflammatory (NSAID) drugs, which suppress the inflammatory histamine action. One of the problems with antihistamines is that they not only suppress allergy symptoms in the body, but also have a systemic inhibitory effect in the brain, which is experienced as drowsiness, fuzzy thinking, and delayed motor action.

One of the curious aspects of the endogenous neurochemical substances in the brain is that not all of them are found exclusively within the cellular bodies of neurons, dendrites, or the synaptic terminals. Indeed, some are found operating outside the neural membranes in the vast sea of astrocytes. The most important of these extra-cellular substances is adenosine triphosphate (ATP). ATP has been called the "molecular unit of currency" of intracellular energy transfer.[21] ATP is instrumental in the activation of blood flow to neural networks. As we will see in detail in Chapter 4, the ebb and flow of ATP is central to regulating the ultradian rhythms of the brain. In that fashion, it has a systemic effect on the awake/rest/sleep cycle, not only of the brain but also the various systems of the body. Because astrocytes play such a critical role in the regulatory regime of critical neural networks, they become the target for neurofeedback, albeit indirectly.

1.3.1 Neuropsychiatry: The Pharmacological Breakthroughs

Prior to the 1950s, psychiatry often had to rely on psychoanalysis, hospitalization, or psychosurgery for conditions of mental illness. There were only a few medications available and those were for severe conditions like schizophrenia and bipolar disorder. "All prototypes of modern psycho pharmaceuticals (chlorpromazine, meprobamate, imipramine, and chlordiazepoxide) were discovered in a period of about 10 years" from 1948 to 1958.[22]

Part of the excitement of that period in the new field of neurophysiology was the discovery and identification of the function of the growing numbers of the chemical NTs. With that came intensive research on how either over- or under-production of specific NTs, or dysfunctions at the synapse level, could negatively impact brain functioning. For example, norepinephrine (noradrenaline), an excitatory NT, is produced in the locus coeruleus in the pons of the brain. In response to arousal stimuli, the locus coeruleus distributes norepinephrine to various centers in the brain to regulate the body's physiological arousal response via long axon connections. One of the conditions associated with overproduction of norepinephrine is post-traumatic stress disorder (PTSD), in which the limbic system is in a constant state of over-arousal due to hypervigilance. On the other hand, if too little norepinephrine reaches key cortical areas involved in cognitive processing and emotions, then attention, motivation, decision- making, learning, and memory are likely to be degraded or depressed (as in ADHD). For over-production, the pharmaceutical industry came up with anxiolytics; for under-production, the answer became stimulant medication.

A dysfunction common at the synapse level is related to re-uptake. Generally, NTs only stay in the synaptic gap for a fraction of a second before being reabsorbed into the pre-synaptic axon terminal, in what is known as re-uptake. When a mood regulating NT like serotonin is released into the synaptic gap, it needs to connect to the post-synaptic serotonin receptor sites instantly before being reabsorbed into the pre-synaptic axon terminal. However, if there are too few post-synaptic receptors, or they are not functioning well, the serotonin may be reabsorbed into the pre-synaptic vessel before it can pass on its neuromodulating message. Low serotonin levels are associated with depression, and once this mechanism was discovered, the major pharmaceutical companies raced to produce a solution. Each came up with its own formulation of selective serotonin re-uptake inhibitors, designed to keep the serotonin in the synaptic cleft longer to force itself into whatever post-synaptic receptors are functioning.

The seemingly great success of the early psychopharmaceuticals like the benzodiazepines, the monoamine inhibitors, and the tricyclics for depression – and later meprobamate (Miltown) and again the benzodiazepines (Librium and Valium) for anxiety – spurred the pharmaceutical industry to devote major resources to exploring what other neurochemical brain dysfunctions could be solved with medications.

A major problem with most psychoactive drugs is that they lack specificity in targeting (i.e., they often have effects in other parts of the brain or the central nervous system where their effects are either not needed or they produce negative effects). For example, the main target of stimulant medication is to raise the norepinephrine level in the prefrontal cortex of a person with ADHD. However, the stimulant action affects the whole central nervous system and may produce heart palpitations, high blood pressure, and dizziness (as well as inhibiting appetite). Another point is that most mood-modulating drugs are only slightly more effective than placebos.[23, 24]

The psychiatric profession, for the most part, welcomed and embraced the appearance of pharmaceutical "solutions" to the problems of psychiatric disorders. The profession adopted the "neurochemical paradigm" of functioning of the brain and became the purveyors of the drugs designed to correct the neurochemical imbalances that were said to be at the root of most psychiatric disorders.[25] The pharmaceutical industry had a strong vested interest in promoting the prescribing of psychoactive medications not only by psychiatrists, but also by general medical practitioners. Towards this end, the industry spent hundreds of billions of dollars on advertising and used a system of direct marketing to doctors by "drug reps," who gave away free samples. Big Pharma has profited enormously and therefore has a strong incentive in upholding the neurochemical paradigm, and thus maintaining its influence over the treatment of mental and physical health conditions. The health insurance industry also embraced the neurochemical paradigm, because treatment of symptoms with psychoactive drugs tends to be cheaper in the short run than long-term, face-to-face talk therapy that might be undertaken to resolve the underlying causes of mental health problems.

1.4 Moving to a New Paradigm

The preceding review was designed to show how we arrived at seeing brain functioning through the lens of the neurochemical paradigm. As we have seen, the neurochemical paradigm was deeply rooted in the discovery process of the physical components and functions of the nervous system and the brain. It led to a focus on the neurochemical interactions at the synaptic cleft between neurons at the microscopic level and was a mechanistic view of functioning at the micro level. Less attention was paid to the functioning of the brain at the macro level.

The neuroelectrical paradigm models the whole brain as a self-organizing system. Neurons organize into functional assemblies and execute their functions through collective action, all the while also retaining their individuality of expression. This complementary perspective is absolutely necessary in order to understand brain function.

This has been recognized as far back as the turn of the 20th century, when Camillo Golgi described in his 1906 Nobel Prize acceptance speech:[26]

> Far from being able to accept the idea of the individuality and independence of each nerve element, I have never had reason, up to now, to give up the concept which I have always stressed, that nerve cells, instead of working individually, act together ... However opposed it may seem to the popular tendency to individualize the elements, I cannot abandon the idea of a unitary action of the nervous system.
>
> (Golgi, 1906)

It is apparent that Golgi was standing apart from the views prevailing at the time, and in fact that split stayed with us longer than the controversy about the "Soups" and the "Sparks". In his autobiography, titled *In Search of Memory*,[27] Eric Kandel recalls accepting the mandate of his mentor, Harry Grundfest: "Study the brain one neuron at a time." This absolutely needed to be done and that was the right time to do it, but this was not the key to understanding brain function that had been hoped for. It did not yield the "neural code" by means of which the brain encodes "information."

Observe that the collective action of neurons was understood as a necessity by Golgi even before the discovery of the electroencephalogram (EEG) in the 1920s. Once the EEG was understood as reflecting the electrical activity of neurons, of course, their collective mode of action was immediately apparent, even if the functional implications were not yet understood. However, this did not make much difference at the time. First of all, these two perspectives on the brain remained largely invisible to each other. When looking at the EEG, the action of individual neurons is no longer apparent, and when looking at the action of individual neurons, their participation in group activity is not evident. It is as if one only got to hear the timpani instead of the whole orchestra. Worse than that, neurons can be part of several different choruses at the same time, and each of these choruses is non-local, involving the whole brain. In short, the brain yielded its secrets only reluctantly.

In the absence of a formal theoretical model for self-organizing systems, the approach to the EEG was predominantly phenomenological for most of the 20th century.

The brain's neuroelectrical function was described in terms of rhythmic activity whose ebb and flow reflected the self-regulatory activity of the neuronal network. This electrical activity takes place in distinct wavebands that are distinguishable in terms of their temporal properties and spatial distribution, reflecting their distinct functional roles. In the 1960s, the availability of the first digital signal averagers gave impetus to the study of evoked potentials, which turned out to be a mere perturbation on the passive baseline EEG. It was apparent that the bulk of brain electrical activity related to the brain's self-regulation of states, which was only marginally affected by interaction with the outside world. As it happens, the evoked potential research bore only limited fruit at the time. The brain really had to be understood in terms of its organization in baseline.

The mathematical formalism for the understanding of networks did not become available until the 1990s. The brain is perhaps the most elaborate exemplar in the known universe of what is known as the "small-world" model of networks. This is a combination of high local connectivity – composed of the dendritic tree on the input site and the axonal branching network on the output side – and of high distal connectivity. The latter follows from the fact that every cortical pyramidal cell participates in the communication with distal networks by means of axons that jointly constitute the cortical white matter. By virtue of the globally connected network of pyramidal cells, the brain is drawn into a unitary functional entity, with every part communicating with every other part more or less directly. As the National Institute of Health (NIH)-sponsored Human Connectome Project has shown, our brain is so interconnected that any synapse in the cortex is no more than three synapses away from any other synapse in the cortex.[28]

Because long-distance communication is mediated by the action potential, the entire communication scheme is subject to very specific timing constraints. This is where we find the nexus between the microcosm of the individual neuron and the behavior of the neural assembly. The initiation of an action potential is dependent on the coincidence of synaptic firing events at the receptor neuron. This makes neuronal action contingent on cooperativity, and that imposes a fundamental timing constraint. By virtue of distal communication, the timing constraint ultimately applies to the entire nervous system.

Coincidence at the neuron level translates into simultaneity at the level of the neuronal assembly, which in turn is observable as local synchrony in the EEG. In this manner, the exquisite timing control exercised by the brain at every frequency becomes directly visible to us in the EEG. By the same token, deviations in appropriate timing and network synchronization become evident as well.

Given the dependence of good brain function on universal timing integrity throughout the brain, we have identified a potential failure mode that could, in principle, account for mental dysfunctions, either directly or indirectly. A variety of internal and external factors, like stroke, brain injury, or toxins, can disrupt or inactivate normal patterns of communication among neural networks through structural disruption of neural integrity. Others, like emotional or physical trauma or various mental deficiencies, can emerge out of chronic patterns of electrical instability and/or over- and under-activation in parts of the brain. The dysregulation of brain timing would be expected to yield what we call soft failures, rather than the hard failures we might see in a stroke. The functional deficits are on a continuum and they exhibit variability and dependencies on a variety of factors. This is just what we observe.

We can measure or document these patterns of dysregulation by way of quantitative encephalograms (QEEG), functional magnetic resonance imaging (fMRI), or single-photon emission computerized tomography (SPECT). The QEEG is most closely identified with measuring the actual patterns of the distinct wavebands in various regions of the brain, whereas fMRI and SPECT measure activity by blood flow patterns, which correspond to neuroelectrical activation.

So, let us take a look at the individual elements of this neuroelectrical paradigm. The 19th century German anatomist Korbinian Brodmann divided the cerebral cortex into 47 distinct regions, based entirely on the differences in cellular structure. As study of the brain shifted from purely structural classification to functional classification, it was found that the areas Brodmann had identified, by mere inspection of differences in appearance and texture of brain tissue, corresponded almost exactly to specific brain functions.[29] For example, Brodmann's areas 17–19, located at the occipital pole, contain the visual cortex. The strip of grey matter that runs across the brain from ear to ear – Brodmann area 4 – is known as the motor cortex. It controls our muscular movements and our sense of where we are in space. None of the 47 areas performs its specific function in isolation. All rely on heavy neural interconnectivity with other regions of the brain. This interconnectivity has been graphically demonstrated with the stunning images from NIH-sponsored studies at various research centers, collectively called the Human Connectome Project.[30] The color-coded renderings show axonal connections running vertically from the cortex down into the brainstem and laterally from one side of the brain to the other, as well as from front to back and back to front. One of the precepts of the neuroelectrical paradigm is that this vast net of interconnectivity between different functional networks is achieved through patterns of signaling that are near instantaneous. Neurofeedback practitioners using the infra-low frequency (ILF) approach have learned that this interconnectivity often produces surprisingly global effects. Clinical experience has shown that by targeting a specific Brodmann area with electrode placement on the scalp produces a spillover effect into more distal parts. Thus, for example, calming over-arousal in the right hemisphere also tends to move the whole brain towards balance and optimal self-regulation via this inter-connectivity. (See Chapter 5 for details on how this is done clinically.) This interconnectivity also explains how different regions of the brain interact to perform self-regulatory functions. To help us understand how these self-regulatory functions can become dysregulated, and how we can apply neurofeedback to restore the balance, we can use a simple model of the central nervous system. The basic building blocks from the bottom up are the spinal cord, the brainstem, the subcortical nuclei, and sitting on top of that, the cortex.[31] The spinal cord provides input and output to the body and coordinates some reflexive functions. The brainstem is involved in core physiological functions vital to life. It relays information to and from the spinal cord and also controls our basic sleep/wake cycle. Between the brainstem and the cortex are many functional groups of cells, also known as subcortical nuclei. There are fluid-filled ventricles and a sea of astrocytes among the subcortical nuclei, as well as many vertical connections up to the cortex and down through the brainstem. The limbic system, as part of the subcortical areas, manages and drives emotions. This is where we assess and react to internal and external dangers. It is where our learned fears and reactions to trauma reside. It is also where our priorities and motivations are embedded in our reward centers.

The cortex mediates detailed analysis of sensory input from the structures below and then selects and modulates behavioral output. The cortex, as the most developed part of the brain, also exercises inhibitory control over the subcortical areas and emotional impulses from the limbic area. Indeed, inhibitory control is an important factor in how different levels of the central nervous system work together. Cortical areas process and filter incoming information in the associational areas of the hindbrain and then send that information forward for decisional output by the frontal parts of the cortex. Of specific importance in this process is the prefrontal cortex, the most highly developed region of our brain. The prefrontal cortex moderates (inhibits) impulses from the lower regions of the central nervous system and the automatic and reflexive reactions originating there.

In the ideal of a well-functioning brain, this model is descriptive of what happens. In the perspective of the brain as a self-regulatory system, however, this hierarchy is upside down. The neurofeedback model considers several types of dysregulation. The first is tonic and phasic physiological arousal, which is under brainstem control, where the reticular formation establishes the setpoint and can also activate a total body alarm response. Shifts in arousal levels have specific impacts on the brain's overall level of functioning. In temporary emergencies, high arousal is useful as we need to react reflexively for safety and survival. But chronic stress or trauma can lead to an impairment of the prefrontal cortex's inhibitory control, as the limbic system and brainstem keep us in a state of hypervigilance and over-arousal. For example, for persons with PTSD, novel incoming stimuli, instead of being handed off by the thalamus to the right hindbrain for processing, are routed into the limbic system and brain stem for survival mode.[32] In this switch from thalamo-cortical processing to thalamo-limbic processing, the top-down inhibitory control gets hijacked by the activation of overpowering emotions, like fear, anger, rage, and disinhibited fight–flight–freeze behaviors. At the other side of the arousal curve is under-arousal. This may manifest as depression, low physical energy, and lack of interest. It may slow and impair our decision making and dull our responses to stimuli.

The brain may also experience instability of state, which manifests as symptoms that arise chaotically or with shifts in arousal. Hyper-excitability can lead to paroxysmal symptoms as the brain flies out of control.[33] An electroencephalogram would show that, in the case of extreme instabilities, whole regions of neural circuitry may be firing synchronously (i.e., in-phase), which is characteristic of a seizure. At a slightly lesser extreme, we can see that instabilities indicate a loss of internal control, as in the mood swings of bipolar disorder. These basic regulatory functions constitute the priority in cerebral regulation and are therefore also the therapeutic priority. In the practice of neurofeedback, a 150-item symptom rating form is used to ascertain the type and severity of the above types of dysregulation and then the training strategy is adjusted accordingly (see Chapter 5).

Let us examine another macro element of neuroelectrical functioning. In the neurochemical "Soup" paradigm, we saw that chemical changes in charge build up an electrical charge that travels down the neuron through to the next synaptic gap. We know that the electric potential generated by an individual neuron is far too insignificant to be picked up in an electroencephalogram.[34] EEG activity therefore always reflects the summation of the synchronous activity of thousands or millions of neurons distributed over different networks.[35] Measurable scalp EEG activity shows that these synchronous activities oscillate in wavebands of specific frequency ranges and spatial distributions across the brain. Certain frequency bands are associated with different states of brain functioning (e.g., waking and the various rest or sleep stages). The oscillations of these frequencies are measured in Hertz (Hz) (i.e., how often an electrical wave crosses a midline in one second). In the United States, we tend to be familiar with the 60-Hz cycle of our standard 110-volt household current. In the brain, we have a wide range of frequencies that are usually measured in wavebands of about 4-Hz bandwidths from 0.5 to 40Hz. Until recently, the lowest of these commonly measured was 0.5Hz.

However (as will be elaborated in Chapters 2 and 3), with new instrumentation we can now target Slow Cortical Potentials (SCP), even at extremely low frequencies. These are appropriately termed infra-low frequencies (ILF), but are also sometimes referred to as ultra-low frequencies (ULF). The ILF domain reflects the slow regulatory activity of the nervous system, in which astrocytes play such a dominant role. As David A. Kaiser explains in Chapter 4, these ILF oscillations are the dominant features in state regulation of the brain, meaning that they are critical in managing the functional connectivity of our resting-state networks, as well as managing the hemodynamics of activation. They are highly responsive at the micro level, while being resistant to disruption on the larger scale. As will be elaborated in Chapter 3, this is why they have become instrumental in the ILF approach to neurofeedback work.

1.5 Traditional Wave Bands

Although ILF training directly engages the low frequency bands below 0.1Hz, the other wavebands still play their respective roles in neurofeedback. We also know that targeting the training in the ILF domain has an impact on the higher frequencies that can be measured by pre- and post-QEEGs.

The first traditional 4-Hz band is the delta frequency from 0.5 to 4Hz. Delta waves are predominant during sleep, which is a restorative rest state for the brain. However, if excessively present during waking states, delta can interfere with cognitive and emotional processing. The theta frequency band extends from 4 to 8Hz. It is dominant when we enter into the pre-sleep hypnogogic, dream-like state. We can also enter into this trance-like state while daydreaming or undergoing hypnotherapy. It is the default resting frequency for the prefrontal cortex. Problems arise when there is too high theta (and delta) amplitude pre-frontally. This condition can give rise to distractibility, an inability to focus or pay attention, and poor inhibitory control – all characteristics most often associated with attention deficit disorder (ADHD).

The next frequency band, alpha (8–12Hz), is associated with being awake but relaxed and not processing much information. It is the default resting frequency for the occipital (sensory processing) area. It should be noted that as soon as we close our eyes and cut off input to the visual cortex (Brodmann areas 12–17) we tend to automatically generate alpha as that area goes into its default resting mode.

Our sensory motor cortex (Brodmann area 4) runs in a band from one ear across the top of the cortex to the other. It operates primarily in the 12–15Hz range. This band is called either low beta or the sensory motor rhythm (SMR) band. Activity in this frequency range is associated with monitoring our body in space and movement (proprioception) and also activating or inhibiting muscle actions. It is involved in regulating emotional stability, energy levels, attentiveness, concentration, and impulsivity.

Mid-range beta waves (15–18 or 20Hz) are noticeable during focused cognitive processing. They usually indicate alert external attention and are critical in executive functions. In the right hemisphere, the processing of new stimuli and social-emotional issues are done in this mid-range beta wave band. Activation of high-level mental processing is usually done in the high beta range. Depending who is defining it, high beta at the low end starts at either 18 or 20Hz and extends up to 22–27Hz. High beta can also be present when there is chronic over-arousal from emotional trauma, which prevents key areas in the brain from returning to their default resting mode (see Chapter 13).

More fascinating are the gamma waves (40Hz and up), though what we know of their function is based on relatively scant research evidence.[36] The 40Hz frequency is said to be associated with the binding of elements of cognitive processing via a wave that sweeps the brain from front to back, 40 times per second, drawing different neuronal circuits – including the associational areas in the hindbrain, the memory areas of the hippocampus and the cerebellum – into synch, thereby bringing them into the attentional and decision-making frontal area of the brain.[37] The hypothesis is that when these neuronal clusters oscillate together during these transient periods of synchronized firing, they help bring up memories and associations to create new syntheses of ideas and notions, and possibly a changed self-awareness.[38] As we learn in Chapter 9, in autism spectrum children, where this associational function of the gamma waveband seems not to be functioning well, we see an inability to generalize from one social situation to the next. Thus, gamma waves play an essential role in the acquisition of knowledge from experience and applying it to new situations. Indeed, we can infer that this integrative function of gamma waves is critical to the functioning of the brain as a self-regulating system.[39]

As award-winning neuroscientist Nancy Andreasen has shown in her imaging studies, high levels of activation of these associational areas via the gamma waves are seen in persons of unusually high creativity.[40] Another curious aspect of high amplitude gamma waves is that they have been observed in experienced Buddhist monks in deep meditative states.[41] It has been proposed that the activities in the gamma frequency may be a bridge into the very essence of our own spiritual self.[42] Gamma training has been used by some neurotherapists in the prescriptive training mode for ADHD and other conditions, but, in general, gamma training has not been utilized widely in neurofeedback. This may be changing as Synchrony training is being explored by some prominent researchers.[43]

1.6 Conclusion

The 60-year-long debate between the "Soups" and "Sparks" was resolved by breakthroughs in technology that allowed identification of the action of neurotransmitters at the synaptic cleft in the 1950s. This launched the drive to uncover the biochemical regulation of human behavior, mood, thought, and functioning. For the seven decades since then, a period longer than the "Soups" and "Sparks" debate, the neurochemical paradigm has reigned supreme, while the bioelectrical regulation of human behavior, mood, thought, and functioning has been either ignored or denigrated by those who deal with the brain, i.e. psychiatrists and the medical profession in general.

Today, breakthroughs in technology comparable to the invention of the micropipette and the electron microscope, are allowing us to address the bioelectrical properties of brain functioning with much greater specificity. Stunning advances in both hardware and computer software have given us the capability to use neurofeedback to influence the brain's self-regulatory functions at the very foundational level of the brain's self-organizing activities (see Chapter 3). With current computer capacities that were unimaginable even 20 years ago, scientific interest has turned once again to an investigation of practical applications for a bioelectrical method of re-establishing healthy patterns of electrical activity in the human brain and body, as one whole functioning bioelectrical being. This new edition of the book has added data from documented clinical experience by neurofeedback practitioners that were not available when the first edition was being written in 2013–2014. They have firmly established that our current understanding of the neuroelectrical properties of the brain already suffices to train the brain into balanced self-regulation.

As shown in Part II, various medical specialties have already begun to incorporate neurofeedback into their integrative medicine practice successfully. When the larger scientific community, untethered from the singular focus on the neurochemical paradigm, accepts this understanding of the neuroelectrical functioning of the brain, we can make another leap in human health. Neurofeedback is becoming a core competence in efforts to redress the pressing mental health concerns facing our society.

Notes

1 Cited from Foreword to Fisher S. 2014. *Neurofeedback in the Treatment of Developmental Trauma: Changing the Fear-Driven Brain*. New York: Norton, p. xvi.

2 Norden J. 2007. Historical underpinnings of neuroscience. In *Understanding the Brain*. The Great Courses six disc video DVD. Chantilly, VA: The Teaching Company.

3 Mazzarello P. 1999. *The Hidden Structure: A Scientific Biography of Camillo Golgi*. Oxford, UK: Oxford University Press.

4 Shepherd G.M. 1991. *Foundations of the Neuron Doctrine*. New York: Oxford University Press.

5 Acrimony developed between the two men as Golgi refused to acknowledge the validity of Cajal's research. Ironically, both men were awarded the Nobel Prize in 1906 for their contributions.

6 Sherrington C.S. 1906. *The Integrative Action of the Nervous System*. New Haven, CT: Yale University Press.

7 Golgi evidently was so upset over having to share the 1906 Nobel Prize with Cajal that he used his acceptance speech to attack Cajal's neuron doctrine.

8 Bennett M. 2001. *The History of the Synapse*. Australia: Harwood Academic Publishers.

9 Loewi cited in Clarke E., O'Malley C. D. 1968. *The Human Brain and the Spinal Cord*. Oakland, CA: University of California Press, p. 252.

10 Dubois-Reymond cited in Valenstein E. S. 2005. *The War of the Soups and the Sparks: The Discovery of Neurotransmitters and the Dispute Over How Nerves Communicate*. New York: Columbia University Press, p. 6.

11 Ibid., p. 122.

12 We may regard some of the early terms, such as "neurohumoral substances," as quaint. It needs to be remembered that modern terms such as neuroscience, neurophysiology, and even neurotransmitters did not come into regular use until the 1950s.

13 Dale had met many of the leading German Jewish scientists working at the cutting edge of neurotransmission at international conferences in Europe prior to the rise of Hitler. When the Nazis took over and they lost their jobs, he, with the assistance of the Rockefeller Foundation, brought some of them, including Otto Loewi and Wilhelm Feldberg, to work with his group in Britain.

14 Valenstein, op cit.

15 Brock L. G., Coombs J. S., Eccles J. C. 1952. The recording of potential from motor neurons with an intracellular electrode. *J Physiol* 117: 431–460.

16 Eccles, after his "conversion," became an active proponent and researcher of neurochemical transmission. He was knighted by the Queen in 1958 and received the Nobel Prize in 1963.

17 Shepherd G. M. 2010. *Creating Modern Neuroscience: The Revolutionary 1950s*. New York: Oxford Press.

18 Norden J. 2007. Neurotransmitters. In *Understanding the Brain*. The Great Courses six disc video DVD. Chantilly, VA: The Teaching Company.

19 Knowles J. R. 1980. Enzyme-catalyzed phosphoryl transfer reactions. *Annu Rev Biochem* 49: 877–919.

20   Watanabe M., Maemura K., Kanbara K., Tamayama T., Hayasaki H. 2002. GABA and GABA receptors in the central nervous system and other organs. *J Internat Rev Cytol* 213: 1–47.
21   Ibid.
22   Spiegel R. 1996. *Psychopharmacology. An Introduction* (3rd edition). Somerset, NJ: John Wiley and Sons, p. 45.
23   Kirsch I. 2010. *The Emperor's New Drugs: Exploding the Antidepressant Myth*. New York: Basic Books.
24   Angell M. 2011. The illusions of psychiatry. *New York Review of Books* July 14, 58: 12.
25   Shepherd. 2010. Chapter 15 – Neuropsychiatry: The Breakthrough in Psychopharmacology. In *Creating Modern Neuroscience: The Revolutionary 1950s*. Oxford, UK: Oxford University Press.
26   Golgi C. 1967. The Neuron Doctrine – Theory and Facts, Nobel Lecture 11 Dec 1906. In *Nobel Lectures: Physiology or Medicine 1901–1921*. London, UK: Elsevier, p. 216.
27   Kandel E. 2006. *In Search of Memory: The Emergence of a New Science of Mind*. New York: W. W. Norton & Company.
28   See www.humanconnectomeproject.org/. Accessed on August 15, 2019.
29   Garey L. J. 2006. *Brodmann's Localisation in the Cerebral Cortex*. New York: Springer, retrieved from Wikipedia http://en.wikipedia.org/wiki/Brodmann_area#References on August 15, 2019.
30   Relationship Viewer at www.humanconnectomeproject.org/data/relationship-viewer/.
31   See also Zimmer, C. 2014. Secrets of the brain. *National Geographic*, February 2014.
32   Othmer S. F. 2019. *Protocol Guide for Neurofeedback Clinicians* (7th edition). Woodland Hills, CA: EEG Institute.
33   Nunez P. L., Srinivasan R. 2006. *Electric Fields of the Brain: The Neurophysics of EEG* (2nd edition). New York: Oxford University Press, pp. 518–523.
34   Fehmi L., Robbins J. 2001. Mastering our brain's electrical rhythms. *Cerebrum* 3(3).
35   Othmer S. 2013. *The Role of Infra Slow Oscillations in Infra Low Frequency Training*. PowerPoint presentation of April 2013. Woodland Hills, CA.
36   Bird B. L., Newton F. A., et al. 1978. Biofeedback training of 40-Hz EEG in humans. *Biofeedback Self Regul* 3(1): 1–12.
37   Melloni L., Molina C., Pena M., Torres D., Singer W., Rodriguez E. 2007. Synchronization of neural activity across cortical areas correlates with conscious perception. *J Neurosci* 27(11): 2858–2865.
38   Buzsaki G. 2006. Cycle 9, The Gamma Buzz: Gluing by oscillations in the waking brain. In *Rhythms of the Brain*. Oxford, UK: Oxford University Press. Retrieved from the web June 27, 2014.
39   Andreasen N. C. 2014. The secrets of the creative brain. *The Atlantic* July/August, pp. 62–75.
40   Lutz A., Greischar L., Rawlings N.B., Ricard M., Davidson R. J. 2004. Long-term meditators self-induce high-amplitude synchrony during mental practice. *Proc Natl Acad Sci USA*, 101: 16369–16373.

41 Fehmi L., Robbins J. 2008. *The Open Focus Brain: Harnessing the Power of Attention to Heal the Body and the Mind*. Boston, MA: Shambala Publications

42 Dobbs d. 2005. Zen Gamma, in *Scientific American Mind.*

43 Gamma Wave. 2019. Wikipedia cites 27 separate articles on research projects and also cites a previous survey of research from 2009. See https://en.wikipedia.org/wiki/Gamma_wave#Contemporary_research.

Chapter 2

History of Neurofeedback

Siegfried Othmer

2.1 The Scientific Antecedents of Neurofeedback

The discovery of therapeutic EEG biofeedback in the 1960s was dependent on three principal antecedents. These were the discovery of the EEG by Hans Berger, the development of classical conditioning by Ivan Pavlov, and the establishment of operant conditioning under B.F. Skinner. The original discovery of the EEG was the result of determined effort by Hans Berger over the course of nearly two decades. He was set upon this path by a personal experience of mental telepathy, which redirected his career into medicine, where he was determined to find a physiological basis for the phenomenon. In this enduring side project, undertaken while serving as clinical director of a neurology and psychiatry clinic, he failed. But despite the limitations of primitive electronics he was able to find the miniscule EEG signal. In the face of his own uncertainties it took five years for him to publish his findings, in 1929, and then it was his colleagues' turn to be skeptical (Berger, 1929).[1] It took another five years before Adrian and Matthews (1934)[2] replicated his work in England, which served to change the conversation. These authors were also the first to observe the effects of synchronous visual stimulation on alpha band activity in the EEG, although Berger had first identified this prominent EEG rhythmic bursting pattern, which subsequently came to be labeled the Berger rhythm.

Berger must be considered one of the pioneers of the nascent discipline of psychophysiology, and he is credited with coining the term. Although he did observe EEG phenomenology in epilepsy, he was not oriented toward the medical utilization of the EEG. For decades, as a matter of fact, the principal utility of the EEG in neurology remained with those features that were obvious on mere visual inspection of the clinical EEG. This had the effect of consolidating a rather modest appraisal of the utility of the EEG, one that would prove difficult to dislodge. The usefulness of the EEG in psychophysiology remained modest as well. The full exploitation of the EEG would have to await the availability of new tools of both measurement and of analysis, as well as new understandings.

Ivan Pavlov received his Nobel Prize for his work on the digestive system of dogs rather than for his work in classical conditioning. But one set the stage for the other. In studying salivation he observed that it often occurred well before the food arrived, the response triggered by some correlated preliminary activity. The classical conditioning experimental design placed these observations in a rigorous framework. He called the anticipatory salivation the conditional response. Pavlov also studied the anticipatory reaction to aversive stimuli such as foot shocks, and in one design combined both food reward, signaled by one tone, with the occasional delivery of a foot shock, indexed by another tone. When the two tones were slowly brought together so that the dogs could no longer reliably distinguish between them, the dogs tended to give up on the whole experiment. Some of them even went to sleep.

2.2 The Foundations of Neurofeedback in Animal Studies

Six decades later, Pavlov's study inspired M. Barry Sterman, a research psychologist at the UCLA School of Medicine and at the Sepulveda Veterans' Administration Hospital, in his own investigations of sleep onset. Pavlov's dogs had absented themselves from the task even in the face of the aversive foot shocks. Sterman took this as a paradigm for the voluntary withdrawal of behavioral responding that we all undertake once the head hits the pillow with the intention to fall asleep.

An operant conditioning design was set up in which cats were trained to expect a food reward upon a bar press whenever a light came on in their experimental chamber. The trained cats were then taught that whenever a tone was present, food would not be available. They would simply have to bide their time until the tone stopped. A behavioral state had thus been induced in which cats had to withhold their natural tendency to pounce on the bar whenever the light came on.

The cats had all been fully instrumented for EEG measurements with electrodes surgically implanted beneath the skull but external to the dura. These measurements now revealed a bursting rhythm at the sensorimotor cortex that Sterman named the sensorimotor rhythm. It was present only during periods of motoric stillness, and bore a strong resemblance to the sleep spindle that characterizes Stage II sleep in both cats and humans.[3] Just as the alpha spindle tends to be prominent during eyes-closed conditions, the SMR spindle occurred only during periods of de-activation of the motor system. It was centered at nominally 13Hz, just above the alpha band (at about 10Hz).

Once this association was firmly established, Sterman made the food reward conditional on the appearance of such an SMR-burst. All the cat had to do was to compose itself in a state of quiet anticipation. As hunters, this comes naturally to them. Beautiful learning curves were acquired over a period of some weeks to months. Reinforcement on the waking SMR spindles was found to increase sleep spindle density and improve sleep efficiency.[4] Controlled experiments followed, with both a balanced reversal design and an extinction design, to prove unambiguously that operant conditioning of the SMR bursting pattern had occurred.

The reversal design was the first to demonstrate that suppression of the SMR bursting response could also be trained. This must necessarily occur by an indirect pathway. The cat is fed at regular, brief intervals as long as SMR bursts are not observable. Even this task could be readily learned. The behavioral response to the training was that the cats became physically restless and twitchy, indicating a heightened level of motoric excitability, in contrast to the SMR-conditioned cats who exhibited a general calming. The sleep of the SMR-trained cats also changed. It became more efficient and the sleep spindle density increased with the training. In fact the experiments relied upon the sleep spindle density as the salient index of change, simply because there was no chance that it might be affected by the cat's mood of the moment. The reversal design was implemented with two groups of cats undergoing training in an opposite sequence of reinforcement and suppression.

The extinction design simply involved tracking the SMR bursting behavior upon cessation of the reward. This is illustrated in Figure 2.1 for the reinforcement condition. Shown is the total time in which SMR bursting activity was present within successive 20-second intervals. Almost immediately upon the cessation of the reward, the bursting density increases substantially, signaling an attempt to re-establish the food supply. Once again learning curves were obtained, as illustrated in Figure 2.2, for a cat that had been trained for three months, for comparison with the response after one month. The case for learned behavior, in consequence of the operant conditioning procedure, had been firmly established.

The extinction design also made it clear that the conditioned SMR response had to be understood as a brain response rather than as a volitional response on the part of the cat. All the cat could contribute to the project of obtaining food was its motoric stillness, which was not sufficient by itself. This observation is foundational to the entire field of neurofeedback. The process must be understood in the perspective of the brain and of its engagement with the sensory environment, one that now also includes the feedback signal that bears directly on its own activity.

Subsequently, Sterman had the opportunity to research the low-level effects of the toxic rocket fuel monomethylhydrazine (MMH), for which his instrumented and well-characterized cats were highly suitable. The MMH effected the depletion of GABA, the primary inhibitory neurotransmitter, over the course of about an hour, after which the cats predictably went into seizure. The animals responded

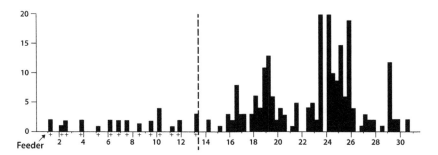

Figure 2.1 Time course of SMR-bursting activity in the extinction design. Shown is the amount of time spent above threshold in SMR amplitude in successive 20-second epochs. Triggers of the feeder are shown as plus signs. After cessation of the feeder response at 13 minutes, the SMR bursting activity increases significantly after a brief latency period, in an apparent attempt to elicit the feeder response. [5]
Source: The figure was redrawn on the basis of Sterman, Wyrwicka, & Roth, 1969.

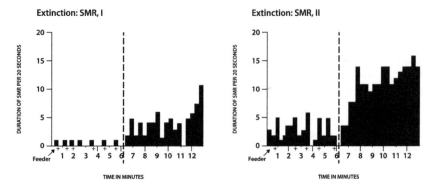

Figure 2.2 Time course of SMR-bursting activity in the extinction design. Performance after three months of training at a rate of three sessions/week is compared with performance after one month. Bursting activity is increased with the additional training both during the regular performance phase and the extinction phase. [6]

Source: The figure was redrawn on the basis of data from Wyrwicka & Sterman, 1968. This figure was recently re-published in Sterman & Egner, 2006.

with a high degree of uniformity until the end stage, at which point the population bifurcated, with a subpopulation showing substantially delayed seizure onset.

The seizure susceptibility was completely predicted by their assignment to cohort in the reversal design that had taken place some months earlier. Those who had received the SMR reinforcement last were selectively resistant to seizure onset. There must have been a carryover effect from the earlier training. Learning must have occurred that was not subject to the usual extinction that attends operant conditioning designs after reinforcement ceases. This experiment, which was quite unambiguous in its implications, was the signal experiment that established the direction and thrust of development in the field of neurofeedback.

Quite unintentionally, the above experiment met all the criteria one would impose on a fully controlled design. For their part, the cats could not have been subject to a placebo response in this case, and the researchers were obviously not biased in that they were totally blind-sided by the outcome. The bifurcation of the response was problematic with respect to the objectives of the research for which they were funded. The experiment had been a totally placebo-controlled and fully blinded design and the implications of the findings were not equivocal. In follow-up experiments, cats could be characterized in terms of their native seizure suscep-tibility, trained in the SMR paradigm, and then re-tested to evaluate their newly heightened tolerance. The results for 30 cats (10 experimental subjects, 10 surgical controls, and 10 naive) are shown in Figure 2.3.[7] The combination of anesthesia and surgery heightened seizure susceptibility, which could then be reduced again with the SMR training. A distribution in seizure risk is seen in the surgery-naïve group, which makes it appropriate to compare cats of the same rank in the rank ordering. On that basis, an average improvement factor of 1.97 (range of 1.34–2.80) is found

Relative Seizure Risk

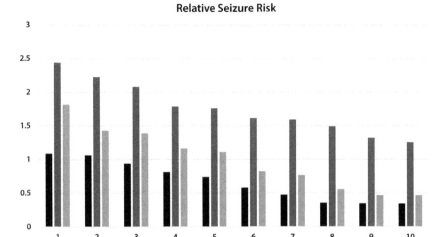

Figure 2.3 Individual results are plotted for seizure risk, expressed as the reciprocal of seizure latency, for three groups of ten cats, after administration of monomethylhydrazene. Cases are presented rank-ordered according to risk factor. The least risk is associated with the naïve, unoperated cats. The largest risk is associated with the operated cats. Intermediate risk is associated with the operated and SMR-trained cats.
Source: Underlying data were taken from Sterman, Goodman &, Kovalesky, 1978.

between the surgical controls (which received either sham neurofeedback or none at all), and the SMR-trained cats. The trained cats remained in deficit by an average factor of 1.5 +-0.12 (range of 1.36–1.67) with respect to the surgery-naïve cats. This factor is tightly distributed, which further justifies handling the data in this rank-ordered fashion. These results were subsequently confirmed by studies on rhesus monkeys as well.[8] The efficacy of SMR reinforcement in diminishing surgery-induced and chemically enhanced seizure risk had thus been established in animal work.

2.3 Evaluation of SMR Reinforcement with Human Subjects

2.3.1 Seizure Disorder

Sterman turned his attention to human trials. An employee in his laboratory suffered from nocturnal seizures and offered to be the first trainee. Training for only 34 sessions over four months resulted in the observation of a near elimination of seizures, which led promptly to a publication,[9] although it took several years of training to render the person entirely seizure-free, to the point where she qualified for a California driver's license. An exploratory outcome study on four participants, all of whom benefited from the training, was published in 1974.[10] By 1972, Sterman's research had attracted the interest of Joel Lubar, Professor of Psychology at the University of Tennessee in Knoxville. His research group published an outcome study on eight participants, seven of whom benefited from the training.[11, 12] Controlled studies followed, using either the reversal design or sham training as an ostensibly neutral control condition. All participants in this research were medically refractory seizure patients whose condition was stable. Whereas the initial target was motor seizures, eventually the scope encompassed complex partial seizures as well.

The first study utilizing an ABA design involved eight participants.[13] Two reinforcement bands were evaluated: 12–15Hz and 18–23Hz. For the reversal phase, Sterman used reinforcements in the 6–9Hz band. This avoided the lower EEG frequencies which, if reinforced, could potentially aggravate seizures. Results were remarkable. Six of the eight improved significantly in their seizure incidence, with an overall improvement of 74 percent. This was despite the fact that half the time had been spent training in the wrong direction, where seizure incidence did indeed mostly get worse. One of the eight became entirely seizure-free, another very nearly so.

A second such ABA study was published by Lubar's group.[14] It was the first to use a double-blind design. This study also involved eight participants. The reversal phase utilized a 3–8Hz spectral band. As feared, seizure incidence could be exacerbated in this manner, and indeed one participant had to be withdrawn from this phase of the training for that reason. Average reduction in seizure incidence in the cohort was only 35 percent. Referenced to the five of eight who were considered 'responders,' the mean reduction was 49 percent, a clinically significant improvement.

In Sterman's sham-controlled study, 24 participants with complex partial seizures were divided into three groups: a passive seizure-tracking group, the sham-training group, and the veridical feedback group. After an initial six-week training program, at a rate of three sessions per week, the two control groups were given the chance to train for another six weeks. All were weaned off the training over the course of four weeks, and a six-week follow-up period was allowed for. An overall improvement in seizure incidence of 60 percent was found in post-testing.[15] The study also included extensive neuropsychological and neurocognitive evaluation, and these results were published subsequently.[16] Those who improved the most in terms of seizure incidence also tended to improve more on the mental skills testing, as well as on the Minnesota Multiphasic Personality Inventory (MMPI). Results also correlated with improvements observed in the clinical EEG. Of the 17 who exhibited typically abnormal EEG patterns, nine normalized their EEGs, and of this subset, three brought their seizures fully under control.

In this same time frame replications were also undertaken as far away as Scandinavia and Italy. There appeared to be a groundswell of interest in the method for a time. The results of all the early studies were reviewed by Sterman in 2000.[17] Some 24 studies were evaluated, which collectively involved some 243 participants. Twenty of these were group studies, and thirteen of those included competent controls. Collectively, 82 percent of all the participants improved their seizure incidence by at least 30 percent, with the average improvement being greater than

50 percent. A more recent reflection on the status of this clinical approach was published in 2006.[18]

A meta-analysis of the epilepsy studies has brought the appraisal up to date.[19] Some 63 studies were evaluated for inclusion, but only ten survived the screen. These involved some 87 participants. The analysis confirmed 'significant' reduction in seizure incidence. The review included one study that trained only on the Slow Cortical Potential (SCP).[20] Strictly speaking, then, the review consolidated the case for the use of EEG-derived cues in a behavioral strategy of seizure reduction. This relatively recent meta-analysis reflects the diversity of approach that came to characterize the field. This is described further below.

2.3.2 Attention Deficit Hyperactivity Disorder

A second principal area of clinical interest developed early around what is now called Attention Deficit Hyperactivity Disorder (ADHD), but at the time was still thought of mainly in terms of hyperkinesis. This thrust was led throughout by Joel Lubar. This interest was initially kindled by the observation that a child undergoing training of seizure control also experienced a subsidence of his hyperactivity,[21] with this observation also confirmed in other such cases. Since the training was targeting the motor strip, it seemed reasonable to assume that hyperactivity was being tamed as well. Formal evaluation followed with children who were not afflicted with a seizure condition.

The first case study was soon published.[22] It was postulated that EEG training would be helpful with those children who were responsive to Ritalin, in which case the training would be expected to yield additive benefits. The study involved a 14 year old who was placed on 10mg of Ritalin for the duration. Six no-drug and six drug-only baselines were obtained on behavioral and EEG assessments. A training sequence of 78 sessions of SMR reinforcement, combined with inhibition on excessive 4–7Hz activity, was followed by 36 sessions of reversal phase training, which in turn was followed by another 28 sessions of the design protocol. Placement was bipolar on left hemisphere sensorimotor strip.

Learning curves were acquired for the incidence of rewards relative to baseline conditions, and electromyographic (EMG) activity at the chin was tracked as an index to muscular tone. Both reward incidence and EMG trends reflected the prevailing protocol to a statistically significant degree. Over the sessions, reward incidence increased by factors up to three or four over baseline. It regressed equally strongly during the reversal phase. Regression was also noted during a two-week break in the training.

Some 13 behavioral categories were tracked by two independent observers monitoring classroom behavior. Eight of these were found to be responsive to the training. Six of these categories had already shown improvement with Ritalin, but further improvement was observed with the EEG training, and countertrends were observed during the reversal phase. Five additional categories included four social behaviors plus self-talk, and these showed no improvement with the SMR training. In fact, benefit that had been observed with Ritalin was reversed with the training.

The above was the first of four cases treated using the same study design.[23] Two children responded much like the first, and one was non-responsive to Ritalin as well as the EEG training. In a final phase added to the program, the three children were successfully weaned off the Ritalin while continuing to train, and behavioral gains were maintained. Years later, Lubar revisited a number of clients whom he trained during those early years and found that the gains had been retained over the longer term.[24]

Other studies followed. Tansey was successful in remediating a case of hyper-activity, developmental reading disorder, and ocular instability with a sequential combination of EMG and SMR training.[25] He utilized a placement on the midline. Normalization of highly elevated EMG levels was achieved, and substantial increases in SMR amplitudes were observed over the course of 20 training sessions. Success was achieved with respect to all three symptoms and status was maintained over a two-year follow-up period.

2.3.3 Learning Disabilities and IQ

Lubar pursued the growing interest in application to learning disabilities with extended training of six boys.[26] In this work, beta1 training (16–20Hz) was added for enhanced focus of attention and arousal regulation. All improved in their academic performance, and all exhibited learning curves with respect to SMR and beta amplitudes, EMG levels, theta-band amplitudes, and gross movement indicators.

The promise of benefit for learning disabilities eventuated in an investigation of SMR training of eight mildly neurologically impaired children by Tansey.[27] The average improvement in Full Score Wechsler IQ score (WISC-R) was found to be 19 points. If either verbal or performance IQ lagged the other by more than 14 points, the deficited variable improved by an average of 40 percent more than the other. This epoch-making study was followed by one on 24 comparably impaired children. The average improvement in WISC-R score was found to be 19.75.[28, 29] Moreover, this was achieved with an average of 27 training sessions, delivered at the rate of one per week. Both the number of sessions and the pace of training would now be considered sub-optimal, and yet the results were stunning.

Tansey's extraordinary findings led to a replication in our own clinic using a left-lateralized protocol and reinforcement at beta1 frequencies (15–18Hz) rather than at 14Hz on the midline. Fifteen children with ADD features and/or learning disabilities were trained just as if they had been in ordinary clinical practice. Independent testing and evaluation were relied upon exclusively.[30] Average improvement in WISC-R score was found to be 23 points. The profile of average change scores for the subtests of the WISC bore a remarkable similarity in the two studies. This is shown in Figure 2.4. Strong improvements in performance were also registered on the Benton Visual Retention Test, the Wide Range Achievement Test, and the tapping subtest of the Harris Tests of Laterality. Not subject to quantitative assessment were the subsidence of oppositionality, general improvement in sleep quality among those where it was deficient, and the relief from persistent stomach and head pain.

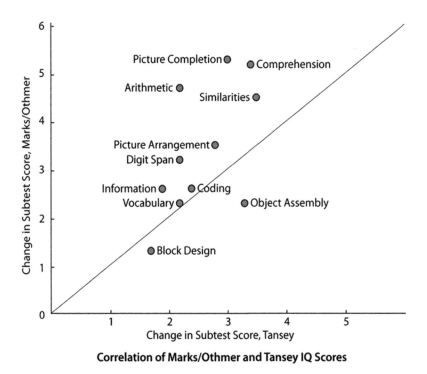

Correlation of Marks/Othmer and Tansey IQ Scores

Figure 2.4 Comparison of WISC-R subtest improvement scores for the Tansey and Marks/Othmer studies on SMR and beta training, respectively. Despite differences in sample populations, in protocols, in instrumentation, and in training procedures, a correlation between the two data sets is apparent.

2.3.4 Comparison of SMR Training with Stimulant Medication

Since stimulant medication was already recognized as a treatment for ADHD, the practical question faced by the medical practitioner is whether neurofeedback is in fact comparably effective. This essential question was answered in a study comparing 23 children in each arm.[31] Comparison of outcomes was by means of the T.O.V.A.® (Test of Variables of Attention), a continuous performance test (CPT). Results were comparable in both arms, with both methods showing essential normalization of inattention and impulsivity, accompanied by more modest improvements in mean reaction time, but with substantial improvement in variability. The comparison is illustrated in Figure 2.5.

Rossiter repeated the same design some nine years later, with thirty participants in each arm of the study. Results were better than they had been in 1995.[32, 33] Both medication management and neurofeedback protocols had improved in the interim, and the two approaches were now even more closely matched. Most likely the neurofeedback strategies benefited particularly from adding pre-frontal

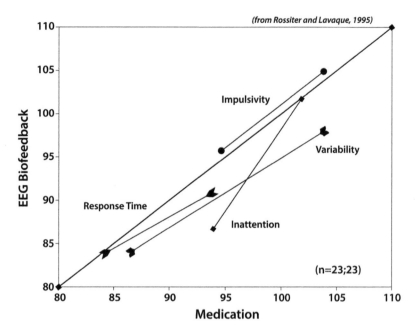

Figure 2.5 Results of a comparison of SMR-beta neurofeedback with stimulant medication are shown here for cohorts of 23, using the TOVA CPT as a measure. Comparability between the two is indicated by parallelism with the 45 degree line. Both impulsivity and variability are cases in point.
Source: Data are taken from Rossiter & LaVaque, 1995.

placements to the standard protocol. The comparison is shown in Figure 2.6. By now at least six studies have been published that compare standard SMR-beta neurofeedback with stimulants, all showing essentially comparable outcomes for pharmacotherapy and SMR/beta neurofeedback.[34, 35, 36, 37]

The largest of these studies involved 100 participants and used the Lubar protocol.[38] By 1991 Lubar had adopted the 'theta-beta ratio' as a criterion of functioning in the ADHD population, based on the observation that the most prominent change observed in the EEGs of these children with training was a decline in theta-band amplitudes. An increase in SMR/beta amplitudes was not observed as consistently. Lubar had also adopted Cz as a standard placement for the SMR training, on the basis that the theta/beta ratio was typically largest at this site.

Lubar was the first to make excess theta-band amplitudes an explicit target of a down-training strategy, which gives additional salience to the theta-beta ratio criterion. This made for a two-pronged training strategy of rewards and inhibits that has become standard. (Sterman had introduced the inhibit strategy originally, but it was for the sole purpose of assuring that there would be no 'false rewards' for SMR-bursts that were corrupted by excess theta-band or upper beta band excursions.) In consequence of the above, the protocol has also been referred to as the 'beta/theta' or 'theta/beta' protocol.

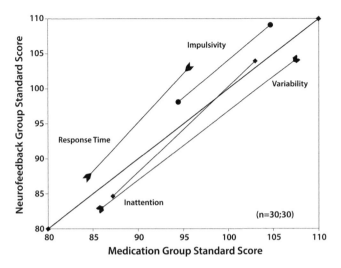

Figure 2.6 Results of the same comparison as in Figure 2.5 are illustrated for a similar comparison study conducted nine years later with cohorts of 30. Outcomes were considerably better than the earlier data, as both neurofeedback protocols and medication management had improved in the intervening years. Comparability between the two therapies is apparent in the data.
Source: Data taken from Rossiter, 2004.

Participants in this large-scale, long-term outcome study were selected on the basis of the theta/beta criterion, among others.[39] All were medicated to a level at which performance on the TOVA CPT was optimized, with the result that both groups normalized their TOVA subtest scores. EEG training was undertaken with the neurofeedback cohort until the theta-beta ratio normalized. This required an average of 43 sessions. Over the course of training behavioral variables normalized for the EEG training cohort, whereas they remained in the clinical range for the medication-only comparison group.

After a year of the above regimen, medication was discontinued for a week to allow the children to be evaluated under no-medication conditions. The neurofeedback contingent held gains on both the TOVA and the parent/teacher ratings, while the comparison group fell back into the clinical range on the TOVA, and remained in the clinical range on behavioral ratings. A clear advantage had been demonstrated for the neurofeedback approach using multiple independent criteria, and medication was not required to sustain the gains.

In 2000, we published on a large-scale survey of outcomes with ADHD children.[40] The objective here was to assess just how well the SMR-beta protocols were working out in actual clinical practice. Some 32 clinics were included in the survey. By the time this was done, the TOVA CPT had become a standard assessment tool within our practitioner network. The most revealing parameter in the CPT is impulsivity, based on commission errors. The results for impulsivity are shown in Figure 2.7 for all those whose initial standard score was 85 or less (i.e., below the 16th

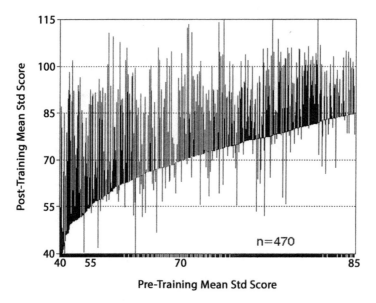

Figure 2.7 Individual case data are shown for impulsivity, as measured with the TOVA CPT, for the 470 cases that scored below 85 in standard score in the survey of 32 practices utilizing SMR-beta protocols. Data refer to reassessments after nominally 20 sessions. The data comparison suffers from the fact that among school children the retests often took place in the afternoon, whereas the test is normed for the morning hours.
Source: Kaiser & Othmer, 2000.

percentile). The results were satisfying indeed. They refer to the outcomes after the first twenty sessions of training.

In 2009 a meta-analysis was published that reviewed the research status of neurofeedback in application to the ADHD spectrum.[41] The unsurprising conclusion was that neurofeedback treatment for ADHD can be considered 'efficacious and specific,' with large effect sizes for inattention (0.81) and impulsivity (0.69), and a medium effect size for hyperactivity (0.4). Fifteen studies were included in the evaluation and these comprised some 476 participants in the controlled studies and some 718 in the pre/post evaluation.[42]

Ironically, the Monastra study was excluded from the above compilation because the effect size was so large (2.22) that it failed the test for homogeneity of the sample of studies. Of course, it did so for the best of reasons. The participants had been picked on the basis of an EEG criterion, the theta-beta ratio, which no doubt selected for those most likely to do well with a protocol tailored to that criterion. Readers unblinkered by foolish consistency will appreciate this illustration of what is possible when the training protocol is matched to the target population.

By 2009, then, meta-analyses had confirmed the efficacy of SMR/beta neurofeedback in application to epilepsy and ADHD, respectively. Both reviews had also included studies employing slow-cortical potential training. In 2013, PracticeWise, a research agency for the American Academy of Pediatrics, appropriately recognized neurofeedback as having met Level I criteria (the highest) for research support in application to ADHD.[43]

2.4 Neurofeedback in Application to Addictions

A third major clinical interest emerged in the late eighties around neurofeedback in application to alcohol dependency. This topic also takes us back to the very beginnings of the field. The original discovery of EEG biofeedback had in fact been made by Joe Kamiya in the course of his research on the alpha rhythm of the EEG. Kamiya had originally intended to investigate the relationship of the EEG to psychophysiological states, and in that quest was testing whether an individual was able to discriminate the presence of an alpha burst in his occiput at a given moment. Fortuitously, he had in his chair someone who was able to learn that task perfectly in just four sessions, over which Kamiya gave him simple verbal feedback on whether or not he was correct whenever he was prompted by an occasional tone. By the fourth session, the trainee had an unbroken run of 400 successful trials. Kamiya never again had such a good subject, but the field was launched. This work took place in 1958 at the University of Chicago, within four years of Kamiya obtaining his Ph.D. there.

Within a few years operant conditioning of the alpha rhythm was undertaken in Kamiya's laboratory.[44] Application to anxiety reduction followed.[45] Just as happened with the work of Sterman with epilepsy, as soon as therapeutic benefit of the training experience was insinuated, the whole procedure was subjected to heightened scrutiny. It did not help that the alpha training had been brought to broad public awareness through an interview with Kamiya that was published in *Psychology Today* in 1968. Kamiya saw no harm in responding to the interview request, as he viewed his work to be fundamental research rather than a steppingstone to a therapeutic modality. His findings resonated with the Zeitgeist of the psychedelic age, however, and alpha training became popular in certain circles as a way of inducing an LSD-like experience without the attendant risks. In the same timeframe, Barbara Brown discovered alpha training independently, and then worked diligently to bring it to broader awareness within the culture through her books and lectures.[46,47] She also edited *The Alpha Syllabus*, which covered more than one thousand publications on the topic.[48]

Several replications by teams of academics failed to support Kamiya's findings, and suddenly the nascent field of biofeedback, which had organized itself formally in 1969 around this new method of promoting self-regulation, found itself on the defensive. In particular, one controlled study used alpha-down-training as a control condition and found that both conditions resulted in improved anxiety control.[49] As the original hypothesis was not supported, alpha training was deemed a nullity. This is understandable in terms of the theories of the day. A more modern perspective would hold that both kinds of training can lead to learned self-regulation. Indeed, bi-directional training has become commonplace in biofeedback.

A second blow was struck with the report that subjects sitting in subdued lighting under eyes-open conditions were unable to increase their alpha amplitude with training above their own eyes-closed baseline.[50] Since this served as a replication of an earlier negative finding the issue was considered settled, and this caused academics to abandon the research into alpha training wholesale. It was soon pointed out that the negative outcome studies had been riddled with methodological flaws. For example, Lynch et al. based their negative findings on the basis of a single training session. By the time of the sober reappraisal by Ancoli and Kamiya,[51] however, it was too late.

The biofeedback community reconstituted itself around the use of peripheral physiology to effect improved self-regulation. Reliance on finger temperature, galvanic skin response, and electromyographic activity as indices of physiological state at least had the benefit of face validity. Fortunately, the alpha and theta-band training continued among a variety of independent groups that included, in particular, one at the Menninger Foundation that was originally organized by Elmer Green at the invitation of Karl Menninger himself. The interests in this group lay with the study of dimensions of the human experience, not with the amelioration of mental disorders. However, their work did inspire such pursuits by others. One early study yielded promising outcomes in application to alcoholism, and that kindled a new focus for the field.[52]

This initial study of the application of alpha training to addictions, among other influences, led Eugene Peniston to apply the method to his alcoholic veterans at the Fort Lyon VA in Colorado.[53] His first study involved ten Vietnam era veterans who had a minimum of four prior treatment failures. The controls received only the regular VA treatment. The experimentals received some initial exposure to temperature training in order to acquaint them with the process of training toward self-regulation. That was then followed up with 30 sessions of what was now called Alpha-Theta training. This training utilizes reinforcements in both the alpha and theta bands. The principal purpose here is not brain training per se but rather the induction of a state that is conducive to the encounter with the core self, and hence represents a pathway to personal transformation.

That is indeed what happened. The results were stunning. Initially eight of the ten experimentals sustained abstinence after release from the program. The remaining two, having contemptuously dismissed the EEG training as a meaningless exercise at the time, soon found out that they had lost their tolerance for alcohol, and perforce became abstinent as well. All the controls stayed true to their prior pattern and all were re-admitted to treatment within 18 months. The experimentals were followed up for more than eight years. All retained their sobriety; one died of cirrhosis of the liver.

In his subsequent replication study, Peniston chose to use the MMPI as a progress measure, despite the fact that it was never intended to be used as a change index. First of all, it is entirely dependent on self-report, and secondly it was thought to reveal aspects of personality that were deemed to be stable, not subject to substantial alteration. In light of that, the changes identified by Peniston were compelling. They are shown in Figure 2.8 for both arms.

Peniston's intriguing research was not welcomed by the biofeedback community when it was first presented in 1990 because it threatened to rekindle the original controversy about alpha training. Thought leaders of the field muddied the

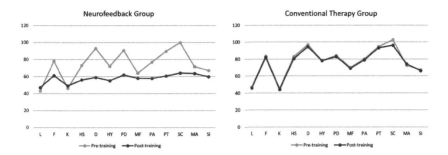

Figure 2.8 MMPI data are shown for the second published study on recovery from alcoholism and PTSD by Peniston and Kulkosky (1991), which was designed as a replication of the first. The differences between the treatment and control groups are dramatic and compelling. [54]
Source: Peniston & Kulkosky, 1991.

waters to the point that the stunning MMPI data was never seriously appraised. When findings are as unambiguous as these they must be taken seriously, or else the source must be discredited. That is, unfortunately, what happened. Nevertheless, Peniston followed with yet another successful replication, and other groups did as well. He summarized his research in 1995[55] and described his method in a book chapter.[56] One major criticism was the limited size of the studies, even though they were clearly sufficient in light of the large effect size.

Following in Peniston's wake, a large-scale study was undertaken in 1994 at an addictions treatment center in Los Angeles. A total of 121 participants were entered into a controlled study in which the control was the regular Minnesota Model in-patient treatment program.[57] Our SMR/beta protocol was inserted in place of the temperature training, but the emphasis again remained on the Alpha-Theta component. One-year post-treatment it was determined that the experimentals were sustaining sobriety at a rate three times that of the controls, at nominally 75 percent. After three years, the control group had mostly relapsed, while the experimentals had largely maintained sobriety—albeit with maintenance of group participation that was a key part of the 12-step-based program. Ongoing sobriety was highly correlated with continued participation in the group, which in turn was highly correlated with the prior EEG training experience. Neurofeedback became standard treatment at this center upon completion of the study. It took six years to get the study published.

What came to be known as the Peniston Protocol was then also evaluated in a multi-faceted program in Houston to rehabilitate homeless crack users. This program was ongoing when Alpha-Theta neurofeedback was introduced. With some 430 eligible to participate, there was 50 percent attrition before completion of 30 training sessions. The 178 who completed the program stayed an average of 103 days longer than those who did not get neurofeedback. Length of stay correlates well with ultimate achievement of relapse-free status. One-year follow-up with 87 participants revealed that 50 percent had retained non-use status and, of those who relapsed, 80 percent had used cocaine fewer than nine times over the year. Graduation rate from the program (meaning non-using, housed, no criminal justice system involvement, and either employed or in student status) rose from 12 per year to 12 per month upon the introduction of neurofeedback. While it is not possible to parse just how much the neurofeedback contributed to this outcome, those involved clearly saw it as the heart of the therapeutic dimension of this comprehensive program.[58]

2.5 Slow Cortical Potential Training

Whereas all of the above developments took place in the United States, a very different method of neurofeedback was being developed by a research group under Niels Birbaumer in Tübingen, Germany. The discovery in 1964 of the Contingent Negative Variation (CNV), a transient negative excursion of the surface potential in preparation for a response, soon led to further observation that the CNV could be subjected to voluntary control. That, in turn, led to successful control of the baseline SCP through operant conditioning techniques.[59] As the SCP appeared to reflect cortical excitability directly, the method was applied to the management of medically uncontrolled seizures, migraine, and even schizophrenia. The emphasis in research, however, has been on ADHD, as in the case of EEG band training.[60]

The clinical claims were not welcomed in Europe any more than they had been in the United States, so research focused increasingly on the use of this method to allow locked-in patients to communicate. Voluntary control of excursions in the SCP could be used in a selection scheme for letters of the alphabet. At a minimum, the success in this application proved the method to be quite capable of yielding real-time control of the SCP. Given the cognitive demand, the training could not be done with very young children, but in other respects the method was straightforward. A single placement at Cz was universally used, and there aren't many nuances to the protocol. Bi-directional training of the SCP has been adopted in order to train for better regulation in general. At each trial during the session, the trainee is given the direction in which the SCP is to be moved.

2.6 New Departures in Neurofeedback

2.6.1 The Beginnings of QEEG-informed Training

Up to the early nineties all of the principal neurofeedback protocols were grounded in physiological models, and hence could be referred to as mechanisms-based. SMR up-training was targeting the down-regulation of motoric excitability. The accompanying theta-band down-training was targeting the improvement of thalamocortical regulatory control. Alpha-band up-training moved trainees to lower arousal levels and to residence in calmer states. SCP training reduced cortical excitability directly.

The beneficial consequences could be observed over a variety of clinical conditions, ranging from migraines to insomnia to pain syndromes, even to those that had not been specifically targeted. Cognitive function was often enhanced as well.

The generality of effects could be best seen in application to minor traumatic brain injury, where benefits could be noted for the entire range of classic symptoms characteristic of such injury. At the same time, there was no reason to assume that a physically-injured brain should necessarily respond in the same way as other brains.

In the early nineties it became practical and affordable to acquire a 19-channel digital EEG capability even in a private clinic, and to subject the EEG to quantitative analysis for comparison against norms. This made it possible to tailor the training to the specific conditions prevailing in a particular brain. That in turn could, for the first time, yield the kind of protocol specificity that researchers sought in order to validate the technique. Finally, this new capability gave neurofeedback the same 'deficit-focus' that characterizes psychiatry and psychology. This need was keenly felt as neurofeedback still lacked general acceptance within the health professions.

One consequence of this orientation to the quantitative EEG is that it placed clinical considerations into the background. Deviation from norms provided the rationale for the protocol rather than any specific symptom or diagnosis. In practice, the observed deviations were often arbitrarily attributed to whatever diagnosis the person came in with, in order to make the case for neurofeedback to the client. Effectively, however, the target was the deviation from norms. Training could now be done at any site and at any EEG frequency, and this resulted in a ramp-up of the collective body of experience and of the learning curve within the practitioner community. Aiding this endeavor further was the fact that this exploration was taking place in hundreds of individual clinics without any central direction. The downside was that this collective effort would not yield the kind of research that would be persuasive to academics or journal editors and hence neurofeedback would retain its outsider status even in the face of this aspiration to a scientifically grounded procedure.

There was yet another problem. Neither the field of neurology nor that of psychiatry had yet adopted digital EEG analysis to guide therapies, so the neurofeedback field had just multiplied its challenges of persuading the mainstream rather than reduced them. It did not help that individual neurofeedback clinicians were typically not credentialed in EEG diagnostics. Hence there was the messenger problem. Further, in its early days, the whole field of digital EEG analysis was riven with controversies because many issues had simply not yet been resolved. Expert analysis of clinical cases rarely corresponded between experts. Then there was also a fundamental problem lying at the root of the whole enterprise, namely that EEG deviations sometimes reflect accommodations rather than deficits, which complicates targeting. EEG deviations were often so numerous that clinical judgment was required to establish the appropriate hierarchy of targets, and, perhaps worst of all, the state dependence of the EEG (the very thing that makes it a good training variable) argues against its use as a diagnostic. The EEG varies substantially with ultradian rhythmicity, for example, a topic dealt with in Chapter 4. Meanwhile, the promise of professional guidance toward reliable prescriptions for training protocols served to attract weak players into the field.

It also transpired that in the new regime, in which normalization of EEG parameters became the objective, the up-training of presumptive deficits in the EEG band amplitudes was found to be much more problematic than the inhibition of excesses.

The latter either worked or it didn't, but it rarely caused a problem. The promotion of higher EEG amplitudes, on the other hand, often led trainees into further distress. In consequence, quantitative EEG-based (QEEG-based) training came to be focused largely on inhibiting excesses. For the reward-based training, clinicians typically defaulted back to the standard protocols that had carried the field to its initial success. In this manner, the information yielded up from the full-head EEG was more clearly additive to what could be done with only single-channel derivation. QEEG-based training had found its proper niche.

Just how is this differential effectiveness of reward- and inhibit-based training to be understood? The inhibit-based training is typically accomplished with threshold-based withholding of the rewards. Nothing is actually being inhibited. This kind of cueing elicits a rather non-specific response on the part of the brain. The reward-based training, on the other hand, is much more specific in its appeal to the brain, and the specifics matter. So in the dual targeting approach one combines a very general, nonspecific appeal to the brain with a very specifically targeted objective. It is obviously the latter that focuses the clinical mind.

2.6.2 The Evolution of Mechanisms-Based Training

In our own implementation of the SMR/beta protocols we consistently observed a preference for higher frequency training on the left hemisphere than the right. This finding came about in an interesting way. We had started out with left-hemisphere training in the beta1 band, 15–18Hz, following Margaret Ayers, who had been a graduate student of Barry Sterman. Ayers had found the higher band to be more consistently helpful for her head-injury and stroke patients.[61] We then added SMR-band training at Cz, following Tansey and Lubar, for the ADHD children. SMR training was done at 12–15Hz. A move from Cz to C4 then led to much more hemisphere-specific effects. Thus, our standard protocol became a combination of 'C3beta and C4SMR,' with the two protocols titrated as needed. This approach became broadly popular within the field and was adopted by several thousand practitioners over the years. This was the protocol employed in our large practitioner survey on ADHD.[62]

By the mid-nineties, even our standard mechanisms-informed, protocol-based training was subjected to evolution. It was observed that trainees who happened to be particularly sensitive to the training responded in a highly frequency-specific manner. (This could not be discovered earlier because we had fixed-frequency filters in the instrument we had developed.) The training needed to be individualized with respect to the rewards as well as the inhibits. First the intermediate frequency of 15Hz was provided. Then adjustment in 0.5Hz steps was provided for. Eventually, even finer frequency divisions turned out to be advantageous. Such a high frequency-specificity has never been adequately explained.

This surprising finding led to our adoption of an optimization strategy for each client, one in which the best reward frequency needed to be determined through sequential A/B comparisons. The optimization had to be accomplished by tracking the sometimes subtle responses of the client through each session and from session to session. It could not be done by merely inspecting the EEG. This finding sheds light on the difficulties that had been encountered earlier with the QEEG-based training, because the requisite discrimination of the optimum target frequency is just not possible on the basis of the EEG.

The discovery of the frequency-specificity of reward-based training gave permission for the migration of the reward frequency beyond the standard bands in pursuit of the optimum training frequency. In fact, for many individuals it became mandatory. This, together with the liberation from the standard training sites that had already been accomplished with the adoption of digital EEG analysis, led to yet another period of protocol evolution. Looking back on this period, however, it is apparent that every step into the unknown was undertaken cautiously. Every incremental step forward was thoroughly consolidated in empirical support before additional steps were taken.

With the availability of 19-channel data for the display of spatial maps, attention shifted to site-specific data, and away from the bipolar derivation that had been customary in clinical EEGs. In the conceptual frame of targeting EEG anomalies it had also become obligatory to undertake single-site training. This is referred to as referential placement. That means only a single active electrode is placed over cortex, with the other active electrode, referred to as the reference, placed on a quasi-neutral site such as an ear lobe. This meant the abandonment of the bipolar montage that had been standard for Sterman and Lubar—even for the standard Sterman and Lubar protocols.

In our own work we had found the Sterman and Lubar protocols to be quite adequate for our purposes, and with the impetus to move beyond the sensorimotor strip we returned to bipolar montage so that we could at once explore new sites while keeping one foot planted, so to speak, on the familiar turf of the sensorimotor strip. By moving the other electrode off the strip, we were training the relationship between the two sites. Training effects were enhanced nicely by virtue of the incorporation of frontal and pre-frontal sites, but likely also by virtue of the return to bipolar montage.

The increase in sensitivity of the training that was purchased with bipolar montage brought about a heightened awareness of the frequency specificity. This was particularly an issue with those who responded very sensitively to the training, such as migraineurs and fibromyalgia clients. It was the challenge of sensitive responders that led us progressively to new placements and new regions of the EEG spectrum. Over the course of some years, the entire conventional EEG spectrum, from 0.5Hz to 40Hz, was eventually encompassed. During this initial exploration, we found the distribution of optimum target frequencies to cover the entire spectrum, albeit with a bias toward the lower frequencies.

2.6.3 The Migration to Lower Frequencies

The greatest challenge we confronted in that time frame (1999–2004) was the progression to ever lower frequencies. We proceeded into this terrain with some trepidation because of the known hazards of training at low EEG frequencies that Lubar and Sterman had already exposed. The difference was that we were now armed with the knowledge that training had to take place under very specific conditions. We therefore actually had complete consistency between the new and the old findings. The problem that had been identified by Lubar was that up-training toward greater EEG synchrony was potentially a risk, particularly in conditions such as epilepsy where excess synchrony is a known hazard. Under specific conditions, however, that could now be managed. The use of bipolar montage biases the training toward desynchronization of the target frequency between the two active sites.[63] Lubar had used bipolar montage as well, but that was not enough to render the training benign in his early study on seizure disorder. With careful adjustment of the training frequency, however, the effects were not only favorable but rather more powerful than we had been accustomed to. This led to breakthroughs with clinical conditions that had not yielded to the earlier higher-frequency training. These positive developments encouraged further exploration and that led, eventually, to the entry into the infra-low frequency regime.

2.7 Status of the Principal Approaches to Neurofeedback

Before that topic is taken up, however, a perspective on the context in which this development took place is in order. Progress was being made in all of the principal ways of doing neurofeedback that have been described. QEEG-based training evolved in the direction of targeting the coherence between two sites rather than amplitudes at a single site. This made for more dynamic, more impactful training, just as we had found when moving from referential back to bipolar training in our own approach. Representative studies that reflect the state of the art of this approach exist for migraine,[64] TBI,[65] and schizophrenia.[66]

Site-specific targeting also evolved further. This approach could be aided with the use of LORETA, a program that constructs a source distribution of virtual dipoles that is consistent with the prevailing EEG at the 19 sites. With the application of physically realistic constraints, the infinity of such 'inverse' solutions that exists in principle can be reduced to just one. This procedure can be used to refine targeting and to focus on sources at depth within the cerebrum. It can also be useful in pre- and post-evaluation of training procedures.

Inhibit-based training also matured as a stand-alone approach in two principal manifestations. In the first, the brain is regarded as a non-linear dynamical system, and the EEG is seen to reflect those properties. This means that the EEG cannot be properly analyzed in terms of Gaussian distributions. On the contrary, EEG parameters are known to exhibit scale-free statistics, or very broad distributions that may be well approximated by power laws. In the Gaussian perspective that we continue to press into service, it would be said that there are long tails, but that misrepresents the state of affairs. In addition, stationarity of the EEG cannot be assumed. What is measured at one moment is not necessarily replicable at another moment. Hence fixed thresholds are contra-indicated. In the particular approach at issue, excursions into dysregulation are detected dynamically at two bilateral sites (C3 and C4) on the sensorimotor strip and the brain is cued with respect to these excursions. All the drama that attends reward-based training because of the decision-making involved is avoided. Since no clean boundary between function and dysfunction is discernible in the EEG, the tactical choice is made to inhibit only the extrema in the tracked variables. This increases the likelihood that the fouls being called on the brain are indeed episodes of dysregulation. A study has been published in which this method was used in the recovery from 'chemo-fog'.[67]

The second approach seeks to enhance the reliability in the discrimination of dysregulation by force of large numbers. By tracking a number of EEG parameters (band amplitudes and site-to-site coherences) for several sites over time, advantage is taken of the fact that correlation between the measures increases as the brain enters a state of dysregulation. Superposition of all the measures then yields a collective index to the instantaneous state of dysregulation of the whole system. The reliability of this index increases further as the brain reaches extremes of dysregulation. In practice, the trainee is simply exposed to the time course of this index, which serves as an incremental guide to more regulated states and, ultimately, to clinical success. Since this method is typically based on deviations from normative behavior, it is referred to as Z-score training.

Despite the proliferation of approaches over the years, the bulk of the work in the clinical realm is still being done with variations on the standard SMR/beta protocols, combined with one inhibit strategy or another. Placement is either on the midline at Cz, straddling Cz on the midline in bipolar montage, or using the traditional lateralized placements such as 'C3beta/C4SMR', which likely remains the most common choice.

Alpha-Theta training has also been adopted quite broadly as a complement to the SMR/beta training. The thrust here is very different. Whereas the intellectual frontier in this field has all along been the challenge of functional normalization, there has remained a persistent need to redress the psychological residue of prior traumatic experiences or of a traumatic early childhood. This can be accomplished with Alpha-Theta training, and more effectively after a measure of physiological stabilization has been achieved. The Alpha-Theta training quietens the outer-directed faculties that keep one rooted in the present moment and calms the fear-driven self. Hence it allows the journey to the interior realm, where historical traumas can be resolved while the person is resident in a perceived calm and safe place. The intent in this training is entirely experiential.

For many who encounter this training, the effect is transformational. In particular, it is those who come with a traumatic history who find this experience healing, and that can go a long way toward explaining the early reports of dramatic spiritual experiences with alpha training that were so off-putting to the academic community originally. Having fled their families, those youngsters who were drawn to Haight-Ashbury and the drug experience were likely also those who would respond powerfully to Alpha-Theta training. By the same token, those same experiences would not easily be replicated with research subjects plucked from among engineering students to populate studies at the psychology department. Such 'extraordinary' claims for alpha training have been confirmed in clinical experience.

Alpha training has also played a large role in training toward functional normalization and the enhancement of our attentional capacities. This is the work of Lester Fehmi, which also had its origins in the early days of discovery of alpha training. Fehmi relies heavily on the language of attention, thus recruiting the individual actively into the task of self-regulation practice. The objective is to move from narrow and objective focus to a broader, more inclusive focus, and from a separate to an immersive presence. This shift is accompanied by a lowering in arousal level, albeit with maintenance of alertness. Reinforcement on alpha-band activity supports this shift, and it does so even more strongly when the training promotes whole-brain synchrony (read coherence) of the alpha signal explicitly.[68]

Jim Hardt has also relied on the promotion of alpha synchrony for most of his work. His engagement with this field extends all the way back to his days as a graduate student of Joe Kamiya, given impetus by his own impactful first alpha training experience. And he had been an engineer. Hardt offers intensive programs in alpha training that also incorporate group therapy to support personal transformation. More advanced training is offered with emphasis on the theta band.[69]

Yet another approach that had an early start is one that emphasizes 40Hz training. This training was first investigated by Sheer, targeting cortical function.[70] The 40Hz region is one where EEG synchrony is commonly observed in the engaged brain, meaning that bursts of such narrow-band activity are readily discernible above background noise. As with other Synchrony training, the protocol is experienced as both calming and alerting, but the subjective response is typically distinct for each of these frequencies in that different network configurations are being appealed to in each case.

2.8 Toward a New Departure in Feedback

The range of clinical conditions that are presently addressed with one or more of these methods now extends to nearly the entire spectrum of psychiatric conditions, plus many neurological conditions. The best evidence indicates that neurofeedback can be far more effective than pharmacotherapy alone, or psychotherapy alone. The best evidence in this case is to be found in the clinical realm, where clients typically come to neurofeedback late in their clinical trajectory and are already getting treatment to current standards.

The implications are clear. Psychiatric and neurological conditions involve learned brain behavior that cannot readily be undone by means of pharmacotherapy or talk therapy alone, and yet this learned behavior is accessible to us through methods of re-learning. It is appropriate, therefore, to think of neurofeedback as a modality of rehabilitation, by analogy to physical rehabilitation. Just as there is a complete continuum between physical therapy and training for optimum functioning in the athletic realm, there is complete continuity between feedback-based rehabilitation and optimal mental capability—not only in the cognitive realm but the affective realm as well.

This core reality has been somewhat obscured by the fact that neurofeedback has had to find its space within the framework of our disease- and disorder-focused health care model. Within that model, problems need to rise to a given level of severity before they get any attention and, in line with that model, neurofeedback strategies have been favored that maximally emulate the prevailing focus on discrete disorders. This becomes obvious in the focus on features of the EEG that manifest the dysregulation status. The immediate target is not the disorder itself but rather the landmarks of disorder, implicitly the dysregulation status per se. Without question, this approach has borne abundant fruit, and therefore its validity is not in question. The approach, however, does remain incomplete. Alas, some of the most disturbing and intractable mental disorders cannot be discerned in the EEG at all by current methods. The personality disorders are a case in point. These are also the conditions that first take root in the course of early development. Dysregulation status is not reducible to what can be readily detected in the EEG—a different approach is needed to complement what we already have.

Throughout our work with neurofeedback over one third of a century, we were always stymied by the most intractable end of the distribution of severity, irrespective of the particular diagnosis involved. This might involve migraines, fibromyalgia, depression, anxiety, Tourette Syndrome, OCD, or substance dependency. Furthermore, there were the conditions that had remained relatively refractory to remediation, such as chronic pain syndromes, the developmental disorders of childhood, Borderline Personality Disorder, Dissociative Identity Disorder, the addictions, and the dementias. Almost all of these most challenging and even intractable cases had in common a problematic early childhood history, with a preponderance of emotional trauma. We were confronting dysfunctions that had had a whole lifetime to be elaborated and consolidated. In other cases, a vulnerability appears to have been created that was later exposed through further physical or emotional traumas.

Since 2006 inroads have been made with a new clinical approach that allows us to address even the most challenging cases that are seen in psychiatry outside of institutional settings. This method is a radical departure from all existing approaches and it cannot be understood in terms of the existing models. It is not deficit-focused; it is not prescriptive. It is not a close-order drill to micro-manage the brain and teach it how to behave. This method allows the brain to acquire new capacities for self-regulation in the same way it learns other skills. Even in the face of all that has already been accomplished with various methods of neurofeedback, this new approach is deserving of special treatment, and for that reason this book is largely devoted to this one approach. We now turn to the further elaboration of the development of this method.

2.9 The Development of Infra-Low Frequency Training

By 2004 we had explored the EEG spectrum across the entire 'conventional' range, from 0.5Hz to 40Hz, and found individuals who optimized in all regions of this spectrum. We were constrained, however, by our software, which limited us to a 3Hz bandwidth. This meant that the lowest center frequency we could dial in was 1.5Hz. Over time, client data piled up to the point where it was obvious that the lowest frequency was preferred by more clients than any other. This motivated the investigation of yet lower frequencies, which transpired in 2006.

We found software that allowed us to extend the range to 0.1 Hz, expecting of course that those who had optimized at 1.5 Hz would now distribute themselves over this wider range. Instead we observed that the new distribution was even more strongly skewed toward the lowest value than had been the case before. In fact, some two-thirds of all of our clients exhibited a preference for the lowest frequency of 0.1 Hz. This frequency was too low for our conventional methods of signal-handling, and accommodations had to be made.

In the conventional EEG frequency range, the narrow-band signal was rectified and smoothed in order to yield the magnitude of the EEG in the particular frequency band. At 0.1 Hz that process is too slow for good feedback, so instead we simply had the trainee watch the EEG signal go up and down with its periodicity of ten seconds. This actually worked quite well. That was not entirely unexpected, however, because we had already been feeding the continuous band magnitude back to the client over all these years to accompany the discrete rewards. The dynamics of the magnitude were displayed with a bandwidth of 0.3 to 0.5 Hz, which the eye can easily accommodate. The intent all along had been to promote engagement of the client with the process, but the brain was clearly also deriving information from the ongoing signal stream, meaning it was more engaged with the process for that reason as well. The continuous signal was information-rich by comparison to the discrete rewards, and as such was responsible for the exquisite frequency sensitivity of the training that we had already observed. The same thing was now happening with the actual signal. The brain got all the information it needed for the low frequency training from the time course of the continuous signal. This struck us as remarkable on first encounter, but at another level it was also not unexpected—after all, we had undertaken this initiative in the expectation of success.

In the low-frequency region, the simple expedient of tracking the actual signal instead of the amplitude envelope meant that the discrete rewards no longer made sense. Thresholds had lost their meaning in the new context. We would have threshold crossings once every cycle and they would not convey significance. With the abandonment of discrete rewards, it also became clear that we had entirely cut our moorings to the operant conditioning model that had been a central pillar of the entire development of clinical neurofeedback. The operant conditioning model had been our lodestone. Indeed, Sterman's cat data stands as an elegant exemplar of that kind of learning. Now another explanation was clearly needed. We will return to this conundrum later.

In the clinic the path was clear. With clients piling up at the lowest frequency, the range obviously needed to be extended further. It was extended another order of magnitude, to 0.01 Hz, early in 2008. We were now dealing with a rather slowly changing signal and yet the brain seemed to handle it much as it had before. Over time, the same pattern we had observed before was once again repeated. About two-thirds of the clients optimized at the lowest frequency. The range was hastily extended yet another order of magnitude to 1 milliHertz, or 1 mHz, later in 2008. Yet the same pattern emerged over time as we became acquainted with this new regime: cases piled up at the lowest frequency available. Finally, as the range was extended in 2010 to 0.1 mHz, a similar pattern once again developed. Some two-thirds of clients eventually ended up preferring the lowest target frequency.

A frequency of 0.1mHz implies a period of 10,000 seconds, or a period of 2.8 hours.We did not have to be told that training a frequency this low is an absurdity on its face, and yet the brain was responding as promptly as ever. In fact, the overall training process was even more demanding than it had been before, quite simply because it was stronger in its impact, which called for more vigilance on the part of the clinician. It needed to be done right, which meant in particular that the choice of target frequency was critical, and also the placement. But just how did the low frequency enter the picture? How is this kind of training even possible?

In the conventional signal analysis perspective, an outside observer would have to track the signal for a good part of a whole cycle in order to know the precise frequency being represented, and yet the brain was responding quickly and it was doing so in a way that was very frequency-specific. Even a 10 percent deviation might matter. The laws of nature—or at least the principles of signal processing—appeared to be violated. On top of everything else, the actual signal did not even appear sinusoidal. It was merely quasi-periodic, which means that the signal unfolding on the screen is not helpful in discerning the target frequency.The only evidence for the optimal response frequency we have is in the actual experience of the client.

2.10 Toward an Understanding of Covert, Continuous ILF Neurofeedback

At this point I would hate to deprive a certain kind of reader of the challenge of figuring out how a rapid and frequency-specific response to extreme low-frequency signals is even possible. So for these people it is recommended that they stop reading at this point and see if they can puzzle this out on their own. For everyone else, and for those who gave up trying to figure this out, what follows is the explanation for what is happening in this process. It is best to start with an anecdote that makes matters concrete: at a professional training course an attendee had just been wired up to experience the training for the first time, in a demonstration of the process. After mere minutes of training (i.e., less than ten) she finds herself feeling distinctly different than before but has no idea why. She is urged to report how she feels because this is the beginning of the process of hunting for the optimum response frequency. Everything was happening as expected, except of course for the particulars that related to this person.A psychologist in the audience—thoroughly steeped in the operant conditioning model—leapt out of his chair at that point and blurted out with finality:'this is not operant conditioning!'

Indeed it is not; he had that absolutely right. So we do have something to explain here.The brain had gone into action on the basis of the information that was being provided, and the clinician had nothing to do with the specifics of that response. To understand this process, matters have to be regarded from the perspective of the engaged brain, not that of an outside observer—or of the client. The low-frequency filter shapes the information going back to the brain about the Slow Cortical Potential so that it contains mainly low-frequency information. Higher-frequency information is sharply attenuated. This would appear to preclude a rapid response on the part of the client, but, even though the frequency response is slow, the transient response is not, and therein lies the explanation. In mathematical terminology, one needs to get the Fourier transform and the transfer functions of narrow-band filters out of one's head and invoke the Laplace transform instead in order to understand the transient response. The transient response is substantially attenuated by the filter but it is still present. Significantly, it is still present in real time, without any delay. Even slow brain rhythms must respond to environmental demands, both internal and external, and they must do so promptly, at the speed of life. The signal processing does not obliterate that information. It does not delay it. It merely attenuates it—so it remains available for detection. In sum, then, the brain is engaging with the real-time behavior—the dynamics—of a regulatory process that is organized at extremely low frequencies.

As soon as the brain recognizes that the signal on the screen somehow reflects an aspect of its own activity, it ceases to be the naïve observer of an innocuous signal. Rather, the brain relates to the signal as its own output and assumes responsibility for the signal going forward. The brain is able to detect the subtle changes in the signal because it is expecting them, and is therefore looking for them. The particulars of the relationship, however, remain obscure, at least at the outset. The brain goes into a hypothesis-testing mode. It attempts to antici-pate, control, and manipulate the signal. This is just how the brain deals with infor-mation about its interaction with the world through movement. Movement that the brain cares about is always the execution of an intention, and then the brain renders an ongoing judgment about whether its intentions are being successfully executed. It takes corrective action such as fine adjustment of the activity. All the elements are there: prediction, comparison to expectation, and correction, although there is no implication that there are brain modules to implement those functions, or even that these activities are sequential. They are all happening con-currently in a process referred to as 'circular causality.' The 'movement' of the SCP signal is treated analogously to the manner in which the brain treats actual movement of the body.

The EEG/SCP signal is a correlate of brain activity, and the same holds true for the dance reflected in the mirror at the dance studio. The brain is directly in charge only of its own neuronal activity, but it adjusts its responses on the basis of the correlates that implement or reflect that intrinsic activity—in the EEG/SCP or in the mirror, respectively. Clearly the regulation of movement has become a highly refined skill on the part of our brain. All that is required to understand Infra-Low Frequency Neurofeedback is to realize that this entire repertoire of refined regulatory control can also be applied to the brain's internal activity, as reflected in the EEG and the SCP. That capability extends to every function that is subject to regulatory control by the brain and can be rendered 'visible' to the brain through its EEG or SCP. The brain relates to the outside world as agent, and the feedback allows the brain to encounter its own EEG and SCP also as agent. Since the brain has been placed explicitly in charge of its own regulatory regime, just as it is explic-itly in charge of learning a motor skill, it seems reasonable to view this kind of neurofeedback process as one of skill learning.

With the above explanation of the process, a certain separation has been achieved between the domain of the target frequency and the associated dynamics that are grist for the brain's engagement. The latter lie at higher ILF frequencies where they can readily capture the attentions of the brain. The former lies beneath the range where it can be grasped and appraised by the brain. Yet the dynamics being revealed characterize the deeper rhythm at issue. A way has thus been found to make even extremely low biological frequencies available to a feedback paradigm. Once that separation has been cognized, it can obviously serve for any target frequency, and thus it may be safe to say at this juncture that the progression to low target frequencies recited above was not yet the end of the story.

Even lower frequencies were found to be useful, down to the region of the circadian rhythm. With every successive decadal descent into the extreme low frequency domain, the clinical reach expanded to more challenging clients; clients responded more wholesomely; and the bar was raised even further on the clinical skill required to manage the process. Clients were now distributed over a broad range of frequencies but with a strong bias toward the lower ranges of frequencies, and in particular to the lowest frequency.

2.11 A Summary Perspective

Tracing the trajectory of development of neurofeedback protocols that emanated from Sterman's original approach has brought us, finally, to a narrow focus on Infra-Low Frequency Neurofeedback. Both methods have all of the essential elements in common: fixed-frequency targeting; bipolar montage; and placement driven by considerations of functional neuroanatomy. Yet, the two methods could hardly be further apart. One is an exogenous, goal-driven method with the therapist in charge, and the other is an endogenous approach in which the brain takes the lead. Since this technique is an extreme outlier in so many respects, when regarded in the perspective of the more conventional approaches to neurofeedback, a strong case must exist to justify it—particularly given the clinical and instrumental challenges involved. The empirical case is made in the remainder of the book. A theoretical model in support of this approach is presented in the next chapter.

The argument can, however, be presented here in broad outline. In the perspective of the sociology of scientifically guided therapeutic practice, neurofeedback had to be introduced into the mid-twentieth century world in the manner that Sterman pursued. There was an animal model; there were blinded controlled studies; there was an established mechanism. Sterman's method carved the first road into the jungle, so to speak, and gave us permission to place electrodes on people's heads with a therapeutic intention. A prescriptive remedy such as he offered was within the Zeitgeist of the therapeutic disciplines, with a deficit focus and with fealty to the prevailing localization hypothesis. Yet that singular protocol turned out to be a fecund point of departure for intervention with a wide range of conditions. The status of our own work as of 1993 is shown in Figure 2.9. (This is the original slide from 1993, as testified to by the misspelling of tinnitus.) The figure illustrates how clinical practice broadened over time, radiating out from the core issues of epilepsy, ADHD, minor Traumatic Brain Injury, and insomnia, for which there was early literature and clinical support.

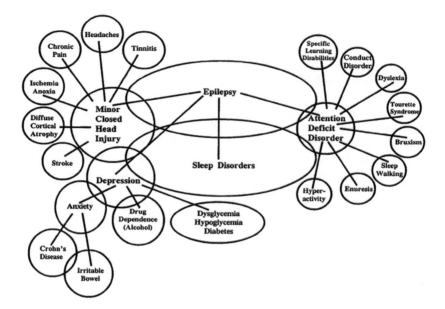

Figure 2.9 This figure shows the state of the art in early 1993, as the clinical reach expanded from the original focus on epilepsy to an ever increasing number of diagnostic categories.

Already at this point it was apparent that the training was not, as Sterman had assumed, targeting a specific mechanism at a particular site and with a standard frequency. Instead we were engaging with a highly integrated regulatory system, one that was affected in broad generality. Functionality improved across various domains, including in areas not in deficit. The clinical realities were outrunning our models, as it was difficult to shed self-imposed boundaries on what was deemed to be possible. A systems perspective was called for.

How is a complex, self-regulatory system best approached in the spirit of clinical research? It is by trial and error—the incremental shedding of boundaries within an established framework. The entry into QEEG analysis first opened up the spatial domain, and the discovery of the principle of the optimum reward frequency then opened up parameter space in the frequency domain. Exploring the spatial domain was problematic, however, in that there was no good way to systematize disparate client data in numerous individual offices. By contrast, the frequency optimization procedure lent itself much more readily to trial-and-error learning. An A-B research design was now inherent in the optimization procedure with every client, made possible by the rapid response of the client to any change. Further, it facilitated a collective learning curve, as it was implemented by way of standard protocol schema and validated by a large practitioner network utilizing the same clinical decision tree. That, in turn, led compellingly to ever lower target frequencies. This could not have been accomplished in a formal research setting, with its narrowly framed hypotheses and fixed experimental designs. Clinical complexity had to be confronted forthrightly, and that could only have happened in a clinical setting.

With the clinical conditions for which benefit was derived over the years, there was always a subset of individuals that could not be substantially helped. These challenging individuals forced the agenda toward protocol innovation and optimization, which in turn drove us to the infra-low frequency regime. QEEG-based training had already loosened the connection between the targets of training and the client complaints. The target was whatever dysregulation status was observable in the EEG. The infra-low frequency training now took that further, addressing dysregulation that did not necessarily feature any localized cortical representation or had any direct tie to the clinical complaints. The quality of cerebral regulation was being addressed in its broadest generality, namely at the foundations of the regulatory hierarchy within the frequency domain.[71]

It is now recognized that the population that was refractory to earlier neurofeedback interventions largely consisted of those reporting Adverse Childhood Events (ACE's), and of those about whom that assumption could reasonably be made (orphans, adoptees, and foster care kids). The ILF training had given us the means to re-normalize the neural network relations that are disturbed by early developmental misdirections, by whatever cause. It turned out, however, that the vast majority of clients benefited from having the training agenda begin with attention to the low-frequency domain, not only those who were identified as victims of early childhood trauma. There was a clear payoff for beginning the project of functional optimization at its foundations. The particulars are taken up in the next chapter, supported by recent findings from neural imaging.

Notes

1   Berger, H. (1929). Über das Elektroenkephalogramm des Menschen. *Archiv für Psychiatrie und Nervenkrankheiten*, 87, 527–570.

2   Adrian, E.D., & Matthews, B.H.C. (1934). The Berger Rhythm: Potential changes from the occipital lobes in man. *Brain*, 57(4), 355–385. doi: 10.1093/brain/57.4.355.

3   Wyrwicka, W., & Sterman, M.B. (1968). Instrumental conditioning of sensorimotor cortex EEG spindles in the waking cat. *Physiology & Behavior*, 3(5), 703–707.

4   Sterman, M.B., Howe, R.C., & Macdonald, L.R. (1970). Facilitation of spindle-burst sleep by conditioning of electroencephalographic activity while awake. *Science*, 167, 1146–1148.

5   Sterman, M.B., Wyrwicka, W., & Roth, S. (1969). Electrophysiological correlates and neural substrates of alimentary behavior in the cat. In *Neural Regulation of Food and Water Intake*. Annals of the New York Academy of Sciences, 157: 723–739.

6   Sterman, M.B., & Egner, T. (2006). Foundation and practice of neurofeedback for the treatment of epilepsy. *Applied Psychophysiology and Biofeedback Journal*, 31(1), 21–36.

7   Sterman, M.B. (1976). Effects of brain surgery and EEG operant conditioning on seizure latency following monomethylhydrazine intoxication in the cat. *Experimental Neurology*, 50, 757–765.

8 Sterman, M.B., Goodman, S.J., & Kovalesky, R.A. (1978). Effects of sensorimotor EEG feedback training on seizure susceptibility in the rhesus monkey. *Experimental Neurology*, 62(3), 735–747.

9 Sterman, M.B., & Friar, L. (1972). Suppression of seizures in epileptic following sensorimotor EEG feedback training. *Electroencephalography and Clinical Neurophysiology*, 33, 89–95.

10 Sterman, M.B., Macdonald, L.R., & Stone, R.K. (1974). Biofeedback training of the sensorimotor EEG rhythm in man: Effects on epilepsy. *Epilepsia*, 15, 395–417.

11 Seifert, A.R., & Lubar, J.F. (1975). Reduction of epileptic seizures through EEG biofeedback training. *Biological Psychology*, 3, 157–184.

12 Lubar, J.F., & Bahler, W.W. (1976). Behavioral management of epileptic seizures following EEG biofeedback training of the sensorimotor rhythm. *Biofeedback and Self-Regulation*, 1, 77–104.

13 Sterman, M.B., & McDonald, L.R. (1978). Effects of central cortical EEG feedback training on incidence of poorly controlled seizures. *Epilepsia*, 19(3), 207–222.

14 Lubar, J.F., Shabsin, H.S., Natelson, S.E., Holder, G.S., Woodson, S.F., Pamplin, W.E., & Krulikowski, D.I. (1981). EEG operant conditioning in intractable epileptics. *Archives of Neurology*, 38, 700–704.

15 Sterman, M.B. (1984). The role of sensorimotor rhythmic EEG activity in the etiology and treatment of generalized motor seizures. Chapter 7 in Elbert, T.S., Rockstroh, B., Lutzenberger, W., & Birbaumer, N. (eds), *Self-Regulation of the Brain and Behavior*. Springer, Berlin, 95–106.

16 Lantz, D., & Sterman, M.B. (1988). Neuropsychological assessment of subjects with uncontrolled epilepsy: Effects of EEG feedback training. *Epilepsia*, 29(2), 163–171.

17 Sterman, M.B. (2000). Basic concepts and clinical findings in the treatment of seizure disorders with EEG operant conditioning. *Clinical Electroencephalography*, 31(1), 45–55.

18 Egner, T., & Sterman, M.B. (2006). Neurofeedback treatment of epilepsy: From basic rationale to practical implication. *Expert Review of Neurotherapeutics*, 6(2), 247–257.

19 Tan, G., Thornby, J., Hammond, D.C., Strehl, U., Canady, B., Arnemann, K., & Kaiser, D.A. (2009). Meta-analysis of EEG biofeedback in treating epilepsy. *Clinical EEG and Neuroscience*, 40(3), 173–179.

20 Kotchoubey, B., Strehl, U., Uhlmann, C., et al. (2001). Modification of slow cortical potentials in patients with refractory epilepsy. *Epilepsia*. 42, 406–416.

21 Lubar, J.F., & Bahler, W.W. (1976). Behavioral management of epileptic seizures following EEG biofeedback training of the sensorimotor rhythm. *Biofeedback and Self-Regulation*, 1, 77–104.

22 Lubar, J.F., & Shouse, M.N. (1976). EEG and behavioral changes in a hyperkinetic child concurrent with training of the sensorimotor rhythm (SMR): A preliminary report. *Biofeedback and Self-Regulation*, 3, 293–306.

23 Shouse, M.N., & Lubar, J.F. (1979). Operant conditioning of EEG rhythms and Ritalin in the treatment of hyperkinesis. *Biofeedback and Self-Regulation*, 4(4), 299–312.

24 Lubar, J.F. (2003). Neurofeedback for the management of attention-deficit/hyperactivity disorders. In M. Schwartz & F. Andrasik (eds), *Biofeedback: A Practitioner's Guide*. Guilford Publishing Co., New York (3rd ed.), 409–437.

25 Tansey, M.A., & Bruner, R.L. (1983). EMG and EEG biofeedback training in the treatment of a 10-year old hyperactive boy with a developmental reading disorder. *Biofeedback and Self-Regulation*, 8, 25–37.

26 Lubar, J.O., & Lubar, J.F. (1984). Electroencephalographic biofeedback of SMR and beta for treatment of attention deficit disorders in a clinical setting. *Biofeedback and Self-Regulation*, 9, 1–23.

27 Tansey, M.A. (1985). Brainwave signatures–An index reflective of the brain's functional neuroanatomy: Further findings on the effect of EEG sensorimotor rhythm biofeedback training on the neurologic precursors of learning disabilities. *International Journal of Psychophysiology*, 3, 85–89.

28 Tansey, M.A. (1990). Righting the rhythms of reason: EEG biofeedback training as a therapeutic modality in a clinical office setting. *Medical Psychotherapy*, 3, 57–68.

29 Tansey, M.A. (1991). Wechsler (WISC-R) changes following treatment of learning disabilities via EEG biofeedback training in a private practice setting. *Australian Journal of Psychology*, 43, 147–153.

30 Othmer, S., Othmer, S.F., & Marks, C.S. (1992). EEG biofeedback training for attention deficit disorder, specific learning disabilities, and associated conduct problems. *Journal of the Biofeedback Society of California*, September, 24–27.

31 Rossiter, T.R., & LaVaque, T.J. (1995). A comparison of EEG biofeedback and psychostimulants in treating attention deficit hyperactivity disorder. *Journal of Neurotherapy*, 1(1), 48–59.

32 Rossiter, T.R. (2004). The effectiveness of neurofeedback and stimulant drugs in treating AD/HD: Part I. Review of methodological issues. *Applied Psychophysiology & Biofeedback*, 29(2), 135–140.

33 Rossiter, T.R. (2004). The effectiveness of neurofeedback and stimulant drugs in treating AD/HD: Part II. Replication. *Applied Psychophysiology & Biofeedback*, 29(4), 233–243.

34 Fuchs, T., Birbaumer, N., Lutzenberger, W., Gruzelier, J.H., & Kaiser, J. (2003). Neurofeedback treatment for attention-deficit/hyperactivity disorder in children: Acomparison with methylphenidate. *Applied Psychophysiology & Biofeedback*, 28(1), 1–12.

35 Monastra, V.J., Monastra, D.M., & George, S. (2002). The effects of stimulant therapy, EEG biofeedback and parenting style on the primary symptoms of ADHD. *Applied Psychophysiology and Biofeedback Journal*, 27(4), 249.

36 Duric, N.S., Assmus, J., Gundersen, D., & Elgen, I.B. (2012). Neurofeedback for the treatment of children and adolescents with ADHD: A randomized and controlled clinical trial using parental reports. *BMC Psychiatry*, 12, 107. doi: 10.1186/1471-244x-12-107.

37 Meisel, V., Servera, M., Garcia-Banda, G., Cardo, E., & Moreno, I. (2014). Neurofeedback and standard pharmacological intervention in ADHD: A randomized controlled trial with six-month follow-up. *Biological Psychology*, 95, 116–125.

38 Lubar, J.F. (1991). Discourse on the development of EEG diagnostics and biofeedback treatment for attention deficit/hyperactivity disorders. *Biofeedback and Self-Regulation*, 16, 201–225.

39 Monastra, et al., see note 35.

40 Kaiser, D.A., & Othmer, S. (2000). Effect of neurofeedback on variables of attention in a large multi- center trial. *Journal of Neurotherapy*, 4(1), 5–15.

41 Arns, M., de Ridder, S., Strehl, U., Breteler, M., & Coenen, A. (2009). Efficacy of neurofeedback treatment in ADHD: The effects on inattention, impulsivity and hyperactivity: A meta-analysis. *Clinical EEG and Neuroscience*, 40(3), 180–189.

42 Ibid.

43 American Academy of Pediatrics: http://pediatrics.aappublications.org/content/125/Supplement_3/S128.full.pdf

44 Kamiya, J., & Noles, D. (1970). The control of electroencephalographic alpha rhythms through auditory feedback and associated mental activity. *Psychophysiology*, 6, 76.

45 Hardt, J.V., & Kamiya, J. (1978). Anxiety change through electroencephalographic alpha feedback seen only in high anxiety subjects. *Science*, 201, 79–81.

46 Brown, B.B. (1974). *New Mind New Body*. Harper and Row, New York.

47 Brown, B.B. (1977). *Stress and the Art of Biofeedback*. Harper and Row, New York.

48 Brown, B.B., & J.W. Klug (eds) (1974). *The Alpha Syllabus: A Handbook of Human EEG Alpha Activity*. Charles C. Thomas, Publishers, Springfield, IL.

49 Plotkin, W.B., & Rice, K.M. (1981). Biofeedback as a placebo: Anxiety reduction facilitated by training in either suppression or enhancement of alpha brainwaves. *Journal of Consulting & Clinical Psychology*, 49, 590–596.

50 Lynch, J.L., Paskewitz, D., & Orne, M.T. (1974). Some factors in the feedback control of the human alpha rhythm. *Psychosomatic Medicine*, 36, 399–410.

51 Ancoli, S., & Kamiya, J. (1978). Methodological issues in alpha biofeedback training. *Biofeedback and Self-Regulation*, 3(2), 159–183. doi:10.1007/BF00998900.

52 Passini, F.T., Watson, C. B., Dehnel, L., Herder, J., & Watkins, B. (1977). Alpha wave biofeedback training therapy in alcoholics. *Journal of Clinical Psychology*, 33, 292–299.

53 Peniston, E.G., & Kulkosky, P.J. (1989). Alpha-Theta brainwave training and beta endorphin levels in alcoholics. *Alcoholism: Clinical and Experimental Results*, 13(2), 271–279.

54 Peniston, E.G., & Kulkosky, P.J. (1991). Alpha-Theta brainwave neuro-feedback therapy for Vietnam Veterans in with Combat-related post-traumatic stress disorder. *Medical Psychotherapy*, 4, 47–60.

55 Peniston, E.G., & Kulkosky, P.J. (1995). The peniston/kulkosky brainwave neurofeedback therapy for alcoholism and posttraumatic stress disorders: Medical psychotherapist manual. Certificate of Copyright Office. *The Library of Congress*, 1–25. http://aaets.org/article47.htm.

56 Peniston, E.G., & Kulkosky, P.J. (1999). Neurofeedback in the treatment of addictive disorders. In J.R. Evans & A. Abarbanel (eds), *Introduction to Quantitative EEG and Neurofeedback*. Academic Press, San Diego, CA.

57 Scott, W.C., Kaiser, D., Othmer, S., Sideroff, S.I. (2005). Effects of an EEG biofeedback protocol on a mixed substance abusing population. *American Journal of Drug and Alcohol Abuse*, 31(3), 455–469.

58 Burkett, S.V., Cummins, J.M., Dickson, R., & Skolnick, M.H. (2005). An open clinical trial utilizing real-time EEG operant conditioning as an adjunctive therapy in the treatment of crack cocaine dependence. *Journal of Neurotherapy*, 9(2), 27–47.

59 Lutzenberger, W., Elbert, T., Rockstroh, B., & Birbaumer, N. (1979). The effects of self-regulation of slow cortical potentials on performance in a signal detection task. *The International Journal of Neuroscience*, 9(3), 175–183.

60 Strehl, U., Leins, U., Goth, G., Klinger, C., Hinterberger, T., & Birbaumer, N. (2006). Self-regulation of slow cortical potentials: A new treatment for children with attention-deficit/hyperactivity disorder. *Pediatrics* 118(5), 1530–1540.

61 Ayers, M.E. (1999). Assessing and treating open head trauma, coma, and stroke using real-time digital EEG neurofeedback. In J. R. Evans & A. Abarbanel (eds), *Introduction to Quantitative EEG and Neurofeedback*. Academic Press, New York, 203–222.

62 Kaiser and Othmer, see note 40.

63 Putman, J.A., & Othmer, S. (2006). Phase sensitivity of bipolar EEG training protocols. *Journal of Neurotherapy*, 10(1), 73–79.

64 Walker, J.E. (2011). QEEG-guided neurofeedback for recurrent migraine headaches. *Clinical EEG and Neuroscience*, 42(1), 59–61.

65 Thornton, K.E., & Carmody, D.P. (2008). Efficacy of traumatic brain injury rehabilitation: Interventions of QEEG-guided biofeedback, computers, strategies, and medications. *Applied Psychophysiology & Biofeedback*, 33(2), 101–124.

66 Surmeli, T., Ertem, A., Eralp, E., & Kos, I. H. (2012). Schizophrenia and the efficacy of qEEG-guided neurofeedback treatment: A clinical case series. *Clinical EEG and Neuroscience*, 43, 133–144. doi:10.1177/1550059411429531.

67 Alvarez, J., Meyer, F.L., Granoff, D.L., & Lundy, A. (2013). The effect of EEG biofeedback on reducing postcancer cognitive impairment. *Integrative Cancer Therapies*, 12(6), 457–487.

68 Fehmi, L., & Robbins, J. (2007). *Open Focus*. Trumpeter Books, Boston, MA.

69 Hardt, J. (2007). *The Art of Smart Thinking*. BioCybernaut Press, Santa Clara, CA.

70 Bird, B. L., Newton, F.A., Sheer, D.E., & Ford, M. (1978). Biofeedback training of 40-Hz EEG in humans. *Biofeedback and Self-Regulation*, 3(1), 1–12.

71 Othmer, S., Othmer, S.F., Kaiser, D.A., & Putman, J.A. (2013). Endogenous Neuromodulation at Infra-Low Frequencies, *Seminars in Pediatric Neurology*, 20(4), 246–260.

Chapter 3

Toward a Theory of Infra-Low Frequency Neurofeedback

Siegfried Othmer and Sue Othmer

3.1 Introduction

Infra-Low Frequency Neurofeedback is not readily subjected to formal evaluation by way of group studies in the classic mode. Not only does the procedure have to be individualized to a degree that is likely unprecedented in clinical practice, but the training procedure has to remain adaptive throughout the training process. The multi-dimensional discovery process involved here could only flourish in the clinical realm, and ILF training will likely remain a clinical frontier. Undoubtedly, we are only at the beginning of the exploitation of this new modality.[1]

At the same time, any arbitrary threshold of validity can be met even in this context by the principle of Bayesian inference, without resorting to group studies. The body of knowledge reflected in this book testifies to that. The clinical model evolves incrementally in a manner similar to the growth of the conventional lava flow at Mount Kilauea: plasticity at the frontier of clinical practice, but leaving a trail of progressive solidity behind. Such plasticity is rare and precious in the sciences that bear on human health. ILF Neurofeedback also offers intrinsic tests of validity, by virtue of its parametric specificity in the frequency domain. And finally, supportive evidence is starting to be furnished by more basic studies.

The more intractable barrier to acceptance is at the theoretical level. The scientific mind resists being asked to take seriously data for which there is no agreed upon operative model. The frontier of ILF NF has, at times, challenged our own belief systems, because the clinical findings were so startling that they pushed the limits of our own credulity. Clients respond rapidly and consistently to a relatively featureless low-frequency waveform. How is this to be explained? In consequence, we have only the greatest sympathy for critics outside of the field. If we hadn't been confronted with our own ineluctable case data, and if we had not had a chance to see systematic patterns emerge over the years, we would have been right among them. Our challenge in this chapter, then, is to shape the data into a compelling narrative, and to present a credible theoretical model.

3.2 Categories of Brain Dysfunction

The top-level criterion for a clinical practice on the path to becoming an accepted discipline is that of systemization. Can the basic facts of a field be categorized, systematized, and manualized? In this regard, we face the challenge of working at the bottom of the regulatory hierarchy, intervening with the lowest frequencies at which brain function is dynamically regulated in a frequency-based manner. There are no established terms of discourse for this problem. There are no measures that track the approach to this objective. We are thrust back upon the self-report of clients with respect to their own self-regulatory status. We are reduced to the client's own "observables," by and large. The best we can do, therefore, is to rely on the terminology that is used with clients. In addition, we also take advantage of indices of autonomic function from physiological measures, and whatever we can discern from trends in the EEG. Over the longer term, we can track improvements in cognitive function with formal tests.

We begin by regarding the brain as a generic control system, one that has to satisfy the requirements of any self-regulatory control system. Thinking of the brain in such holistic terms takes us back to the very beginnings of the neurosciences. The neurologist Hughlings Jackson originally propounded the concept of a "cerebral global function" that governs the susceptibility to seizures. The fundamental burden of the brain is to assure its own categorical stability, sufficient to sustain basic functionality. Macro-instabilities violating this criterion include seizures, migraines, panic attacks, asthmatic episodes, and narcoleptic events. These instabilities constitute the primary objective of a training strategy toward functional normalization, as in their presence all subtlety of regulation is lost.

At the second level, the burden is to maintain setpoints of activation with respect to various functional domains. The most global variable in this category is central arousal. This concept also traces back to the origins of the neurosciences. As far back as 1895, Freud and Breuer asserted that "a certain measure of arousal exists in the conductive pathways of the resting, waking, engagement-capable brain." This whole-brain property of necessity could serve only a heuristic function then, and the same holds true now. Central arousal, in turn, modulates sympathetic arousal of the autonomic nervous system, and vigilance, which comprises the alertness of the attentional system, engagement of the executive function domain, and the poise of motor system. None of these can be readily quantified. We are therefore compelled to operate clinically with what is termed "ipsative trend analysis"—the discernment of change induced via the training process in correlates of the categories of interest. In the absence of measures, we are compelled to live with how the client interprets terms bearing on arousal, vigilance, and excitability that the clinician brings into the discussion. In addition, there are terms characterizing the affective state, the state of the autonomic nervous system, the quality of sleep, and the status with respect to drives such as hunger, pain, and cravings.

This unsettling lack of quantifiability notwithstanding, one may still ask the question: Just how are we thinking about terms such as arousal and vigilance? In the early years of our work, we understood the term arousal in the Yerkes-Dodson sense. Central arousal is whatever is under the management of the reticular activating system. (Even Yerkes-Dodson referred to motivation before it became arousal in their famous plot!) That view is coming into some question with the descent into the extreme low-frequency regime. The time constants of responsiveness of the reticular activating system are fairly short—seconds to minutes. Something else seems to be in a controlling role at the longer time constants, and with respect to our clinical agenda, that appears to be the most relevant aspect. One can think of the fast response of the reticular activating system as being precipitated by interactions with the outside world. For our purposes, the more salient issue is the maintenance of the internal milieu, our ambient or so-called resting state, where the time constants are typically longer.

Our clinical experience can be distilled into a primary concern with brain instability and with arousal dysregulation. These two categories are foundational to the whole enterprise of neural regulation, and both benefit from being readily describable by most clients. They map into our two primary protocols for the initiation of the clinical work. This is possible because the entire class of brain instabilities is responsive to the same protocol, or at least to the same class of protocols. Similarly, arousal dysregulation primarily responds to a single protocol.

The context out of which brain instabilities arise tends to be one of neuronal hyper-excitability. The roots of this concept also go back to Freud, who as early as 1894 referred to the "sum of excitation," which he saw as relevant to psychopathologies such as hysteria and hallucinatory psychoses. As we now conceptualize the issue, there is a cellular (synaptic or other membrane) aspect to hyper-excitability, one that is typically addressed by anti-epileptic drugs, and there is a network aspect. The ILF training impinges on the network aspect in first instance, and over time appears to also affect the setpoints of excitability at the cellular level. That proposition is testified to by the observation that often levels of anti-convulsants can be reduced or even eliminated through the course of neurofeedback training.

The context out of which arousal dysregulation arises tends to be trauma-based, where this term is to be regarded in its most encompassing scope. Trauma does not have to be life-threatening (or its equivalent) in order to wreak havoc with the course of early neuronal development or to result in its dysregulation in maturity. The loss of a sense of safety, of personal security, or even of status at any level tends to move the nervous system to a state of over-arousal. This may become so well established as the new ambient that it is not perceived as such. A new comfort zone develops such that a return to calm states may even give rise to a sense of insecurity and loss of safety.

Physical injury, such as concussions and other minor head injuries, also disturb the integrity of neuronal network relations, which likely constitutes their primary failure mode. Commonly, these are also observed to heighten neuronal excitability, particularly among those with that vulnerability. Our greatest clinical challenges are those for whom both arousal dysregulation and neuronal excitability prevail. In the case of the latter, we are typically dealing with a genetically-mediated propensity. Brain instabilities such as migraines tend to run in families, but they may not be evoked until triggered by a minor brain injury or other trauma. That is also the case for seizures, where the vulnerability may well remain latent in the absence of compounding events.

As over-arousal conditions tend to be trauma-related, they are typically environmental in causation. With affect dysregulation and the fear response as mediators, some considerable commonality in the neuronal failure modes is not unexpected. This may in turn account for the fact that a standard protocol goes a long way to resolving these issues. Already noted is that brain instabilities also tend to respond favorably to a single protocol, despite all of the variety in which they manifest, and that, likewise, suggests a common failure mode.

3.3 The Trauma Model

The term trauma is at risk of becoming hackneyed and trivialized from over-generalization. It is particularly at risk when apparently minor traumas are discussed in the same context as major ones. But the fact is that even minor traumas can have major consequences. This holds true for both minor emotional traumas and minor brain injuries. The explanation is the obvious one. When even minor traumas afflict a vulnerable nervous system, it can be tipped into major dysfunction. When we look at personal histories in such cases, a consistent story can usually be told of a progressive vulnerability that finds its origins in early childhood. This means that minor traumas cannot be considered in isolation in the general case, or judged "on their own merits."

This shifts our perspective from minor traumas, which are in fact ubiquitous in our upbringing, to the matter of recovery. What really matters here is the dispersion that exists in the distribution of recovery potential across the population. The wide variation in vulnerability, in the lack of resilience, compels us to see the connection among apparently disparate events. This process, in which a concatenation of apparently minor traumatic events can lead progressively to major dysfunction, we refer to as the "Dysregulation Cascade." Tracing such a cascade to its causal origins commonly takes us back to a perilous environment for early upbringing.

Perhaps the best exemplar of a Dysregulation Cascade is a boxing match, in which the overt objective is the disruption of the neural integrity of the opponent. During the match there is little opportunity for functional recovery, so injury is cumulative. Full functional recovery may eventuate, however, with nothing more than the tincture of time between matches. What matters most in accounting for attrition in the careers of boxers is not the magnitude of the blows received but the variation in recovery capacity. This observation generalizes to the population at large.

This is such a critical issue that it bears further discussion. It has been found that even a single change in domicile in a 14-year-old teenager doubles the cumulative risk (to middle age) of attempted suicide. Roughly the same holds for the increased risk of substance abuse, violent offending, and of any psychiatric diagnosis. What appears to be a minor traumatic episode may, in fact, be quite significant in some children's lives. The only reasonable explanation is that this apparently "minor" trauma has outsize consequences for a subset of the teenage population that is already at risk by virtue of prior history.[2]

What first brought this issue broadly into public awareness was the "Adverse Childhood Experiences (ACE) Study."[3] Here the focus was on overt traumatic experiences or contexts of living: psychological, physical, or sexual abuse, etc. Evaluation of some 9500 adult questionnaires yielded the finding that "Persons who had experienced four or more categories of childhood exposure had 4- to 12-fold increased health risks for alcoholism, drug abuse, depression, and suicide attempt." Even more surprising was the correlation with chronic medical disease: ischemic heart disease, cancer, lung disease, liver disease, and diabetes. With four or more ACE's the relative risk was elevated by about a factor of two.

Results were similar for a Scandinavian study that also evaluated the somatic health impact of psychological stress. In tracking the increased incidence of disability-related pensions post age 65, a dramatic correlation with early psychological stressors was brought to light. 3–7 stress factors yielded a doubling of the incidence of disability-related pension in the subsequent five years. 9–12 stress factors yielded a risk multiplier of four. Overall, "over a quarter of … disability pensions granted for somatic diagnoses could be attributed to psychological distress." Even more concerning, "…even mild psychological distress was associated with later onset of long-term disability."[4]

Our first solid indication of the relationship between early development and general health was furnished by the so-called Grant study on 256 Harvard students that began in the late 1940's.[5] Some fifty years later, the remaining 160 were evaluated for the usual diseases of aging. If the person had grown up in a positive emotional environment, the incidence of such diseases was 25%. If they had grown up in an adverse emotional climate, the incidence was 89%. The risk multiplier was an astounding 3.6. This is a more reliable figure than that furnished by the ACE study, where the more severely impacted may already have attritioned out of the population by the time it was questioned.

The Harvard study, on the other hand, has different limitations. It is representative of the segment of the population that was not in economic straits. Socio-economic status is known to be the largest single risk factor with respect to overall health and mortality. So, a more inclusive view would assign even higher import to emotional wellbeing than is implied in the Harvard study. A later study found that those with "six or more ACE's died nearly twenty years earlier than those without ACE's."[6]

The clear implication is that our general health status—mental and physical wellbeing—are closely correlated with early emotional upbringing. That brings us, then, to the question of mechanisms. We distinguish between event trauma and a steady-state adverse living environment. Event trauma transiently heightens memory function. The salience of an event renders it state-stamped rather than date-stamped. It is registered as a whole-body memory, with cognitive, affective, autonomic, and somatic responses fused into a unitary configuration, bound together with the historical memory of the event. Irrespective of whether the individual is personally at risk or is a mere witness, the event alters the setpoint of the threat response, and it does so relatively permanently. This may well be protective of the individual, but it comes at a cost to the physiology over the longer term. It has implications for the subsequent development of neural network relations, and of neuroimmune and neuroendocrine system activation.

In the matter of steady-state exposure to toxic living environments, we turn to the research of Martin Teicher and colleagues at Harvard. This group uses the term maltreatment trauma to characterize this population, which includes both overt mistreatment and abject neglect, physical as well as sexual and emotional abuse. The impact is so substantial that in the characterization of mental disorders, those with a maltreatment history may well constitute a distinct ecophenotype.[7]

Evidence for altered brain development is now coming into view.[8] Of particular interest to us is evidence for altered functional connectivity, as illustrated in Figure 3.1. The evidence is compelling that in unexposed brains one sees a healthy network under the aegis of the left anterior cingulate, directing a confident

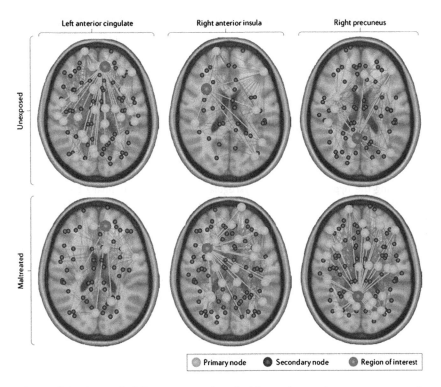

Figure 3.1 Network differences are identified for maltreated versus unexposed young adults. The black dots indicate regions of interest for the left anterior cingulate cortex, the right anterior insula, and the right precuneus. Connectivity analysis yielded the primary nodes that were common within each cohort. These are nodes with direct connections to the region of interest (light-gray dots). Secondary nodes (gray dots) are linked to the region of interest only via the primary nodes. Jointly these linkages determine the 'centrality,' the relative importance, of the three regions of interest for the two cohorts. (See color version in the plate section.)

Source: Teicher, M.D., Samson, J.A., et al, 2016; Original source: Teicher, M.H., Anderson, C.M., 2014.

interaction with the outside world. By contrast, in the exposed case the well-elaborated network emanates instead from the right precuneus, which has primary responsibility for securing safety, in collaboration with the right anterior insula. At the same time, the frontal circuitry is impoverished in comparison with the unexposed individuals. The trauma history, irrespective of its nature, has fundamentally altered how the brain engages with the outside world and manages its internal regulatory regime.[9]

What about the 25% of the remaining Harvard students who suffered chronic disease but had a benign emotional upbringing? If neural network dysregulation, and dysregulation more generally, lies prominently within the causal chain of chronic disease, has something been overlooked? Indeed. It is minor traumatic brain injury, which is an equal opportunity immiserator, afflicting the rich and poor alike. Minor traumatic brain injury has been just as much neglected as minor emotional trauma. Originally, the study of traumatic brain injury was largely a military matter, and those who did not have a bullet in their brain or a skull fracture were assigned to the category of minor traumatic brain injury (mTBI). This tragically misrepresented the clinical realities. mTBI has been a stealth condition that has contributed to declining health status by the same mechanism of neural network dysregulation.

Symptoms often get worse over the first six months post-insult, which means that—just as in the case of emotional trauma—the endogenous remedies that serve a short-term purpose may exact a longer-term penalty, a process referred to as maladaptive plasticity. Symptoms also get worse through cumulative insults, confirming the hypothesis of the Dysregulation Cascade. It is finally being recognized that sub-concussive injury must be taken seriously as well, particularly if it is part of a repetitive pattern, as in soccer play or football.[10] None of these events need to rise to the level of creating organic injury within the brain, as that term is ordinarily understood (i.e., neuronal shearing, etc.). They may not even rise to the level of detectable symptoms. The primary mechanism of injury lies in the functional domain. This proposition is attested to by the finding of a tendency toward hyper-connectivity in mTBI.[11] Rapid recovery effected through neurofeedback training is also persuasive on this point.

3.3.1 ILF Neurofeedback: Rescue Remedy for the Trauma Response

The trend to lower training frequency that has been underway since around the turn of the century has, to all appearances, been driven by the imperatives of working with the traumatized population, which presents the greatest clinical challenge to the neurofeedback clinician. In this project, success has largely been achieved. Whereas there have always been clients who could not be helped with these protocols, that has become largely a non-issue with the available palette of training options, the extension into the deep ILF regime in particular. But a larger reality has also been uncovered. It is not only those who bear the scars of trauma that benefit from the two starting protocols. It is nearly everyone who comes for training.

One must conclude that these protocols are redressing failure modes that our species largely has in common. The tendency is for a challenged nervous system to move toward over-arousal, with hyper-excitability an additional consequence if that is a vulnerability. When that status cannot be sustained, the system may slide into under-arousal or crater into functional collapse. The languor and effort fatigue that we associate with mTBI is a case in point. The time courses seen in the anxiety-depression spectrum are another. Cratering is often masked by the kindling of a disease process, being then naturally associated with the latter rather than with its antecedent.

The prominence of early childhood adverse events in the life history of our most challenging clients implies that neural network development is affected in its earliest stages of development. By working at extremely low frequencies, we are addressing the foundations of the regulatory hierarchy in three aspects: 1) the developmental hierarchy; 2) the regulatory hierarchy; and 3) the hierarchy in the frequency domain. In the latter, the lower frequencies set the context for the dynamics unfolding at higher frequencies, and this hierarchy extends into the gamma range of frequencies. The implication of our clinical success is that even the intrinsic connectivity networks are sufficiently plastic so that re-normalization of function can be mediated by way of ILF Neurofeedback.

Moreover, this appears to be possible at any age. The clinical agenda has become one of re-normalization of the regulatory hierarchy from the bottom up with every client. It appears that the residue of challenges to our early development resides in all of us at some level, and that the mature nervous system can aid its own cause of functional enhancement by way of ILF Neurofeedback at these extremely low frequencies. Higher training frequencies then attend to other levels in the hierarchy, to which the entire history of the neurofeedback field attests.

It may be helpful at this point to draw on a law of physics to elucidate the agenda: "The Law of Least Action." The most efficient operation of the human brain transpires at the levels of central arousal and of sub-system activation just sufficient for the demand, but no more. Experts in the martial arts, meditators, chess and Go players are likely well acquainted with this principle. Clients may become aware of it through the training process, as they experience higher levels of vigilance, of alertness and mental clarity, even as the nervous system is moved toward calmer states within a session.

3.4 Mechanisms of Regulation: Historical Roots of the Slow Cortical Potential

By 1935 the study of the EEG was substantially aided with the introduction of electronic (tube) amplifiers by Hubert Rohracher. This called for capacitive coupling, which blinded us to the slow potentials that lay beneath the cutoff frequency. In consequence, the world of EEG research went dark on the Slow Cortical Potential (SCP) for about three decades. There was a re-awakening in 1964 with the discovery by Grey Walter of the expectancy wave (Bereitschaftspotenzial), and the publication by Nina Aleksandrovna Aladjalova of her extensive animal studies on the tonic SCP in book form[12] (Aladjalova, 1964). The engagement with evoked potentials and contingent negative variation soon followed, all of which focused on the transient properties of the SCP. The tonic SCP was followed up by Joe Kamiya, Karl Pribram, and Juri Kropotov. Intimating its importance, Karl Pribram referred to the tonic SCP as "the second language of the brain."

Aladjalova's research has turned out to be of the greatest relevance to our present purposes. She studied the infra-slow rhythmic potential oscillations (ISPOs) at great length. "A single stimulation of the reticular formation immediately elicits an arousal reaction in the EEG of the cortex, but has no effect on infraslow activity," she writes.

> This reaction is apparently regulated by the rapid regulatory system. Stimulation of the ventromedial part of the hypothalamus ... intensifies infraslow cortical activity within 30–40 minutes. This reaction is presumably regulated by the slow regulatory system.
> ... infraslow activity is intensified by certain actions after a long latency period, 30–100 and 120–200 minutes later. We conjectured that this phenomenon reflects the activity of the slow control system of the brain ... not only to automatically adjust the system to keeping [the] internal environment constant but actively to establish a new level of activity.

It does not take a great leap to connect our training in the deep infra-low frequency region with the slow control system Aladjalova identified. This system appears to be centrally regulated by the hypothalamus, known to govern our internal milieu— autonomic function, sleep–wake cycle, ultradian rhythms, etc. Thus, it makes sense that the ILF training extends down to the circadian frequency.

It should be mentioned in the interest of completeness that the electrical stimulation of other hypothalamic nuclei can also induce rapid state shift—even rapid de-activation—in the same systems governed by the slow control system. For example, torpor could be suddenly induced in a cat with suitable stimulation. This was the work of Walter Rudolf Hess, published in 1954.[13]

ISPOs did not generate much interest again until fMRI imaging refocused attention through the discovery of the intrinsic connectivity networks, or resting state networks, around the turn of the century, some three decades later. They have been an intense area of study over the past fifteen years.[14, 15, 16] Raichle and He have illuminated the connection between the fMRI signal and the slow cortical potential.[17] It is these dynamics, predominantly in the range of 0.005 to 0.2 Hz, that are engaged in ILF Neurofeedback. However, we impinge on this activity indirectly via the contribution the extremely low frequencies make to their generation.

In 2017 we became aware that Giovanni Piantoni, of Mass General Hospital, had identified slow brain rhythms of one to two-hour periodicity in extended recordings on epileptic patients using depth electrodes. He identified these with the Basic Rest and Activity Cycle (BRAC), a hypothesis that we entertained as well until we found it necessary to use even lower target frequencies, and were thus compelled to broaden our perspective. One hypothesis does not necessarily dispose of another. Over the entire ILF frequency range, we are no doubt engaging with a number of core regulatory mechanisms, including, in particular, the BRAC.

3.4.1 The Regulatory Hierarchy

Seen from the vantage point of our neurofeedback challenge, the regulatory hierarchy looks like that shown in Figure 3.2. Early neurofeedback, including our own protocols, conformed to the interests of cognitive neuroscientists by engaging with the attentional and executive function domains, effectively the top of the regulatory hierarchy, as well as the motor system, which was also well characterized. Our adoption of an adaptive procedure for protocol refinement shifted the process from being prescriptive to being observational. That led, ever so gradually, to the brain guiding us to its own priorities, namely the bottom of the regulatory hierarchy, one client at a time, over the course of nearly two decades. This meant a progression to lower training frequencies, which took place at a pace of about one decade in frequency space per year for a number of years. This also meant a shift toward right-hemisphere (RH) rather than left-hemisphere (LH) priority, as right-hemisphere function is the first to develop, and has primary responsibility for personal safety as well as internal integrity and harmony.[18] It is also where the primary vulnerability to psychopathology is lodged.[19]

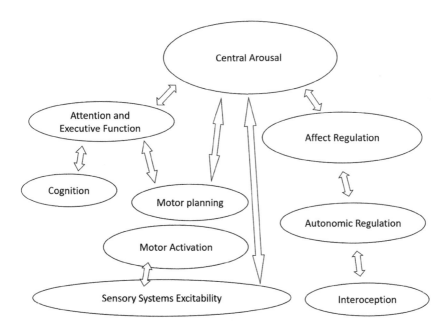

Figure 3.2 The Hierarchy of Regulation as seen in the perspective of the neurofeedback therapist. Of primary interest is central arousal, which is intimately coupled to affective state, sympathetic activation, and interoception. All are seen as principally under the management of the right hemisphere, which therefore demands the earliest attentions. Executive function and cognition lie highest in the hierarchy, and are typically attended to later in the training, if that is still necessary.

The sword-and-shield hypothesis is often invoked to concretize the above dichotomy. The sword is typically wielded by the right hand, governed by the left hemisphere, whereas the shield is borne by the left, governed by the right hemisphere. Left-handers most likely reverse this pattern. A less graphic version is the approach/withdrawal dichotomy. We bestride the world confidently with the left hemisphere in the lead, while the right is doing its best to keep us alive and healthy.

Of course, this simple dichotomy has not gone without challenge, but we spare the reader a recitation of the counter-vailing evidence by reason of the following observation: In ILF Neurofeedback hemispheric reversal has not been observed. This finding has been consistent now for more than a decade, involving hundreds of thousands of clients, all being trained according to the identical schema. We are engaging with the core architecture beneath the level where lateralized dominance—of eye, hand, and foot—is organized. In the early days of exclusively EEG-band training, reversals of right and left were observed with several sets of mirror image twins, as might well be expected. Since entering the ILF regime, however, we have not become aware of work with mirror image twins.

We may well observe a reversal of dominance with the training, and we understand this within the frame of birth trauma. Fetal thumb-sucking is the earliest indicator of laterality, and on that basis a substantial laterality shift with the natural delivery process has been documented (from ~95% right laterality to ~85% post-partum). That shift appears to be reversible with the training at any time in the person's life. The protocols with which that laterality reversal is achieved, however, are themselves invariant with respect to laterality! The resolution of the conflicting data appears to lie in the fact that whatever observables are relied upon to counter the universal assignment of core LH and RH control functions are themselves confounded by laterality issues.

With reference to Figure 3.2, the clinical priority in almost all cases is to train the regulatory arc of interoception, autonomic (sympathetic) activation, affect regulation, and central arousal. All of these are highly correlated, reflecting a high level of functional integration. This objective involves two protocols, targeting the posterior and the anterior aspect of the right hemisphere sequentially. The priority lies with the posterior aspect, by virtue of its coupling to the posterior hub of the Default Mode Network (DMN), which is the first to develop in infancy, and hence the first to bear the scars of a non-nurturing environment.[20] The anterior placement yields our most direct engagement with the Salience Network (SN) and the affective domain.[21]

The posterior placement is the primary site for calming over-arousal of the nervous system—of central arousal and of sympathetic activation. The latter should be demand-responsive, leaving one in the general case in a state of sympathetic–parasympathetic balance, or even of parasympathetic dominance—just as the lions of the veldt have modeled for us. If a steady state of sympathetic over-arousal prevails, it is costly to our physiology, and it is the right parietal placement that allows the system to de-escalate most efficiently and with the greatest persistence.

Brain stability has to be promoted concurrently whenever that issue arises. This calls for inter-hemispheric placement. Here the objective is good regulation, not merely the absence of overt instabilities. This is most readily observable in the autonomic nervous system. Thus, interhemispheric placement is called for not only to redress dysautonomia, or to tame asthmatic episodes (which can be thought of as parasympathetically mediated paroxysms), but to achieve good autonomic regulation more generally. The subtle coordination between the hemispheres turns out to be key to the objective of a dynamic balance between the sympathetic and parasympathetic arms in the steady-state condition, when the organism is not under challenge or duress.

The DMN must be seen as the primary target of ILF NF, in that it is our resting state (i.e., task-negative) network, which governs our level of function and bears our dysfunction.[22] The cortical resources it manages account for nearly all of the energy expended by the brain. The SN is the secondary priority.[23] It mediates between the task-negative and the task-positive control network, the central executive.[24] It has a dual monitoring role, one in which the insula attends to our internal status (interoception), and the anterior cingulate portion tends to the interface with the external world. This activity is largely right-lateralized.[25]

This right-lateralization is most readily demonstrated in the description of Default Mode connectivity relationships by Buckner et al (2008),[26] as shown in Figure 3.3. Observe that the connectivities linked to the right lateral temporal cortex, in the immediate neighborhood of the right insula, are much more elaborated than those to the left. This is the essential point. The lateralized hubs of the DMN (T3 and T4 and P3 and P4) have been our primary training sites, but it should be noted that that has been the case since the late nineties, well before the DMN was first characterized.[27]

Despite the major shift in our clinical priorities over the years, the specific placements have remained substantially invariant over that time. The shift from EEG-band priority to ILF-priority has mainly involved some shift from upper tier to lower tier sites, e.g. from central to temporal sites. But in truth, that shift may well have been more at the conceptual level than the practical. For example, the standard placement for Sterman's and Ayers' early work was C3-T3. So, temporal placement has been in the picture since the beginning of research with human subjects. But the Sterman model concerned the sensorimotor strip exclusively, whereas presently the model concerns itself primarily with the temporal sites, with T3 and T4 present in all lateralized placements.

The rationale for the shift to temporal priority emerged only after the clinical reality had been thoroughly established. The constellation of principal training sites lined up with the multi-modal association areas. This made sense since these areas are the most integrative in character, and they rank highest in terms of functional plasticity. For both reasons, they should therefore rank highest in training efficiency. This integrative character has been nicely demonstrated in a determination of connectivity gradient from the primary sensory areas to the multi-modal sites.[28] This is shown in Figure 3.4, which has been adapted from the original. The connectivity gradient maximizes in the multi-modal association areas. The loci of lighter colors identify our primary training sites: Lateral temporal cortex (T3 and T4); angular gyrus (P3 and P4), and the inferior frontal gyrus (Fp1 and Fp2). At these sites, the DMN is accessible to us at the cortical surface for the purpose of lateralized training.

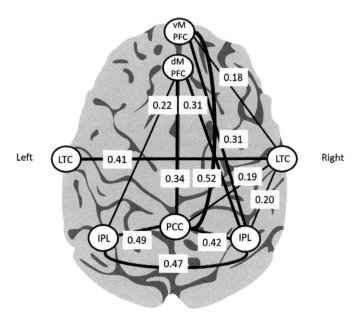

Figure 3.3 The principal hubs of the Default Mode Network are shown with their respective connectivities reflected in the thickness of the lines between them. The right lateral temporal cortex (R LTC) is shown to be more intimately connected to other hubs of the DMN than the left lateral temporal cortex (L LTC). These two sites are involved in all lateralized placements and thus constitute the primary training sites. The other primary training sites are the left and right inferior parietal lobules (L IPL and R IPL). The principal midline hubs of the DMN are the posterior cingulate and retrosplenial cortex (PCC/Rsp) and the ventromedial prefrontal cortex, along with the dorsomedial prefrontal cortex (vMPFC and dMPFC).
Source: Buckner, Andrews-Hanna, and Schacter, 2008.

The Default Mode is accessible to us also at midline sites, and the primary linkage in the DMN, between the posterior and the anterior hubs (The PCC and MPFC in Figure 3.3), beckons for clinical attention. But this linkage turns out to train according to different rules. The differential training with bipolar montage, which was so clarifying in lateralized training, so unambiguous in its imperatives, turned out to be minimally productive when applied to midline sites. This repeatedly sidelined our attentions to this critical linkage for some years. Here the primary need is the enhancement of the coordination of the posterior and the anterior hubs of the DMN. Alpha band Synchrony training, long popular within the field, may already have been serving this objective. To this agenda we have now added Synchrony training in the ILF regime. In some of the most severe cases of early trauma, ILF Synchrony training can be the keystone for functional restoration. In those cases where it is observed to be highly beneficial, it appears also to be indispensable.

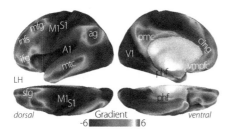

Figure 3.4 The gradient of connectivity exhibits a distribution that maximizes in the multi-modal association areas (light-delineated areas on the external view). These connectivity maxima identify our primary training sites for lateralized training: medial temporal cortex (T3 and T4); angular gyrus (P3 and P4); inferior frontal gyrus (Fp1 and Fp2). They also correspond to the regions in which the Default Mode Network is accessible to us at the cortical surface for lateralized placements. A1, primary auditory cortex; S1, somatosensory cortex; M1, primary motor cortex; V1, primary visual cortex; mfg, medial frontal gyrus; infs, inferior frontal sulcus; sfg, superior frontal gyrus; phf, parahippocampal formation; pmc, posteromedial cortex; cing, cingulate; vmpfc, ventromedial prefrontal cortex. (See a color version in the plate section.)
Source: Daniel S. Margulies et al, PNAS 2016: 133:44:12574-12579.

In the extreme cases of early maltreatment and/or neglect, the intact core self does not have a chance to emerge because it is formed in relationship (the burden of the posterior hub) before it is consolidated in agency (the burden of the frontal hub). Neglect disrupts the orderly maturation of the posterior hub of the DMN in the first year of life, and the early phases of the coordination with the frontal hub. That state of maladaptation is then further consolidated over the course of development. Applying the ecophenotype model to this aspect, the mental health universe can be said to divide between those in whom the front–back axis of the DMN is profoundly dysregulated, and everyone else. Development takes us either on a boot-strapping path of repair and recovery, or of further consolidation of dys-function. The reed bends as it lists, as it were. We end up with a bimodal distribution with little middle ground.

The Harvard group has looked at their bimodal distribution, distinguished as susceptible versus resilient, and, perhaps surprisingly, found the same array of brain abnormalities in both.[29] Reduced nodal efficiencies distinguished the resilient cohort, particularly with respect to the amygdala, and these were deemed to be neuroprotective. From our current vantage point, one is tempted to conjecture that the differences may show up more prominently in the dynamics than in static measures. Our clinical findings indicate that the remedy is to be found there as well, and that whatever brain abnormalities exist do not present a categorical barrier to recovery.

Some progress has recently been made in identifying a possible neurophysi-ological representation of the core self. This emerged out of extensive studies of sleep by Andreas Ioannides and colleagues in Japan.[30] A prominent characteristic of non-REM sleep is the high degree of variability associated with these states. They are not homogeneous in character. In that context, the stability and context-independence exhibited by two small regions attract attention. They are located anteriorly and posteriorly on the left side of the dorsal midline fissure, and are characterized by high levels of gamma-band activity. Curiously, this activity level progressively increases from awake state to light sleep to deep sleep, and maximizes finally in REM sleep.

Ioannides proposes that these two regions constitute the neural representation of the core self. They are identified as the Midline Self-Representational Core (MSRC1 and 2). Evidence for this is provided in the waking state, in which mental activities that are self-referential and autobiographical tend to evoke activity in the penumbra of the MSRC1 and 2. The Default Mode can therefore be characterized as a three-layer onion: The bulk is committed to managing the resting or baseline state of the brain, and is most active when the brain is in a non-engaged state; then there is the penumbra of the core self; and finally there is the core self. The penumbra mediates between the core and the bulk of the DMN. The core self, meanwhile, is preserved from ready alteration, particularly during the waking state.

It is during sleep states, in which the brain is largely non-engaged, that the opportunity maximizes for accommodation by the intrinsic self to new realities that have been assimilated during the waking state. Dreaming may be an essential part of this process. The inherent bias, however, remains one of stability and of resistance to ready alteration on the part of the core self. A threat to the survival or integrity of the self suffices, no doubt, to surmount this barrier to change.

3.5 ILF Neurofeedback in the Frequency Domain: The Frequency Rules

Whereas nearly all of the terms of discourse utilized in connection with ILF Neurofeedback resist rigorous quantification, there is one singular exception, namely the relationships among the optimal response frequencies (ORFs) that prevail at the different training sites.[31] It is found that the ORFs for right-lateralized placements stand in harmonic relationship to the ORFs in left-lateralized placements. The ratio is universally a factor of two, with the left hemisphere at the higher frequency. This is found in the context that harmonic relationships are not commonplace in the EEG world. And indeed, a non-harmonic relationship for the ORFs prevails in the EEG range, where the left hemisphere optimizes at a frequency 2 Hz higher than the right. This is shown in Figure 3.5. Significantly, inter-hemispheric placements follow right-hemisphere rules.

The crossover between the two regions is necessarily where the two criteria converge, which is at a LH frequency of 4 Hz and a RH frequency of 2 Hz. The 2–4 Hz range therefore represents a major transition region between the domains where the ILF rules and the EEG spectrum rules apply. The distinction has long been made between the delta band and the theta band, and 4 Hz has been broadly accepted as the dividing line. So, we now have reason to associate the delta band with the ILF regime in this critical respect.

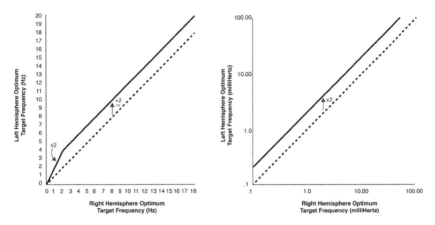

Figure 3.5 The frequency rules governing lateralized training are shown here. A harmonic relationship prevails in the ILF region, whereas an arithmetic relationship applies in the EEG domain. The crossover is necessarily in the 2-4 Hz region of the delta band. Inter-hemispheric placement follows RH rules.

The implications of the frequency relationships for model-building are likely profound, although they can only be intimated at the present state of knowledge. First of all, the fact that inter-hemispheric training follows RH rules confirms RH primacy in organizing the frequency hierarchy. It is therefore more foundational in the regulatory hierarchy. This is consistent with the observed dominance of our right-hemisphere placements with respect to the regulation of the resting state.

Frequency rules have also been discerned for inter-hemispheric placements at homotopic sites. With respect to the central strip sites of C3/C4 and T3/T4 that have garnered most of the clinical attention in the history of EEG neurofeedback, frontal and pre-frontal sites train at ORFs that are 2 Hz lower, and posterior sites train at frequencies that are 4 Hz lower. In the ILF range, a harmonic relationship once again applies, as frontal sites train a factor of two lower than central, and posterior sites a factor of four lower. There has been little opportunity, however, to explore these relationships in the ILF regime. This is for two reasons. First of all, we have the historical circumstance that over most of the period of development of ILF NF, the lowest frequency available in the software ended up being the preferred frequency, rendering submultiples unavailable. The primary reason, however, is that most of the inter-hemispheric training has defaulted the T3-T4 placement, and there has been little incentive to date to explore other homotopic site pairs. This remains a task for the future.

The solidity of the findings with respect to frequency rules more than compensates for the manifest shortcoming of the ORF phenomenology, namely that the entire basis rests on the self-reports of clients. No other evidence in support of the model has ever been found. Nevertheless, the reproducibility of the ORF from session to session, the one just as blinded as the other, places the whole matter beyond dispute, unsatisfactory as that may be in the eye of the critical researcher.

Typically, the ORF only undergoes subtle migration over the course of training. Moreover, one protocol has been found to alter the ORF slightly and, to all appearances, systematically.

The ORFs are dynamically regulated and the ILF training clearly impinges on that process, subtly re-organizing the frequency-based properties of the neural networks. This constitutes the most rigorous proof of validity over the entire frequency regime, in that the observed frequency rules hold consistently over eight orders of magnitude, from 10^{-6} to 100 Hz. Is there anything that renders the unitary quality of our regulatory regime more obvious than this? When it comes to brain function, we are confronted with dynamics on all relevant temporal and spatial scales—a continuous modulation of activation, of successive affiliation and dissociation of neural assemblies—but certain relationships can be invariant and stable, and so they appear to be.

3.6 A Resonance Phenomenon

We first published the observation that the behavior of the training process in the vicinity of the ORF was reminiscent of a resonance phenomenon in 2008, so this model of the process has engaged us for a long time.[32] The usual handicap prevails, namely the limits on performing experiments in clinical settings. The standard resonance curve is shown in Figure 3.6, showing only the real component. It reflects the major features of the clinical experience. The training appears to be more impactful at the center frequency, and also more unambiguously positive, than training at nearby frequencies.

The approach to the ORF in actual practice can be analogized to a piece of music going from dissonance to resolution. In the immediate vicinity of the ORF, the training experience can be more complex, confounding, and even adverse. When this is encountered in a clinical setting, the clinician feels obliged to find resolution in the ORF promptly. One does not linger to establish reproducibility of such a phenomenon. Clients are not research subjects. Once the ORF is found, it is not abandoned for the sake of scientific exploration. Hence the handicap. All of the observations along these lines remain singular events for which patterns of reproducibility could not be established.

The resonance phenomenon does not lend itself to ready evaluation in that it is not being studied in isolation, as would be the case for electronic apparatus, for example. The "system under test," so to speak, is the client's brain in interaction with the signal. We are seeing the response of a control loop with a sentient being in a controlling role. Once signal acquisition occurs, in the sense that the brain has detected the correlation of the signal with its own internal state, the brain undertakes to refine and particularize its response to that signal, an essential part of the learning process. The control loop becomes a function of time, and repeatability is not available to us in any event. As the training proceeds to lower frequencies within the first session in the search for the ORF, a return to higher frequencies yields a different response than was observed before—even after just a few minutes. The process is so impactful that the caution of the Buddhist meditator prevails, to paraphrase: "You never train the same brain twice."

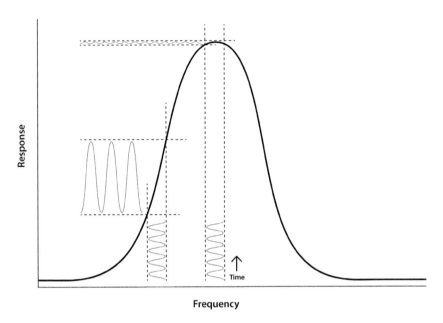

Figure 3.6 A standard resonance curve is shown to illustrate the dependence of the response on frequency with the assumption of an operative biological rhythm at the ORF. Shown also is the effect of perturbations, including in particular fluctuations in the ORF itself. If the spectral filter is mistuned with respect to the ORF, large errors can creep into the signal that the brain may then misinterpret. These error signals are much smaller when the filter is aligned with the ORF.

Yet another confound is that the strongest responses to the training are observed with the most dysregulated brains, which are on their own unpredictable journey—particularly under the provocation of the feedback loop. That is sufficient all by itself to obliterate any expectations of reproducibility. Matters become much more manageable, however, once the ORF is found, and a systematic path forward can usually be charted on the basis of ongoing client reports. This ORF may have to be targeted within 5%, or even less.

What could account for such a degree of parametric specificity? It is the requirement to operate at the very top of the resonance curve, which is flat. Under these conditions the subtle modulations on which the training depends are least compromised by all the confounding factors that prevail in this experimental design. This is illustrated in Figure 3.6, in which an arbitrary perturbation of the system is shown as a sinusoidal excursion on the frequency axis. When the target frequency is mistuned to the skirts of the resonance curve, a large fluctuation is expected in the signal output. At the ORF, the fluctuation is much smaller. This can explain the much greater "turbulence" that prevails when training on the slope of the curve near the peak. A related issue is that of phase, which varies strongly in the vicinity of the resonance peak. This phase combines with the phase shift induced by the filter to yield the phase of the loop response function. A narrow workspace in the frequency domain follows. The resonance curve giveth, and it taketh away—all within the scope of a few percent variation in the training frequency around the ORF.

We are closing in on a model in which dynamically-organized biological rhythms exist within the EEG and ILF realms that play key roles in organizing frequency-based relationships on the large spatial scale—interhemispheric and lateralized. In the ILF realm, they govern resting state dynamics on the longer time scales. Nevertheless, they must be responsive at the speed of life. The resulting modulations are detectable if the brain itself is the detector, and they become meaningful as the brain assigns meaning. The feedback loop effectively becomes internalized, and thus makes possible the subtle refinement of resting state temporal organization "within paradigm," i.e., entirely within the resting state framework.

This process is capable of refining the regulatory regime to the limit of subtlety at which it should ideally function. That cannot be accomplished via externalities such as reinforcers any more than one could hope to improve Hilary Hahn's violin playing by such means. This process is also an answer to Karl Friston's open-ended question back in 2009: Just how does one do experiments on resting state organization (i.e., without disrupting what one is trying to study)?[33] The answer is to let the brain operate within paradigm, absent any external challenge, and just monitor the unfolding process. That is ILF Neurofeedback.

3.7 Implications for Inter-hemispheric Coordination

The case has been made for the primacy of the right hemisphere in managing resting state activation and coordination. All along, however, there has been a latent concern that a shift to right hemisphere priority in the training, along with a shift from the EEG band to ILF, might entail the neglect of what had previously been our priority, namely the training of vigilance with left-central and left-frontal placements. That concern has been laid to rest. Continuous performance tests have been done throughout this period of protocol evolution, and they documented that no price was being paid with the shift in clinical priorities. The quality of resting state organization governs even those functions that we associated with the left hemisphere, and involve the engaged rather than the resting brain.

To illuminate the role of the left hemisphere, we turn to a seminal paper that looks at information flow among the principal hubs of the DMN. These were originally identified in the study of microstates by the Lehman group in Switzerland, well before there was any talk of resting state networks.[34] These are shown in Figure 3.7. Each of the microstates is identified with one of four hubs of the DMN, three in the posterior region and one with an anterior locus. Two are lateralized, and two lie along the midline.

Information flow among these hubs was determined by means of a measure of directed coherence on the alpha and low beta bands, leading to the finding that information flow was dominant from the left hemisphere to the right, as well as

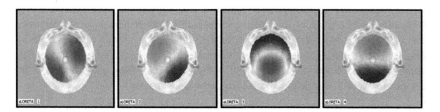

Figure 3.7 Shown schematically here are the four microstates that were originally identified by Lehman et al. Two are lateralized; two are on the midline; three are posteriorly centered; only one has a frontal bias. This tends to support the parietal bias in ILF neurofeedback. (See a color version in the plate section.)
Source: Adapted from Lehman et al, 2014.

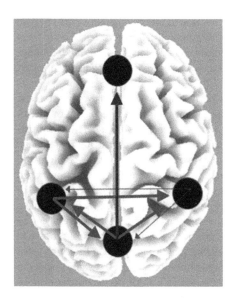

Figure 3.8 The relative magnitude of information flow between the posterior hubs is shown here. This is derived from calculations of directed coherence in the EEG bands of alpha and low beta. The information flow from left to right vastly exceeds that from right to left, which implies that in the EEG range the left hemisphere is playing the dominant role in organizing inter-hemispheric communication. (See a color version in the plate section.)
Source: Adapted from Lehman et al, 2014.

from the left to the midline hub, relative to the flows the other way. The imbalance can be substantial. This is shown in Figure 3.8. The clear implication is that with respect to the regulatory role of the lower EEG bands, the left hemisphere is in a commanding position with respect to the right hemisphere.

A division of responsibilities is indicated. The right hemisphere bears the primary burden of organizing our resting states while the left hemisphere supervises our engagement with the outside world. The ILF regime plays a primary role in organizing the resting state configuration, whereas the EEG regime handles the complexity, coordination, and temporal precision required for our interface with the outside world. The delta band falls in the middle ground.

3.8 Foundational Research in Characterization of ILF Neurofeedback

ILF Neurofeedback has attracted the attentions of Dr. Olga Dobrushina of the International Institute of Psychosomatic Health in Moscow, and of the Treatment and Rehabilitation Center of the Russian Federation, also located in Moscow. Over the last several years they have collaborated on a large-scale study of ILF NF using functional magnetic resonance. The objective was to identify the networks engaged in this process of covert neurofeedback in a comparison of veridical with sham training. 52 healthy volunteers were recruited to a single session of ILF NF under uniform conditions, and resting state fMRI data were acquired immediately prior to, and again following, the session.[35]

Significant changes were observed in both groups, and there were systematic findings among the members of each group, despite their heterogeneity. In the veridical training group, "increased connectivity was observed through a network consisting of the right and left inferior lateral occipital cortex, right dorsolateral prefrontal cortex and striatum nuclei." The sham training group, by contrast, showed increased involvement of the salience network but not of the striatum. The authors proposed that whereas the salience network is responsible for the conscious perception of rewards, the striatum plays more of a role in reward that lies beneath consciousness.

This major study also contributes to the accreting body of evidence testifying to the proposition that sham neurofeedback is not to be considered a neutral process. In order for the control to be meaningful at all, the sham training group has to be given the same instructions as the veridical training cohort. Both enter the study under the assumption of undergoing an active process. In the search for persistent correlations that results, the brains in the veridical group experience closure and get to settle down to an actual feedback process, whereas the brains in the sham remain in a search status, one that is never graced with success. This can account for the greater role of the salience network in the sham group, which is expected to be largest when the salience question on the table cannot be satisfactorily resolved over an extended period of time.

The theoretical aspects of neurofeedback are also starting to attract academic attention.[36] Among the several models for neurofeedback, the skill learning model being proposed here is also dealt with in this treatise.

3.9 Summary and Conclusion

The state of our current thinking with respect to the basic mechanisms underlying ILF Neurofeedback has been presented in narrative fashion, appropriate to the state of knowledge derived largely from clinical practice, which does not lend itself to experimentation for ethical and other reasons. The basis has been laid for further fundamental studies of the ORF phenomenology using the ILF feedback scheme as a probe of resting state functional organization.

ILF Neurofeedback is likely the most prominent exemplar of endogenous neuromodulation—i.e., covert and continuous neurofeedback—in clinical practice. Whereas in the ILF frequency domain there is no alternative, the advantages carry over to EEG-band training as well. After all, it was in the EEG range that the ORF principle was first discovered more than twenty years ago—also by way of covert, continuous feedback that was provided for within the then-standard operant conditioning design. This approach allows the brain to assume control through internalization of the process. Only endogenous neurofeedback can take the process to the limits of subtlety and refinement at which brain regulation must necessarily take place.

This skill learning modality, for which there is no known alternative, has import for the entire realm of human functioning that involves the nervous system. It holds the greatest significance for those contending with severe functional deficits acquired in the early stages of development. Moreover, it offers a remedy available at any age when a need for the training is identified, even down to early infancy. This is possible because the training imposes no cognitive demand and is not contingent on conscious awareness on the part of the trainee.

Notes

1 Othmer, S., Othmer, S.F., Kaiser, D.A., Putman, J. (2013). Endogenous neuromodulation at infra-low frequencies. *Seminars Ped Neurol*, 20(4), 246–260.
2 Webb, R.T., Pedersen, C.B., Mok, P.L.H. (2016). Adverse outcomes to early middle age linked with childhood residential mobility. *Am J Prev Med*, 51(3), 291–300 doi: 10.1016/j.amepre.2016.04.011.
3 Felitti V.J., Anda R.J., Nordenberg D., et al (1998). Relationship of childhood abuse and household dysfunction to many of the leading causes of death in adults: The adverse childhood experiences (ACE) study. *Am J Prevent Med*, 14, 245–258.
4 Rai, D., Kosidou, K., Lundberg, M., et al (2011). *J. Epidemiol Heal*, doi:10.1136/jech.2010.119644.
5 Vaillant, G., Mukamal K. (2001). Successful aging. *Am J Psyc*, 158, 839–847.
6 Brown, D.W., Anda, R.F., Tiemeier, H., Felitti, V.J., Edwards, V.J., Croft, J.B., Giles, W.H. (2009). Adverse childhood experiences and the risk of premature mortality. *Am J Prevent Med*, 37(5), 389–396 doi: 10.1016/j.amepre.2009.06.021.
7 Teicher, M.H., Samson, J.A. (2013). Childhood maltreatment and psychopathology: A case for ecophenotypic variants as clinically and neurobiologically distinct subtypes. *Am J Psyc*, 170, 1114–1133.
8 Teicher, M.H. Samson, J.A., Anderson, C.M., Ohashi, K. (2016). The effects of childhood maltreatment on brain structure, function, and connectivity. *Nat Rev/ Neurosci*, 17, 652–666.
9 Teicher, M.H., Anderson, C.M., Ohashi, K., Polcari, A. (2014). Childhood maltreatment: Altered network centrality of cingulate, precuneus, temporal pole and insula. *Biol Psych*, 76, 297–305.

10   Talavage, T.M., Nauman, E.A., Breedlove, E.L., Yoruk, U., Dye, A.E., Morigaki, K.E., Feuer, H., Leverenz, L.J. (2014). Functionally-detected cognitive impairment in high school football players without clinically-diagnosed concussion. *J Neuro*, 31, 327–338 doi: 10.1089/neu.2010.1512.

11   Muller, A.M., Virji-Babul, N. (2018). Stuck in a state of inattention? Functional hyperconnectivity as an indicator of disturbed intrinsic brain dynamics in adolescents with concussion: A pilot study. *ASN Neuro*, 2018, 1–17 doi: 10.1177/1759091417753802.

12   Aladjalova, N.A. (1964). *Slow Electrical Processes in the Brain*. Elsevier Publishing Company.

13   Hess, W.R. (1954). *The Diencephalon: Autonomic and Extrapyramidal Functions*. Grune and Stratton, New York ASIN: B015AFG0SU.

14   Vanhatalo, S., Palva, J.M., Holmes, M.D., Miller, J.W., Voipio, J., Kaila, K. (2004). Infraslow oscillations modulate excitability and interictal epileptic activity in the human cortex during sleep. *Proc Natl Acad Sci USA*, 101, 5053–5057.

15   Monto, S., Palva, S., Voipio, J., Palva, J.M. (2008). Very slow EEG fluctuations predict the dynamics of stimulus detection and oscillation amplitudes in humans. *J Neurosci*, 28, 8268–8772.

16   Palva, J.M., Palva, S. (2012). Infra-slow fluctuations in electrophysiological recordings, blood-oxygenation-level-dependent signals, and psychophysical time series. *NeuroImage*, 62, 2201–2211.

17   He, B.J., Raichle, M.E. (2009). The fMRI signal, slow cortical potential and consciousness. *Trends Cogn Sci*, 13(7), 302–309.

18   Chiron, C., Jambaque, I., Nabbout, R., Lounes, R., Syrota, A., Duklac, O. (1997). The right brain hemisphere is dominant in human infants. *Brain*, 120, 1057–1065.

19   Schore A.N. (1997). Early organization of the nonlinear right brain and development of a predisposition to psychiatric disorders. *Develop Psychopathol*, 9(1997), 595–631.

20   Gao, W., Alcauter, S., Smith, J.K., Gilmore, J.H., Lin, W. (2014). Development of human brain cortical network architecture during infancy. *Brain Struc Func*, 1–14 doi: 10.1007/s00429-014-0710-3.

21   Sridharan, D., Levitin, D.J., Menon, V. (2008). A critical role for the right fronto-insular cortex in switching between central-executive and default-mode networks. *Proc Natl Acad Sci U S A.*, 105, 12569–12574.

22   Broyd, S.J., Demanuele,C., Debener,S., Helps, S.K., James, C.J., Sonuga-Barke, E..J. (2009). Default-mode brain dysfunction in mental disorders: A systematic review. *Neurosci Biobehav Rev*, 33, 279–296.

23   Menon, V. (2011). Large-scale brain network and psychopathology: A unifying triple network model. *Trends Cogn Sci*, 10, 483–506.

24   Menon, V., Uddin, L.Q. (2010). Saliency, switching, attention and control: A network model of insula function. *Brain Struct Funct*, 214(5–6), 655–667 doi 10.1007/s00429-010-0262-0.

25   Sridharan D., Levitin D.J., Menon V. (2008), op. cit.

26   Buckner, R.L., Andrews-Hanna, J.R., Schacter, D.L. (2008). The brain's default network: Anatomy, function, and relevance to disease. *Ann N Y Acad Sci*, 1124(1), 1–38.

27 Raichle, M.E., MacLeod, A.M., Snyder, A.Z., Powers, W.J., Gusnard, D.A., Shulman, G.L. (2001). A default mode of brain function. *Proc Nat Acad Sci U S A*, 98(2), 676–682 doi: 10.1073/pnas.98.2.676.

28 Margulies, D.S., Ghosh, S.S., Goulas, A., Falkiewicz, M., Huntenburg, J.M., Langs, G., Bezgin, G., Eickhoff, S.B., Castellanos, F.X., Petrides, M., Jefferies, E., Smallwood, J. (2016). Situating the default-mode network along a principal gradient of macroscale cortical organization. *Proc Nat Acad Sci U S A*, 113(44), 12574–12579 doi: 10.1073/pnas.1608282113.

29 Ohashi, K., Anderson, C.M., Bolger, E.A., Khan, A., McGreenery, C.E., Teicher, M.H. (2018). Susceptibility or resilience to maltreatment can be explained by specific differences in brain network architecture. *Biol Psyc.* doi: 10.1016/j.biopsych.2018.10.016.0.

30 Ioannides, A.A. (2018). Neurofeedback and the neural representation of self: Lessons from awake state and sleep. *Front Human Neurosci*, 12, 1–20 doi: 10.3389/fnhum.2018.00142.

31 Othmer, S., Othmer, S.F. (2017). Toward a frequency-based theory of neurofeedback. *Chapter 8 in Rhythmic Stimulation Procedures in Neuromodulation*, James R. Evans and Robert A. Turner, Eds, Academic Press, London, pp. 254–307.

32 Othmer, S. (2008). Neuromodulation technologies: An attempt at classification. *Chapter 1 in Introduction to QEEG and Neurofeedback: Advanced Theory and Applications* (Second Edition), Budzynski, Helen Kogan Budzynski, James R. Evans, and Andrew Abarbanel, Eds, Elsevier, pp. 3–26..

33 Friston, K..J. (2009). Modalities, modes, and models in functional neuroimaging, *Science*, 326(5951), 399–403 doi: 10.1126/science.1174521.

34 Lehmann, D., Pascual-Marqui, R.D., Milz, P., Kochi, K., Faber, P., Yoshimura, M., Kinoshita, T. (2014). The resting microstate networks (RMN): Cortical distributions, dynamics, and frequency specific information flow. Available from: http://arxiv.org/abs/1411.1949.

35 Dobrushina, O.R., Pechenkova, E.V., Vlasova, R.M., Rumshiskaya, A.D., Litvinova, L.D., Mershina, E.A., Sinitsyn, V.E. (2018). Exploring the brain contour of implicit infra-low frequency EEG neurofeedback: A resting state fMRI study. *Int J Psychophysiol*, 131S(2018), S69–S184 doi: 10.1016/j.ijpsycho.2018.07.217.

36 Sitaram, R., Ros, T., Stoeckel, L., Haller, S., Scharnowski, F., Lewis-Peacok, J., Weiskopf, N., Blefari, M.L., Rana, M., Oblak, E., Birbaumer, N., Sulzer, J. (2017). Closed-loop brain training: The science of neurofeedback. *Nature Rev Neurosci*, 18, 86–100.

Chapter 4

Astrocytes and Infra-Low Frequencies

David A. Kaiser

4.1 Introduction

Imagine a world with 25 times more people than today: Los Angeles would be a city of 90 million people, New York City a metropolis of 200 million, and there would be 7 billion Americans in total. At 25 times current population density, our world begins to resemble the complexity of our brain. Our brain is 25 times bigger than the world, it has 25 times more inhabitants than we currently have on Earth. Human society in all its complexity amounts to a tiny fraction of that which characterizes our internal workings. To rival cerebral complexity we must either consider all of human history, every human ever born, to obtain cerebral numbers – or we look to the stars. Astroglia and neurons rival the number of stars in our galaxy and galaxies in our sky. Both neurons and astrocytes amount to around 85 billion each.[1] With billions of these organisms competing and getting along, our brain is an arena of cosmic-scale politics of neurons, glia, and capillaries.

Glia, Greek for *glue*, are interwoven as they were throughout the brain. At first, most considered these star-shaped cells as not relevant to behavior, suggesting they may do little more than fill empty spaces between neurons – provide structural support for neurons.[2] Recent research identified functions of astroglia far more numerous and more complex than anticipated. Among many duties, astroglia facilitate the creation of new synapses (synaptogenesis), a necessity for neuronal survival and vital to cortical networks.[3,4,5,6,7,8] Astroglia manage network excitability through capillary blood flow, directing blood flow to currently active networks and away from inactive sites, a process called *cerebral hemodynamics*.[9,10] As pyramidal neurons also communicate long distance between cortices and astrocytes, together they regulate, coordinate, and organize mood and goal behaviour, including language.[11,12,13,14,15,16,17,18]

For most animals, brains are more neuronal than glial: one astrocyte for every 25 neurons in the leech, one for every six in the round worm, and one for every three in rats and mice.[19] Human neocortex ranges ratios between one glia for two-plus neurons down to one-to-one neurons to astrocytes. When oligodendrocytes (white matter) and microglia are factored in, glia make up 90% of the volume of our cortex.[20] Oligodendrocytes wrap around axons, insulating them electrically and speeding electrochemical signal velocity by a factor of 3,000 by virtue of faster (saltatory) propagation and quicker refractory phases.[21, 22, 23, 24] Microglia constitute a first line of defense for our central nervous system (CNS). Through release of glutathione and ascorbate, they protect neurons from oxidative damage,[25] and they are critical for our protective blood-brain barrier.[26] Through phagocytosis they clean up inter-cellular space, disposing of neuronal waste products, as well as toxins that make it across the blood brain barrier.[27, 28, 29]

It is the emergence of novel functions of astrocytic networks that have spurred most mental and behavioral advances of our species. Human astrocytes are larger and signal other glia ten times faster than rat astrocytes.[30] When healthy, they send different messages to different neurons, laying the groundwork for a well-regulated brain. However, when immature or diseased, they send the same signals to all neurons they attend.[31, 32] Hence, it is no surprise that functional disturbances in astrocytic networks are common to most mental health conditions, including Attention Deficit Disorder (ADD), depression, bipolar disorder, autism, schizophrenia, epilepsy, Alzheimer's, Parkinson's, and Multiple Sclerosis.[33, 34, 35]

4.2 Rhythmicity of the Brain and Energy Cycles

Far from being passive structural support that sheathes axons or fills space between different elements of the brain, we recently learned that astroglial cells have a variety of complex regulatory functions essential to the health and smooth functioning of our brain. Neurons and glia interact dynamically at the molecular level to process information. Astrocytes modulate the *tone* of neuronal activity through capillary management and timed releases of Adenosine Triphosphate (ATP).[36, 37, 38, 39, 40] Tone is the level of activity (or inactivity) of neuronal assemblies subject to internal and external demands, as well as to our daily cycles of rest and engagement. In this regard, astroglia regulate cortical excitability and plasticity via both short-term and long-term rhythmic fluctuations in ATP release, which in turn affects glutamate and calcium availability which is vital to neural firing.[41, 42] A synapse can be considered as a communication link among an astrocyte and two neurons.[43, 44, 45, 46] Astrocytes provide a feedback loop on synaptic transmission, integrating activity of connected neurons.[47, 48, 49, 50, 51, 52]

Astrocytes are also implicated in our daily (circadian) and hourly (ultradian) cycles of rest and activity.[53, 54, 55, 56] Ultradian rhythms can be described as an alternation between a reduction or insensitivity in sensory processing, i.e., a trough of activity, followed by a peak of activity and receptivity. Each cycle varies by person from between 90 minutes to 3 hours: periods of less activity, followed by more activity, in repeating cycles. Ultradian rhythms are a signature of life and our brain is replete with them.[57] What interests many neurofeedback practitioners is that ultradians are themselves an infra-low frequency (ILF), around 0.14 milli-Hertz (mHz) on average[58] (see Figure 4.1).

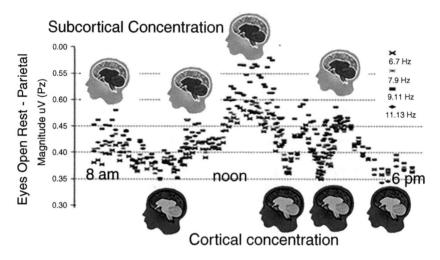

Figure 4.1 Time of day changes in posterior alpha.

4.3 Implications for Neurofeedback

In healthy individuals, ultradian rhythms are reasonably phase-locked to the circadian rhythm, so that of the number of cycles of peaks and troughs within a 24-hour cycle is approximates an integer (10 or 12 as opposed to 13.6 or 8.38 cycles per day). The number of ultradian cycles per person typically ranges from 8 to 15 per day. As stated above, this activity falls into the infra-low frequency range. A frequency of 1 mHz corresponds to a 17-minute ultradian rhythm; 0.18 mHz to a 90-minute cycle; and 0.14 mHz to 2 hours, the general range of our Basic-Rest-Activity-Cycle (BRAC), i.e. how we tend to rest and work in near-two-hour increments.[59,60]

This cycle of cortical excitability is controlled by astroglia. In cases where astroglia are affected by internal genetic anomalies, biomedical factors, or damaged by physical trauma (e.g., traumatic brain injury), the regulation of these cycles is disturbed. Brain functioning degrades due to regulatory loss and mismanagement of energy. This is where neurofeedback in the infra-low frequency domain is used effectively to restore healthy functioning of astrocytic networks, leading to improved brain efficiency.[61] Much of infra-low frequency training is presently conducted in the vicinity of 0.01 mHz, strongly suggesting that we engage and adjust a person's circadian rhythm with ILF training, aligning our wake–sleep cycles with Earth. Recently, ILF neurotherapists have experimented with even slower rhythms, those associated with 48-hour, 72-hour, and weekly rhythms.

Finally, astrocytes organize cortical groups into functional networks, yielding another echelon in the hierarchy of regulation.[62,63] On the largest spatial scale, the corticolimbic system divides into competing networks centered around our resting state network, also known as the Default Mode Network. These core networks organize cortical activity in response to engagement.

Cortical networks are highly active at all times, including during sleep and anesthesia. The default mode network is most active during rest and self-referential tasks including mind wandering, self-judgments, empathy, and envisioning our future. This network deactivates when outward directed attention is needed, in which case task-positive networks, including the dorsal attention and central executive network, engage. A salience network mediates among these networks. Our primary target in Infra-Low Frequency Neurofeedback is usually the Default Mode Network, as all cognition, all coordinated network action and response systems, work in relation to this grouping. Our default network includes the medial prefrontal cortex, posterior cingulate cortex, lateral and medial temporal lobes, and posterior inferior parietal lobule; when it is active, we are at rest, and when other networks, like dorsal attention or central executive, are active, we are at work.[64, 65, 66, 67] Infra-low frequency training typically target regions of the Default Mode, Central Executive, and related networks accessible in surface EEG. One form of neurotherapy that adjusts astrocytic networks with faster frequencies is known as Default Network Training (DNT), which relies on conventional EEG band activity (e.g., alpha, beta) to induce healthy cerebral plasticity. DNT complements and is often combined with ILF training, to great effect on a variety of symptoms and disorders by addressing regulatory activity and connectivity inherent to maturation. Whereas neurofeedback in the corticolimbic rhythm (conventional) range of EEG frequencies (1–100 Hz) engages neuronal assemblies in all of their complexity, Infra-Low Frequency Neurofeedback simplifies the focus to regulatory dynamics, astrocytic mechanisms with a minimum of other influences, the current best explanation for why the brain is able to accomplish so much reorganization on the basis of so little information. This allows the neurotherapist to shape and improve astrocytic networks non-invasively toward patterns of well- being and mental health.

Notes

1   von Bartheld, C. S., Bahney, J. & Herculano-Houzel, S. (2016). The search for true numbers of neurons and glial cells in the human brain: a review of 150 years of cell counting. *J Comp Neurol*, 524, 3865–3895.

2   The Brain from Top to Bottom. Thebrain.mcgill.ca. Retrieved on August 26, 2014.

3   Zonta, M., Angulo, M. C., Gobbo, S., et al. (2003). Neuron-to-astrocyte signaling is central to the dynamic control of brain microcirculation. *Nat Neurosci*, 6, 43–50.

4   Metea, M. & Newman, E. A. (2006). Glial cells dilate and constrict blood vessels: a mechanism of neurovascular coupling. *J Neuro Sci*, 26(11), 2862–2870. doi: 10.1523/.4048-05.2006.

5   Gordon, G. R., Mulligan, S. J. & MacVicar, B. A. (2007). Astrocyte control of the cerebrovasculature. *Glia*, 55(12), 1214–1221.

6   Parpura, V., Basarsky, T. A., Fang, L., et al. (1994). Glutamate-mediated astrocyte–Neuron signaling. *Nature*, 369, 744–747. doi: 10.1038/369744a0.

7   Bezzi, P., Carmignoto, G., Pasti, L., et al. (1998). Prostaglandins stimulate calcium-dependent glutamate release in astrocytes. *Nature*, 391(6664), 281–285.

8   Schummers, J., Yu, H., Sur, M. (2008). Tuned responses of astrocytes and their influence on hemodynamic signals in the visual cortex. *Science*, 320, 1638–1643.

9 Sasaki, T., Kuga, N., Namiki, S., et al. (2011). Locally synchronized astrocytes. *Cerebral Cortex*, 21, 1889–1900.
10 Poskanzer, K. E. & Yuste, R. (2011). Astrocytic regulation of cortical UP states. *Proc Nat Acad Sci USA*, 108(45), 18453–18458. doi: 10.1073/pnas.1112378108.
11 Rossi, E. & Lippincott, B. (1992). The wave nature of being: ultradian rhythms and mind-body communication. In *Ultradian Rhythms in Life Processes: A Fundamental Inquiry into Chronobiology and Psychobiology*, Lloyd, D., and Rossi, E., eds. Springer, New York, 371–402.
12 Attwell, D., Buchan, A. M., Charpak, S., et al. (2010). Glial and neuronal control of brain blood flow. *Nature*, 468, 232–243.
13 Cauli, B. & Hamel, E. (2010). Revisiting the role of neurons in neurovascular coupling. *Front Neuroenerg*, 2(9).
14 Gordon, G. R., Choi, H. B., Rungta, R. L., et al. (2008). Brain metabolism dictates the polarity of astrocyte control over arterioles. *Nature*, 456, 745–749.
15 Zonta, M., Angulo, M. C., Gobbo, S., et al. (2003).
16 Takano, T., Tian, G. F., et al. (2006). Astrocyte-mediated control of cerebral blood flow. *Nat Neurosci*, 9, 260–267.
17 Cauli, B. & Hamel, E. (2010).
18 Pereira, A. Jr. & Furlan, F. A. (2010). Astrocytes and human cognition: modeling information integration and modulation of neuronal activity. *Progress Neurobio*, 92, 405–420.
19 Oberheim, N. A., Takano, T., Han, X., et al. (2009). Uniquely hominid features of adult human astrocytes. *J Neurosci*, 29, 3276–32787.
20 Laming, P. R., Kimelberg, H., Robinson, S., et al. (2000). Neuronal-glial interactions and behaviour. *Neurosci Biobehav Rev*, 24, 295–340.
21 Kang, J., Jiang, L., Goldman, S. A., et al. (1998). Astrocyte-mediated potentiation of inhibitory synaptic transmission. *Nat Neurosci*, 1, 683–692.
22 Araque, A., Parpura, V., et al. (1999). Tripartite synapses: glia, the unacknowledged partner. *Trends Neurosci*, 22, 208–215.
23 Carmignoto, G. (2000). Reciprocal communication systems between astrocytes and neurons. *Prog Neurobiol.*, 62, 561–581.
24 Barres, B. A. (2008). The mystery and magic of glia: a perspective on their roles in health and disease. *Neuron*, 60, 430–440.
25 Barreto, G. E. & Gonzalez, J. (2011). Role of astrocytes in neurodegenerative diseases. In *Neurodegenerative Diseases: Processes, Prevention, Protection and Monitoring*, Chang, R. C., ed. Books on Demand. Retrieved from: https://www.intechopen.com/books/neurodegenerative-diseases-processes-prevention-protection-and-monitoring/role-of-astrocytes-in-neurodegenerative-diseases.
26 Gordon, G. R., Mulligan, S. J. & MacVicar, B. A. (2007). Astrocyte control of the cerebrovasculature. *Glia*, 55, 1214–1221.
27 Tambuyzer, B. R., Ponsaerts, P., & Nouwen, E. J. (2009). Microglia: gatekeepers of central nervous system immunology. *J Leukoc Biol*, 85, 352–370. doi: 10.1189/jlb.0608385
28 Gordon, G. R., Mulligan, S. J. & MacVicar, B. A. (2007).
29 Koehler, R. C., Roman, R. J. & Harder, D. R. (2009). Astrocytes and the regulation of cerebral blood flow. *Trends Neurosci*, 32, 160–169.
30 Oberheim, N.A., Takano, T., Han, X., et al. (2009).

31 Schummers, J., Yu, H. & Sur, M. (2008). Tuned responses of astrocytes and their influence on hemodynamic signals in the visual cortex. *Science*, 320, 1638–1643.

32 Arizono, M., Bannai, H., Nakamura, K., et al. (2012). Receptor-selective diffusion barrier enhances sensitivity of astrocytic processes to metabotropic glutamate receptor stimulation. *Sci Signal*, 5(218), 27.

33 Todd, R. D. & Botteron, K. N. (2001). Is attention-deficit/hyperactivity disorder an energy deficiency syndrome? *Biol Psychiatry*, 50, 151–158.

34 Hines, D. J., Schmitt, L. I., Hines, R. M., et al. (2013). Antidepressant effects of sleep deprivation require astrocyte-dependent adenosine mediated signaling. *Transl Psych*, 3, 212.

35 Nagele, R. G. & Wegiel, J. (2004). Contribution of glial cells to the development of amyloid plaques in Alzheimer's disease. *Neurobiol Aging*, 25, 663–674.

36 Cotrina, M. L., Lin, J. H., Alves-Rodrigues, A., et al. (1998). Connexins regulate calcium signaling by controlling ATP release. *PNAS*, 95, 15735–15740.

37 Pascual, O., Casper, K. B., Kubera, C., et al. (2005). Astrocytic purinergic signaling coordinates synaptic networks. *Science*, 310, 113–116.

38 Parri, H. R. & Crunelli, V. (2002). Astrocytes, spontaneity, and the developing thalamus. *J Physiol*, 96, 221–230.

39 Parri, H. R., Gould, T. M. & Crunelli, V. (2001). Spontaneous astrocytic Ca2+ oscillations in situ drive NMDAR-mediated neuronal excitation. *Nat Neurosci*, 4, 803–812.

40 Parri, H. R. & Crunelli, V. (2001). Pacemaker calcium oscillations in thalamic astrocytes in situ. *Neuroreport*, 12, 3897–3900.

41 Fellin, T., D'Ascenzo, M. & Haydon, P. G. (2007). Astrocytes control neuronal excitability in the nucleus accumbens. *Sci World J*, 7, 89–97.

42 Innocenti, B., Parpura,V. & Haydon, P. G. (2000). Imaging extracellular waves of glutamate during calcium signaling in cultured astrocytes. *J Neurosci*, 20(5), 1800–1808.

43 Kang, J., Jiang, L. & Goldman, S. A. (1998).

44 Barres, B. A. (2008).

45 Araque, A., Parpura, V., et al. (1999).

46 Carmignoto, G. (2000).

47 Parpura, V., Basarsky, T. A., Fang, L., et al. (1994).

48 Bezzi, P., Carmignoto, et al. (1998).

49 Innocenti, B., Parpura, V. & Haydon, P. G. (2000).

50 Zonta, M., Angulo, M. C., Gobbo, S., et al. (2003).

51 Metea, M. & Newman, E. A. (2006).

52 Gordon, G. R., Mulligan, S. J. & MacVicar, B. A. (2007).

53 Halassa, M. M., Florian, C., Fellin, T., et al. (2009). Astrocytic modulation of sleep homeostasis and cognitive consequences of sleep loss. *Neuron*, 61, 156–157.

54 Halassa, M. M., Dal Maschio, M., Beltramo, R., et al. (2010). Integrated brain circuits: neuron-astrocyte interaction in sleep-related rhythmogenesis. *Sci World J*, 10, 1634–1645.

55 Fellin, T., Halassa, M. M., Terunuma, M., et al. (2009). Endogenous nonneuronal modulators of synaptic transmission control cortical slow oscillations in vivo. *Proc Natl Acad Sci USA*, 106, 15037–15042.

56 Lörincz, M. L., Geall, F., Bao, Y., et al. (2009). ATP-dependent infra-slow (<0.1 Hz) oscillations in thalamic networks. *PLoS One*, 2, e4447.

57 Rossi, E. & Kleitman, N. (1992). The basic rest-activity cycle – 32 years later: an interview with nathaniel kleitman. In *Ultradian Rhythms in Life Processes: A Fundamental Inquiry into Chronobiology and Psychobiology*, Lloyd, D., and Rossi, E., eds. Springer, New York, 303–306.

58 Kaiser, D. A. (2013). Infralow frequencies and ultradian rhythms. *Semin Pediat Neurol*, 20, 242–245.

59 Rossi, E. & Kleitman, N. (1992). The basic rest-activity cycle – 32 years later: an interview with nathaniel kleitman. In *Ultradian Rhythms in Life Processes: A Fundamental Inquiry into Chronobiology and Psychobiology*, Lloyd, D., and Rossi, E., eds. Springer, New York, 303–306.

60 Rossi, E. & Kleitman, N. (1992).

61 Othmer, S., Othmer, S. F., Legarda, S. B. (2011). Clinical neurofeedback: training brain behavior: treatment strategies. *Pediat Neurol Psyc*, 2, 67–73.

62 Vanhatalo, S., Voipio, J. & Kaila, K. (2005). Full-band EEG (FbEEG): an emerging standard in electroencephalography. *Neurol Clin Neurophys*, 116, 1–8.

63 Vanhatalo, S., Palva, J. M., Holmes, M. D., et al. (2004). Infraslow oscillations modulate excitability and interictal epileptic activity in the human cortex during sleep. *Proc Natl Acad Sci USA*, 101, 5053–5057.

64 Yates, F. E. & Yates, L. B. (2008). Ultradian rhythms as the dynamic signature of life. In *Ultradian Rhythms from Molecules to Mind*, Lloyd, D., & Rossi, E. L., eds. Springer, London, 249–260.

65 Leopold, D. A., Murayama, Y. & Logothetis, N. K. (2003). Very slow activity fluctuations in monkey visual cortex: implications for functional brain imaging. *Cereb Cortex*, 13, 422–433.

66 Staba, R. J., Wilson, C. L., Bragin, A., et al. (2002). Sleep states differentiate single neuron activity recorded from human epileptic hippocampus, entorhinal cortex, and subiculum. *J Neurosci*, 22(13), 5694–5704.

67 Steriade, M., McComick, D. A. & Sejnowski, T. J. (1993). Thalamocortical oscillations in the sleeping and aroused brain, *Science*, 262(5134), 679–685.

Part II

Neurofeedback in Clinical Practice Settings

Chapter 5

Neurofeedback in Clinical Practice

Meike Wiedemann

5.1 Overview of the Clinical Process and Development of Individual Treatment Plans

A clinician who decides to work with an individualized Neurofeedback approach like ILF training definitely needs sufficient specialized education and preparation for this specific method. This is best obtained in professional training courses with a lot of practicum work and self-training, which allows for discussion time of the training effects by all attendees. As Director of Training for Neurofeedback practitioners in Europe, the author has found it continually fascinating to observe just how variously people react to the same kind of training. The ILF training induces shifts in physiological state.[1] Sometimes these state shifts arise unexpectedly and rapidly. In clients with unstable nervous systems, these sudden state shifts might lead to unwanted training effects that need to be dealt with promptly by the clinician. This can only be done if the clinician knows how to interpret the symptoms and how to react to them in terms of Neurofeedback. Fortunately, these adverse effects are usually transient and can be quickly reversed. The following section will give a short summary of the clinical process and the related decision making. A more comprehensive overview is given in the "Protocol Guide" by Sue Othmer.[2] The following is a distillation of some of that material.

5.1.1 Assessment and Re-assessment: Type of Intake Information Needed from the Client

Before we start training someone with Neurofeedback, a detailed client interview and assessment is performed. As in any other kind of treatment, the clinician has to decide whether Neurofeedback is a promising tool for the issues and goals of the client. From the information gathered at intake the clinician may decide that the client needs to be referred for further medical work-up before Neurofeedback can be integrated into the overall treatment plan of the client (e.g. medication, other medical or psychological treatments). The client should be comprehensively informed about the training process, about the commitment of time and money, and especially about his responsibility to report training effects, negative as well as positive, to the clinician.

The client must be told how often and how long the training should be. The ILF training is a very effective Neurofeedback approach, so it is not unusual for clients to feel state shifts and symptom changes during or after the first session, and to observe noticeable symptom reduction after only very few sessions. Nevertheless, we are talking about a training and a learning process that needs time and repetition. Unless the training process is reinforced by repetition, the brain will tend to fall back into its old patterns. If the training is terminated too early because of initial positive results, symptoms may well return over time. Therefore, it is necessary to explain to the client that at least 20 sessions of training are needed to solidly embed the gains. Generally, after 20 sessions a reassessment is performed, to compare the results obtained so far with the initial assessment and in light of the established goals.

Clinician and client then should decide together whether the training goal has been reached, or whether it would be useful to continue the training and reassess again after another 10 or 20 sessions. This is more easily said than done. Quite commonly, expectations escalate during the training process as progress is experienced. After all, clients usually come to the training with quite modest expectations, and for their part, clinicians do not wish to overpromise. During the initial assessment, the client must also be informed that the training needs to be done intensively, at a rate of at least two or three sessions per week for the first 10 or 20 sessions. If good progress is made during the intensive training phase, the frequency of the training sessions can be lowered to build upon and consolidate the changes. If all symptoms are reduced sufficiently, or even resolved, the frequency of the training sessions can be further reduced to ascertain whether the changes are stable and persist over longer time periods.

To understand the patterns of dysregulation of each client, the clinician needs as much information as possible about the client's function and dysfunction, strengths and weaknesses. We use a specific symptom rating list to look at indicators for different modes of dysregulation. It is not enough to know if a certain symptom exists or not. Symptoms need not only to be rated in severity, but we also need to know the typical patterns of occurrence to gauge the effects of the specific training parameter. For example, it is not enough to know that the client has sleep problems and that they got better after the training session. To decide which training parameters might be useful we need to distinguish between problems of falling asleep, waking up frequently, inability to return to sleep after waking, waking up too early in the morning, sleeping too long but not feeling rested, and so on.

Besides the medical interview and other possible tests and questionnaires (depending upon the clinician's background), there are two very valuable tools to assess symptoms and to judge Neurofeedback training success in the re-assessment: Symptom Tracking and the Continuous Performance Test (CPT).

Symptom Tracking: Most symptoms that clients come with are not measurable objectively. Nevertheless, we need the Symptom Profile as a guide to where and how to train, and also as an indicator of progress of the training effects. For the ILF training, it is important to track as many symptoms as possible in order to form a comprehensive perspective on the client. Reporting all the symptoms can help determine whether the self-regulation of the trained brain is being enhanced with the training. Often clients would choose to describe only a few key symptoms at their own initiative. The Symptom Tracking system helps to fill in the whole picture. The Symptom Tracking system contains a list of 150 symptoms that can be addressed with Neurofeedback. The list is printed out for the assessment and every symptom needs to be rated on a scale from 0 to 10 (0 = no issue, 10 = biggest issue the client can imagine). The symptoms are allotted to seven different symptom categories (sleep, attention and learning, sensory, behavioral, emotional, physical, and pain). We use specific symptoms as indicators for different modes of dysregulation. That doesn't mean that we target symptoms directly; rather we use symptom status to guide us through the training toward better function, which is the real objective. This understanding has great import for our work. For example, if a client suffers from migraine and has no other symptoms to track, the training might seem like a kind of blind flight in its initial stages, especially if the migraine is irregular and only appears every 3–5 weeks. If the migraine itself were the only indicator of training success, one might need to train for many sessions before one knew whether matters were on the right track. Since the objective is really the enhancement of regulatory status, there are always many indicators. At a more subtle level there are usually other symptoms to key on, such as problems of falling asleep, feeling groggy during the day, muscle tension, tension headache, and so forth. In the absence of even such minor issues, one inquires into the perceived level of functionality: alertness, mental sharpness, vigilance, energy level, motivation, and susceptibility to fatigue. By all these means collectively, it is possible to discern whether self-regulatory capacities are being enhanced.

Another reason to use comprehensive symptom tracking is to create awareness in the client about what symptoms can be influenced with Neurofeedback, to motivate them to talk about a variety of symptoms, and to report changes after the training sessions. Clients often start Neurofeedback training because they are seeking relief for very specific symptoms.

Typically, they are not inclined to think about what else could be influenced by the training and, therefore, they may not talk about other symptom changes. In consequence, the clinician might miss something or not be able to interpret the training effect due to missing information. It is a well-known phenomenon that we are only aware of things that we focus on. The client who comes complaining of concentration problems would not necessarily mention his muscle tension or digestion problems unless such information is explicitly sought. Filling out and discussing the Symptom Tracking list helps to motivate the client to observe and report all different kinds of symptoms during and after training sessions. Since good reporting by the client is so critical to the best success, an essential part of the process is educating the client in the role of being a good reporter. Hence there are really two kinds of training going on, that of the brain and that of the client, the latter in the skill of awareness of self and of self-appraisal.

In the assessment and the reassessment, all 150 symptoms, as well as other individual symptoms that are not contained in the Symptom Tracking forms, are recorded in a table. This can be done either in custom software or in an online platform like EEGexpert (www.eegexpert.net). The online platform has the advantage that access can be given to the client, and the client can then type in his own rating via the Internet. Graphs of the time course of severity of all symptoms are created automatically and can be all be shown in one combined graph, as well as in graphs of individual symptoms. Online access to Symptom Tracking forms can also be given to other people such as parents, partners, teachers, etc. to give feedback on the training effects.

We have learned from experience that due to limited self-awareness, one cannot expect that positive training effects will always be noticed by the client or their family, or that they will always be reported. As for adverse effects, they are frequently not recognized as being connected with the training, particularly since in most cases such states are not novel in the client's experience. Often, we learn about some of the client's positive changes haphazardly. Therefore, sometimes it is a good thing to chat for a while and listen very closely. It is also common for symptoms to be forgotten once they subside, so careful probing is called for.

An example may serve: In the training of a long-term bulimic woman, she failed to report that she had not binged-and-purged the day before, a first in about 18 years. She did not feel that it was worth reporting because "I had not felt like binging, so not doing so didn't seem like a big deal." Of course, "not feeling like binging" was the whole point.

CPTs: Symptom Tracking suffers the limitation of being a subjective rating. However, a Continuous Performance Test, such as the T.O.V.A.® (Test of Variables of Attention) or the QIKtest (https://www.eegexpert.net), provide the possibility for quantifying training results objectively. Whereas the T.O.V.A. needs to be done at the computer, the QIKtest is a standalone, hand-held device which allows for the data to be transferred to the computer after testing. The CPTs measure impulsivity, sustained attention, reaction time, and consistency of reaction time. Not only do the results give useful hints as to where and how to train, but any improvements in the measured variables, which can be impressive, furnish objective evidence of progress.

After the assessment the clinician needs to judge if any contra-indications are present. Although there are almost no contra-indications with respect to Neurofeedback itself, there are still clients who should not be trained by just any clinician and in just any setting. Clients with severe psychiatric indications should only be treated by clinicians who are experienced with these clinical presentations. At a minimum, the clinician needs to work within an adequately supportive network environment. It may be that such high-risk clients can only be treated in a safe inpatient environment. Of course, this caution is not specific to Neurofeedback but rather applies for any kind of impactful treatment. Still, one should be aware that Neurofeedback is a particularly efficient clinical tool that needs adequate education, experience, care, and attention in its utilization. There is also the issue of prioritization. In some cases, other interventions should precede, or at least accompany, the utilization of Neurofeedback if it is to be optimally productive.

5.1.2 Protocol Decision Tree – the Art and Science of How and Where to Train

With Neurofeedback the brain is able to witness its own brain activity and use this information for better self-regulation. Better self-regulation promotes better function. We are not treating disorders, nor are we repairing brain wave patterns. Our goal as Neurofeedback clinicians is to help the client's brain to find its own path to better self-regulation and, consequently, better function.

With ILF Neurofeedback we get strong and specific effects. That means it makes a significant difference where we put the electrodes and what frequencies we feed back to the brain. Therefore, we need a model of brain function to understand categories of regulation and of dysregulation. From these patterns we derive where to train and how to train. We can use a very simplified model to understand basic categories of brain regulation and dysregulation. In this model it helps to look at the central nervous system in three axes:

- Top-down and bottom-up axis ↔ cortical–subcortical axis
- Front–back axis ↔ prefrontal and parietal cortex
- Left–right axis ↔ left and right hemisphere

Good balance in all three axes is the basis for good brain function. We will come back to the three axes when we discuss the five training categories. The three-axis model of the Central Nervous System (CNS), together with the five training categories, is a working model that will support our decision making during the whole training process. The model is shaped by clinical Neurofeedback experience over many years, mainly from the group working with Sue Othmer. Finally, modern neuroscience is providing us with theoretical models that may explain why training sites and frequencies that have been found empirically are as effective and specific as they are in clinical practice (see Chapters 2 and 3).

Table 5.1 gives an overview of the five training categories that we have to keep in mind when finding our path through the training process. These basic training categories will correlate with how and where to train with ILF training and Alpha-Theta training. They play a key role in understanding the assessment and the results of each training session. They help the clinician to find the best starting point after the assessment, and also to optimize the training step by step and from session to session.

Let's have a closer look at the different categories:

Category 1 – Arousal indicators: The arousal indicators help us to adjust the response frequency during the training and from session to session. We use symptoms that are related to shifts in arousal to adjust the response frequency for each client.

Physiological arousal is the most basic component of brain state regulation and is related to the cortical–subcortical axis. Core arousal is managed by brainstem nuclei that project widely throughout the CNS. It is the so-called Reticular Activating System (RAS) that manages the different states of wakefulness and alertness. No

Table 5.1 The five training categories of the working model

No	Category	Relation to training process
1	Arousal indicators	Response frequency
2	Instabilities	Paroxysmal symptoms need inter-hemisphericstabilization
3	Disinhibition	Loss of control needs calming and prefrontal control
4	Localized dysfunction	Electrode placements
5	Learned fears and habits	Alpha-Theta

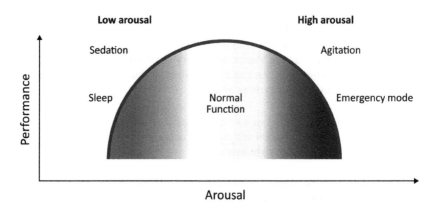

Figure 5.1 The Arousal Performance curve shows different states depending on the arousal level

matter where we place the electrodes on the scalp we will always interact with this system, therefore it is always an issue in the training.

The brainstem sets the tone of the arousal system; this is about how awake the person is, but it is not very specific. On the other hand, it is very specific in how individual persons react to shifts in arousal level. This might affect attention, mood, or physical tension, which involve other, more specific, brain functions. The individual shifts in arousal level guide us to find the optimal, comfortable response frequency for the client.

Arousal level has a crucial influence on the overall level of functioning, which is reflected in the individual Arousal Performance curve (Figure 5.1). It is normal that everyone will move up and down along their own arousal curve during the course of the day. Good self-regulation means flexibility and stability on the arousal curve. That enables us to stay in the middle range for good function, go to the lower end at the close of the day, when we need to sleep, and use the higher end of the curve when we need to react quickly to emergencies, without freezing and without taking time to stop and analyze the situation. However, getting stuck in a state of high arousal without an emergency can lead to significant problems. In an emergency situation we hyper-focus on the emergency and ignore our body and future plans; this can lead to chronic dysregulation in the long run. Low arousal states, on the other hand, are essential for rest and sleep, but are not helpful for good alert function during the day. The first objective with Neurofeedback training is to improve flexibility and stability of state regulation. In Neurofeedback training we use symptoms that indicate arousal shifts to adjust the response frequency. Increasing the response frequency leads to symptoms of high arousal, while decreasing the response frequency leads to symptoms of low arousal.

It is remarkable how sensitive the brain is to even minute shifts in response frequency, which is why it needs to be adjusted carefully for each client. When the response frequency is too high, the brain responds with feeling increased agitation – physical, emotional, mental, or physiological. Training too high might produce increased muscle tension or spasms, hyperactivity or impulsivity, tics or OCD symptoms, increased heart rate or heart palpations. Emotional agitation might show up as increased anxiety, anger, fear, despair, or emotional reactivity. Sleep could be disturbed by nightmares or difficulties falling asleep. Constipation is often a common symptom for people that live in emergency mode. Hence increased constipation could be a sign of training too high. Decreased constipation is often a sign of training in the right direction.

Training with a response frequency that is too low leads to brain responses of feeling too slowed down or sedated. It can be uncomfortable for the client. Training too low might result in feeling dizzy, heavy, nauseated, groggy, or sad. It can also lead to being emotionally sensitive, which is very different from being emotionally reactive, a risk that is normally related to training too high. Another sign of training too low can be a heaviness in the chest that might make it difficult to inhale deeply. This has to be differentiated from chest tension that can result from training too high and producing increased anxiety. Also, symptoms similar to low blood sugar might arise from training too low. With respect to sleep issues, training too low can result in extreme sleepiness and also lack of deep sleep. This might show up in falling asleep easily, but then waking up frequently and not feeling rested in the morning, despite sleeping long enough. Sleepiness during and after training always needs to be looked at closely and is very helpful in finding the right response frequency. Relaxation often leads to comfortable sleepiness and in this case is probably a sign of a good response frequency. With Neurofeedback, we want to calm the brain but not to sedate it. If people feel groggy, sedated, slowed down, or uncomfortable during the session, this is often a sign of training too low. On the other hand, this has to be differentiated from feeling uncomfortably exhausted when training too high, eventually with difficulty keeping the eyes open. Table 5.2 shows an overview of arousal indicators when training too high or too low.

Table 5.2 High and low arousal symptoms

Training too low: Increase Response Frequency	Training too high: Decrease Response Frequency
Sedated, slowed down	Agitated, sped up
Dizziness, nausea	Physical tension, muscle spasms
Groggy, lethargic	Hyperactivity, impulsivity
Heaviness	Tics, obsessive compulsive behavior
Sadness, crying	Heart palpations, tachycardia
Emotional sensitivity	Emotional reactivity
Lack of deep sleep	Difficulty falling asleep
Difficulty waking	Nightmares
Low blood sugar symptoms	Constipation
	Aggressive
	Anxiety, fear, anger, despair

Category 2 – Instabilities: Instabilities result in paroxysmal symptoms as the brain loses control, as in migraines, seizures, panic attacks, narcolepsy, or in radical state shifts as in bipolar mood swings or dysautonomia. The presence of instabilities at any time in a person's life implies a vulnerability that indicates inter-hemispheric training for stabilization with T3-T4 as a part of the training.

At a physiological level, instabilities might be explained as hyper-excitability due to deficient local inhibitory control. Incoming excitation can then set off an escalation of nerve activity that destabilizes the brain. People with instabilities often react very sensitively and reproducibly to changes in response frequency. So, for these persons the response frequency has to be adapted very carefully without too many changes in frequency in one session, because rapid shifts in arousal state, as well as shifting up and down on the arousal curve, can also trigger instabilities. Medically, instabilities are often treated with anticonvulsants, so if clients depend on anticonvulsants for any condition that would be an indication for inter-hemispheric training.

In terms of Neurofeedback, we must differentiate between hyper-excitability, high arousal, and reactivity. Hyper-excitability leads to instabilities with paroxysmal symptoms that need inter-hemispheric training such as T3-T4. Symptoms of high arousal need to be addressed with the response frequency (see Category 1), and reactivity in terms of Neurofeedback is better understood in terms of disinhibition, as is explained in Category 3.

Category 3 – Disinhibition: Disinhibition relates to loss of self-control with stress or boredom, as with tics or impulsivity. This needs prefrontal training for better inhibitory control.

The prefrontal cortex is the most highly developed part of the brain. It develops last, both phylogenetically and ontogenetically. Good brain function depends on inhibitory control from the highest level of the CNS, the prefrontal cortex. Due to its complexity, the prefrontal cortex is vulnerable to loss of function. If we lose good inhibitory top-down control, due to injury, illness, or sedating substances, this might result in disinhibition, with a release of immature and primitive behaviors. With ILF Neurofeedback we can improve prefrontal control substantially, most commonly in combination with parietal training for physical calming. Training the right prefrontal quadrant (T4-Fp2) increases control of emotional reactivity and helps with aggressive, oppositional and fearful behavior. Left prefrontal training (T3-Fp1) increases control of thinking and acting, especially in cases of impulsivity and compulsive behavior/thinking.

Category 4 – Localized dysfunctions: Localized dysfunction might be indicated by reported symptoms, brain injury, by testing, or by brain imaging, all of which is information that can suggest useful training sites.

ILF training has very specific effects, depending on frequency as well as on electrode placement. With ILF training it becomes increasingly important where to place the electrodes, left or right, front or back, intra-hemispheric or inter-hemispheric. The clinician needs to decide if sensory processing in the back of the brain needs to be trained or if circuits creating output in the front need to be involved. Does the right side need to be targeted for big picture awareness or left side for processing of details? Or is there a need to target limbic areas to impact drives and emotions? It is remarkable how rapidly shifts in brain state can occur in response to changes in electrode placements. The change can be observable in mere minutes.

Table 5.3 Training on left and right hemisphere for different issues

Left hemisphere	Right hemisphere
Cognitive routine	Novelty and flexibility
Self-motivated behavior	Environmentally motivated behavior
Top-down control	Bottom-up control
Knowledge and skills	Sensing danger
Competence	Creativity
Later development	Early development

If a new electrode position is incorporated into the training procedure to address specific functions, it is normally obvious within one or two sessions whether or not this new site will be useful in the further training process.

Left and right: The division of the brain into left and right is something neuroscientists don't like to discuss anymore, because of its oversimplification in popular science whereby certain skills have been attributed to only one hemisphere, e.g. one hemisphere for reason and one for emotion, or attributing language function exclusively to the left. Indeed, our cerebral architecture supports the view that we effectively have two brains in our head with quite different functions. But we also must recognize that it is critical that they communicate and cooperate with each other. So key functions, such as language, cannot be assigned to one hemisphere. Nevertheless, the effects of left-side and right-side ILF training are very different and need to be taken into account throughout (see Table 5.3).

We have to consider all the information that we got from the assessment about life history and symptoms to sort out indicators for left- and right-side training. For Neurofeedback training, it is important to be aware of the fact that things that are newly learned are mainly processed on the right side and later, when they have become routine, they are processed mainly on the left side. This has implications, especially for developmental disorders that normally call for a lot of right-side training. The foundations of our regulatory hierarchy are predominantly organized on the right side and that generally gives priority to right-hemisphere training as the point of departure.

Front and back: Besides the left/right decision, the clinician also needs to figure out if training in the back, training in the front, or both is needed. Generally, we assume that training in the back of the head improves sensory processing and training in the front improves executive function. The back of the brain processes input, which means all kinds of sensory information from outside the body as well as from inside. In clinical experience, training the back of the brain has an impact on sensory processing and integration. It improves body awareness and spatial attention to our environment. The frontal region processes output such as moving, speaking, planning, thinking etc. Training over the frontal part of the brain improves executive function and self-control. Training over the frontal sites, especially the prefrontal areas, has impacts on impulsivity as well as on immature and reactive behaviors. It enhances inhibitory control to give the client the possibility of considering how to respond prior to acting.

Table 5.4 The four training quadrants plus inter-hemispheric training sites

Left frontal (T3-Fp1)	Right frontal (T4-Fp2)
Mental calming	Calms emotional reactivity
Planning and organization	Emotional comfort and security
Verbal and written expression	Emotional expression
Logical thinking	Common sense

Left-right (T3-T4)
Stabilizing for instabilities e.g. migraine, headache, seizures, panic, mood swings

Left back (T3-P3)	Right back (T4-P4)
Awareness and processing of detail	Physical calming
Symbolic processing	Body and spatial awareness Sensory
Stored knowledge and skills	integration Orientation to time and space

Multi-modal association areas: The highest level of input and output processing in the CNS are the multi-modal association areas. In these areas sensory input from all different modality-specific areas (visual, auditory, somatosensory, and pre-motor) and output modalities is integrated. This is the basis for making sense out of all the different inputs that finally results in adequate feeling, acting, and behavior, a process that principally involves the right insula and hippocampus. The multi-modal association areas mainly involve inferior parietal, mid-temporal, and prefrontal cortical regions.

Basic training sites: The multi-modal association areas lead to the basic training sites. As described in the beginning of this chapter, the training sites were found empirically but, of course, not without knowledge about neurophysiology. The multi-modal association areas correspond to the basic ILF training sites (T3-T4, T4-P4, T4-Fp2, T3-Fp1, T3-P3). For most of the clients in ILF training only a subset of the basic sites is needed to reach the training goals. To comprise the categories 2–4 in terms of where to train, it is useful to simplify the possible training sites in a picture of 4 quadrants, plus inter-hemispheric (left–right) training and the prospective training effects. This puts together the understanding of front versus back and left versus right training effects in a simplified model.

Inter-hemispheric: Training in one hemisphere (left side or right side) normally has strong and specific effects. In some people with instabilities, training in only one hemisphere might even trigger instabilities. Therefore, a gentler way of training, namely the reliance on inter-hemispheric placements, can be used as an alternative for people with instabilities, particularly for those who do not tolerate left- or right-side training. This process normally starts with T3-T4 to adjust for the optimal response frequency.

More specific training sites: More specific training sites are only used after training with the basic sites, which is often specific enough for most clients. Only in some cases, e.g. in rehabilitation after brain injury or specific learning disabilities, might one take other sites into account to address specific functions. On the left side this may be T3-F7 for word finding and verbal articulation, or T3-T5 for decoding words when reading. On the right side this may be T4-F8 for acquisition of language and emotional expression. T4-T6 might be used to enhance the ability to read facial expressions and body language of others, which is useful with clients on the autistic spectrum. T4-O2 is sometimes an emotionally calming electrode position with traumatized clients.

Localization theory versus network theory: The most useful training sites developed empirically over the years upon observation of the clinical training effects, as well as on available knowledge of functional neuroanatomy, such as the functional differentiation of Brodman areas. However, we should not go back to the localization theory. Rather, we should keep in mind that billions of neurons are working together in complex networks. This interconnectedness of the brain on the structural level is vividly illustrated with images that can be seen online at www.humanconnectome.org. On a functional level, it is interesting that the key electrode montages that were empirically found in the development of ILF training target nodes in the Default Mode Network and the Salience Network.[2] It has been proposed that a number of psychiatric disorders are characterized by significant deviations in the functional connectivity of these control networks, in interaction with the Central Executive Network.[3,4] The list includes Autism, ADHD, and PTSD. Interestingly, these are conditions we are treating very well with ILF training.

Category 5 – Learned fears and habits: Alpha-Theta training is not ILF training but is often a necessary complement to work in the ILF domain. Alpha-Theta training isn't even primarily a brain training procedure. It addresses learned fears and habits, and it does so largely experientially. After physiological calming and stabilizing with ILF training, the Alpha-Theta procedure can then allow the required processing and resolution of traumatic experience while the client resides in a safe and relaxed state. The role of reinforcements in the alpha and theta bands is to serve as cues to the brain, to facilitate state shifts into deeply relaxed, disengaged, and internally directed states. As a deep state training it is only indicated after enough awake state training with ILF has been done to provide a stable foundation for the subsequent experience. Alpha-Theta is one of the older training protocols that can fruitfully complement the ILF training process. It is discussed in more detail below in sections 5.2.1 to 5.2.4, together with other older, but still useful, protocols.

5.1.3 Interaction with the Client – Importance of In-session Communication and Reports from between Sessions for Adjusting Training Protocol

All the above categories help us to design a treatment plan and form a hypothesis of what kind of training sites might be helpful for the client. Training the client can then rather quickly either confirm or invalidate the hypothesis. Training then needs to be adjusted step by step based on the response. The client's response to the training within the session, and even more importantly after the session, guides us through the different training categories above. There is no fixed rule about what to do for how many sessions and when to change parameters, change frequency, or change or add electrode positions. With some clients changes can occur in quick succession, while in other cases multiple changes in short order might lead to outcomes that are difficult to interpret in terms of cause and effect relationships.

Because ILF training is client-oriented, it is a challenge for the clinician and demands close attention. A burden is also placed on the client. This is why it is critically important to have good client–clinician interaction, and a good understanding of the complexity of the training process to be able to recognize and interpret the training responses. This is not an easy job, neither for the client nor for the clinician. Most of the clients are not used to reporting on how they feel and may not be aware of their own state shifts unless they become very uncomfortable. Yet, for the optimization process, we do need to know about the small changes in the client's state and we need to interpret them with the help of the client as symptoms of under-arousal and over-arousal, or as other indications to change or add electrode sites. So how do we accomplish that and how do we proceed in the first session? We have to start somewhere in terms of electrode position and response frequency and then go from there.

First session: For the starting protocol we need to decide between two electrode positions according to the assessment, either T4-P4 or T3-T4, or both. Again, we have to start somewhere, and only after we get the results of the initial training session do we know if we made the right decision. Fortunately, it is not as difficult and uncertain as it seems because we have clear indications for each of the two positions that help with the decision. So, if we follow the indications, they fit most of the clients. We start with one electrode position in the first session and adjust response frequency as needed.

Indications for starting positions (the given starting frequencies are valid for the Cygnet® HD-application):

- **T4-P4** is used as a starting position for clients with early development or attachment issues, chronic disorders, lack of resilience, or trauma history. People with chronic pain, chronic mood disorders (except Bipolar)., chronic insomnia, chronic addictions, etc. generally respond best to T4-P4 as a starting position for physical calming.
  With T4-P4 we start with a response frequency of 0.1 mHz and optimize frequency from there.
- **T3-T4** is used as a starting position for clients where right-side training alone might trigger instabilities. This refers particularly to clients with instabilities (like migraine, seizure, bipolar disorders, etc.) and no indications for T4-P4, or in cases where too much right-side calming without inter-hemispheric stabilization can leave people unbalanced in their function. This might be an issue, for example, with some ADD clients with no strong indications for T4-P4 training. At T3-T4 we start with a response frequency of 0.5 mHz and optimize frequency from there.

For some clients we need to start with **T4-P4 and T3-T4** from the first session. This refers to people with strong right-side indicators such as developmental trauma or addiction, plus significant instabilities (e.g., seizures, panic attacks, or dissociation).

If the decision is made for the starting placement, we need to know the symptom baseline for that day. So, the client needs to describe his current state concerning his symptoms and level of arousal. Most people are not well versed in describing their own state, so in most of the cases they will need some coaching from the clinician. It is best to ask simple questions, starting with general questions and then getting more specific. The questions should always be open-ended and the inquiry should be conducted in a non-judgmental manner.

- How does your body feel?
- Are you tense or relaxed?
- How do you feel mentally?
- Are you tired or awake?
- Do you have any pain or tension at the moment?
- Where do you have this pain/tension, can you show the area?
- Is the pain sharp or dull?
- On a scale from 0–10, where would you judge your pain/tension now?
- From which situation do you know this symptom?
- Do you feel this when you are stressed or when you are relaxed, tired?

Why do we need to ask all these questions? We expect to induce state shifts with the training. To interpret in which direction we shifted the state, we need to know where we started from. Since we must rely on the client to indicate what change has occurred, it is important to benchmark the status at the outset of the session and to place these matters within the conscious awareness of the client.

The next step is to find an appropriate feedback application for the client. For the first session this should be a more or less neutral and comfortable one. Why comfortable? Because if the client feels comfortable with the feedback, it is easier for his brain to engage with the training. Why neutral? Because state shifts should be induced by the brain's response to the signal and not because the client is suddenly agitated or depressed due to the movie or a car race that is too activating. What is comfortable and neutral could be very different for each client. Therefore, it is important to have a variety of options from which to choose.

After the state of the client has been appraised, electrodes are placed in the chosen locations on the head. Then impedance is checked to see if the electrodes have good contact, feedback is chosen, and then the training session can start. The client needs to be instructed that he needs to tell the clinician immediately if he doesn't feel good. Otherwise, the session can be run with the starting frequency for a few minutes, and then the clinician can begin to query the client with regard to state shifts. The interaction starts again with open ended questions to give the client the chance to describe the experience in his own words. In a few cases this might be a detailed description, but most of the time this will be something like "good," "I feel fine," or "no difference." The clinician may need to help with some more detailed questions about the symptoms or the states that were described at the beginning of the session. The questions should be specific but not suggestive or tendentious. For example, we might ask: "In the beginning you described a pain above your right eye with an intensity of 4. Is this still the same or did it change during the training?" Further useful questions might be:

- Do you feel more alert, less alert, or the same?
- Is the tension you described in the beginning more, less, or the same?
- Did your relaxation change? More, less, same, different?
- How do you feel mentally?
- How do you feel emotionally?

In addition to the questions, the clinician of course needs to observe the client and look for changes in physiology, facial expression, voice, posture, and so on. According to the answers of the client and the observations of the clinician, the clinician needs to interpret the results primarily in terms of under- and over-arousal, which speaks to the issue of response frequency, and also criteria that bear on site selection. Low arousal symptoms are typically obvious and uncomfortable for the client. Clients might feel groggy, sedated, nauseous, dizzy, or sad. If the client feels symptoms of under-arousal, the response frequency needs to be increased to relieve symptoms. If high arousal symptoms are induced by the training, the client might feel agitated or physically tense, calling for a decrease in the response frequency to relieve symptoms. Response frequency always needs to be adjusted carefully, and usually slowly and incrementally, guided by the symptoms reported by the client.

In clinical practice it is not always easy to interpret the reported symptoms correctly, therefore, it is always worthwhile to bring the reported symptoms into the context of the individual client, and not just rely on Tables 5.2 and 5.4 like a cook book. If we misinterpret the symptoms and change the frequency in the wrong direction the client might feel worse after the session. This might be explained best with the example of how we interpret sleepiness during the session. Does sleepiness mean we trained too high, too low, or are going in the right direction? It could be any of the three depending on the whole picture of the client. It could be absolutely ok if somebody feels comfortably sleepy and relaxed. A lot of people do experience relaxation as a comfortable sleepiness. If people feel sedated or groggy and uncomfortable, the training frequency was likely too low. But this is often difficult to differentiate from training too high and bringing the client to exhaustion, sometimes in combination with eye strain. Therefore, we need to probe further. A key question is: "Do you know this feeling from certain situations in your life?" If the answer is something like "Yes, I normally feel that way when I am sitting outside in the garden and relaxing," then one would not be concerned. If, on the other hand, the client reports to this question "Yes, I know this from when I am very exhausted after sleeping only 2–3 hours for several days or nights," then the clinician can be sure that the response frequency was too high. In this case, if the clinician misinterprets the sleepiness as the frequency being too low and raises the response frequency, the client might indeed feel more awake during the session but might have more trouble falling asleep that night. In some cases, one can only be sure about the interpretation of sleepiness in consideration of the effect after the session. If the client feels sleepy during the session, refreshed after the session, and sleeps well at night, this is a confirming sign. If instead the client feels sedated, heavy, and groggy after the session, and sometimes even the next day, that is a definite sign of having trained too low. So, one should not rush to judgment prior to having all the information.

Normally we stay with the starting site for a few sessions because we want to be sure of the optimal response frequency and the specific effect of the training site. It becomes the base from which we move in the ongoing training process. Sometimes there might be a need to change starting position in or after the first session. Indications to change the starting site and rethink the original hypothesis might be:

- It is not possible to find a comfortable response frequency at the first site. For example, if even the lowest response frequency is too agitating at T3-T4, electrodes need to be changed to T4-P4 for a more calming effect. Even at the lowest frequency, T3-T4 can be too activating for some people.
- If instabilities are triggered by training T4-P4, then T3-T4 needs to be added or T4-P4 replaced entirely for a more stabilizing effect.
- If there are indications for T4-P4 and headaches are not impacted with the training, this might be an indication for T3-T4.
- In some cases, T4-Fp2 needs to be added for more emotional self-control. T4-P4 is a very calming training but might lead to right/left or back/front imbalance for some people. If there is loss of emotional control due to T4-P4 training, this is an indication for adding T4-Fp2, while keeping T4-P4 in the mix. If there is more ADHD-like immaturity and impulsivity, one needs to move to T3-T4 as a first step on the way to T3-Fp1.

One big advantage of modern ILF Neurofeedback is that clients feel state shifts and changing of symptoms very quickly, often after only a few minutes of training. That makes the process of optimizing response frequency easy. Still, there are some clients who do not feel any difference during the session. That is not a reason to panic or shift response frequency up and down in the search for something better. Even if people do not feel anything during the session, they might have strong and specific effects after the session. If the clinician's hypothesis about the starting position is verified by the client's response to the training, it sometimes still takes a few sessions to optimize the response frequency. So, if lowering the response frequencies yielded a positive result, even lower frequencies should be evaluated. If the response frequency has been optimized at the starting electrode site, but after a few sessions has not impacted all the symptoms, then the next electrode position can be added according to the pattern of dysregulation indicated. In that case several frequency rules have to be considered.

5.1.3.1 Frequency Rules

- Response frequencies for basic sites: All right-side sites train with the same response frequency and the same frequency as T3-T4. The left side, in most cases, needs to be trained higher, normally 2 times as high as the right side and T3-T4.

  Example: If the response frequency is optimized on T4-P4 at 0.4 mHz, then T4-Fp2 and T3-T4 should also be trained at 0.4 mHz. Whereas training on the left side, like T3-Fp1 or T3-P3, should be at 0.8 mHz. *Exception*: If T3-T4 or T4-P4 is already being trained at the lowest frequency (0.0001 mHz), it might be that left-side sites are also trained best at frequencies less than the expected 0.0002 mHz.

- Response frequencies for inter-hemispheric sites: The response frequency for inter-hemispheric training at Fp1-Fp2 needs to be divided by 2 from the response frequency at T3-T4. The response frequency for inter-hemispheric training at P3-P4 needs to be divided by 4 from the response frequency at T3-T4. *Example*: If the response frequency for T3-T4 is optimized at 0.8 mHz, the training frequency for Fp1-Fp2 would be 0.4 mHz and 0.2 mHz for P3-P4. *Exception*: If T3-T4 is already trained at the lowest frequency (0.0001 mHz) the other inter-hemispheric sites might also be trained best with 0.0001 mHz.

Besides these rules, response frequency is always an issue in subsequent training. For some people, the optimal response frequencies can be kept constant during the whole training process; for others they need to be adjusted repeatedly. If response frequency needs to be adjusted at one site, then all other sites likely have to be adjusted accordingly.

In building up the training process step by step, the clinician must be very clear about the rationale for changing training parameters and what effects are expected due to the change. Of course, the expected effects then need to be verified during the training session and, even more importantly, with the results between sessions. For the interpretation of training effects, it is absolutely essential that only one parameter be changed at a time, either frequency or electrode position. Too many steps in frequency within a session can make for difficulties in interpretation of what effects can be attributed to a particular cause. The training parameters and changes need to be documented accurately in order to keep the training process comprehensible. This can't be emphasized sufficiently. The training process needs to be as disciplined as is possible within a clinical setting. At each step we have to document what was changed and why. Did the change of training parameters result in the expected training effects? If yes it could be continued, if not the hypothesis of the clinician needs to be rethought. But of course, the clients do not react like machines. Sometimes this is obvious after one session and sometimes it needs a few sessions to become apparent.

As the training process continues, we have to determine which training sites are useful and which can be dropped. Useful sites are kept in the mix, and sites that bring negative effects or no effects should be skipped. Normally the training will end up with 2–4 useful sites and training time should be divided equally among all sites. The addition of Alpha-Theta training is described in Section 5.2.

End of training:

The training progress should be assessed regularly with adequate tools like the Symptom Tracking system, CPT test, or whatever is appropriate in each case. In most of the cases, successful completion of the training can be achieved in 20, 30, or 40 sessions. If the training goals are reached, or sometimes even exceeded early, the training should not be ended too abruptly. Instead, it is suggested that training sessions be spaced further apart to verify that the effects are long-lasting. There is no risk of training too much; on the contrary there is always room for improvement of function and quality of life.

5.2 Combining the ILF Approach with Proven Older Neurofeedback Methods

5.2.1 Reasons for Doing

If we talk about the ILF approach as formalized in the Othmer Method, the awake state training over all the years has been usefully complemented with Alpha-Theta training. Alpha-Theta training is one of the most impressive training methods from the early days of Neurofeedback. One important principle of the ILF training concerning electrode position is to keep useful sites and skip training sites that are not useful. The same principle holds true more generally for the different Neurofeedback approaches. Alpha-Theta training is one Neurofeedback method that has always been useful and obvious in its effect. It is not alone in that regard. There is ongoing investigation on how other methods that train for enhanced synchrony of the resting rhythm EEG frequencies can support the ILF training effectively as well.

5.2.2 Combining with Alpha-Theta

The Alpha-Theta training addresses the resolution of learned fears and adverse patterns of habitual responding. This training is folded in after physiological stabilization is achieved with the awake state training in the ILF range. Alpha-Theta training has a long history. As early as 1966, Joe Kamiya[5] successfully reinforced the alpha rhythm in the EEG of his subjects by ringing a soft bell every time he observed alpha spindles in the EEG. As a result, the trainees learned to produce more alpha activity. Elmer and Alyce Green from the Menninger Clinic in Topeka also worked with Alpha training, and at their hands this evolved into what we now know as Alpha-Theta training. They saw the alpha component as the stepping stone to the theta experience, which in turn was seen as the entry portal to personal transformation. For more than 20 years they travelled all over the world teaching biofeedback and self-regulation techniques and investigating brainwaves and other bio signals from meditators, shamans, and healers. Some of their experiences from their fascinating journey were published in the book *Beyond Biofeedback* in 1977.[6] Another pioneer in this field is Les Fehmi, who in the late 1960s started with Alpha Synchrony training. Later he combined the EEG training with other techniques, like mindfulness training, for mental and physical health. His more than 30 years of research and professional experience are summarized in his very absorbing book, *The Open Focus Brain* published in 2007,[7] in a perfect combination of theoretical background, practical exercises, and first-hand experiences. As already described in Chapter 2 of this book, several studies where Alpha-Theta training was successfully used in the treatment of addiction and PTSD followed.[8, 9]

5.2.3 How Is Alpha-Theta Training Performed?

Alpha-Theta can be trained with one or more EEG channels. In single-channel mode training a unipolar montage is used. One active electrode is positioned on Pz and the reference behind one ear (mastoid). The ground can go anywhere on the head, but normally the other mastoid is used for the ground. Alpha as well as theta frequencies are rewarded, to allow the client to shift to a relaxed alpha state and, from there, to a hypnagogic state, alternating between alpha and theta dominance. Delta is inhibited to prevent a shift into sleep states.

Beta and high beta are inhibited to allow the brain to calm down. Traditionally, the training is done under eyes-closed conditions. That is because the unloading of the visual system increases the incidence of alpha spindles in the EEG. Modern Neurofeedback systems allow the client to choose from a variety of calming, peaceful scenes like forest, beach, fireplace, etc. For some people a pre-recorded guided imagery routine can be used to help shift attention away from the outside to the inner realm. Of course, clinicians can also use their own personalized imagery scripts that are adapted to the client's needs.

Sensory deprivation can be used to facilitate entry into deep states. The client should sit or lie comfortably and with closed eyes (perhaps aided with eye shades), with auditory feedback delivered via headphones, and cocooned in pillows and a blanket. Training time is normally 20–30 minutes. There is no special introduction to the client, except something like "allow yourself to relax without falling asleep." There is no need for the client to try to influence the different noises and tones from the feedback. Instead, the client should simply accept whatever happens and yield to the sounds. Some clients are already acquainted with special relaxation or meditation techniques, but these should not be used during the Alpha-Theta training. Instead, the brain should be allowed to interact with the feedback signal by itself, without guidance or direction. Normally, if people close their eyes and fall in a light trance the alpha amplitude in the posterior region rises almost immediately. After a while, for most people the alpha drops down within a few minutes, sometimes below the theta amplitudes, and theta might even rise a little bit, indicating a deeper state. Still, the client's experience can never be judged by the trend lines, and if the client had wonderful experiences during the session and positive effects after the session, there is no need to be concerned about producing higher alpha or theta amplitudes! These are mere indices of residence of particular states, and that is what matters rather than the particulars of the waveform.

In Alpha-Theta states cortical control is loosened and dream-like pictures might emerge. It is a state somewhere at the edge of sleep, which is a state of high suggestibility that is optimal for the self-regulation of psychological processes in a manner that is once again totally self-directed. Actually, this is a very natural state but, unfortunately, not very supported in our culture. We all go through these states on our way to sleep or back again to wakefulness. In Western cultures these states are too brief for many people to really enjoy or benefit from. Many clients report feeling that their brain only knows two states: Busy awake state and sleep. Many are not even aware of the variety of states in-between.

The Alpha-Theta training is very helpful in facilitating residence in this undefended state that allows the resolution of traumatic experiences, the finding of solutions to personal crises, and the working out of relationship issues from a position of feeling safe and intact. This is the venue in which the core self finds expression through imagery and visual narrative. The experience can be profoundly healing to the traumatized self in a way that is difficult for the person himself to verbalize.

An Alpha-Theta training session should not be stopped abruptly. Instead, it should be brought to closure gently by fading out the feedback and giving the client sufficient time to come back and reorient. Some clients like to talk about their experience at that time, so there should be enough time for that. Others may need a few minutes of awake state training to restore full alertness promptly.

For most people Alpha-Theta is a very comfortable and useful training, not only for psychological issues but also in terms of peak performance and visualization of goals and the ideal self, or to deepen mindfulness training. Nevertheless, if Alpha-Theta training is used too early in the training process, there might be some uncomfortable reactions. Therefore, it needs to be handled with care and should only be used after enough awake state training has been done. There are a few indications that show the clinician that the client is **not ready** for Alpha-Theta training that we have to keep in mind:

● Persons still anxious, hyper-vigilant, and unable to relax will <u>not</u> benefit from Alpha-Theta training. They will likely report not enjoying the session and might actually feel more anxious. These clients normally need more sessions of awake state calming or stabilization training before they can benefit from Alpha-Theta training later on in the process.
● Some ADD clients and people who are very exhausted fall asleep immediately when they relax. They also need more awake state training until they are able to relax without falling asleep.
● Alpha-Theta training might trigger instabilities in unstable brains because Alpha- Theta enhances synchronous EEG activity. If this happens within the Alpha-Theta session, this can usually be corrected immediately with a few minutes of stabilizing training on T3-T4, if this was tolerated before, or else with their primary awake-state training protocol. Alpha-Theta training should only be tried again later on in the training process, after more awake state training focused on stabilization. For some clients, Alpha-Theta training can be done only if it is balanced with a few minutes of stabilizing ILF training after the Alpha-Theta session. For others with instabilities, it is enough if they alternate Alpha-Theta and awake state sessions.
● In clients with a trauma history, Alpha-Theta training is an important part of the recovery process, but it could lead to abreactions if it is used too early in the training. Although abreaction might be a useful part in several kinds of psychotherapy, it is not an intentional part of the Alpha-Theta training. If it happens during the Alpha-Theta training, there is no need to panic. The clinician should keep calm, stop the feedback and let the client report what is happening. The next steps depend on the clinical background of the clinician. If the clinician is trained in working with abreactions he might want to seize the opportunity. With respect to Neurofeedback, the client should be stabilized with awake state training.

The above listing makes it very clear that the clinician should always know the "parachute" for each client before training Alpha-Theta. What does that mean? The clinician should always know for each client which ILF training position and frequency leads to which effect. If a new training site, or a new kind of training (like the Alpha-Theta training) is added to the treatment plan, the basic stabilizing positions and the optimal reward frequency needs to be known to have the possibility for correction if changing of the training parameters leads to negative effects. Without knowing this parachute it is not advisable to experiment with new training parameters. Neurofeedback effects are strong and specific and need to be handled with care and responsibility. There is no one-size fits all protocol in the ILF training approach, and even Alpha-Theta training might not be suitable for everyone – but it is always worth a try.

5.2.4 Combination with 2 Channel Sum Training

In 2 Channel Sum training, two EEG channels, each with a unipolar electrode montage, are summed to yield the feedback signal. This type of training, which has been done up to now only within the conventional EEG spectrum, promotes common-phase or synchronous activity in the reinforced frequency band. Historically, it has typically been used with the primary cortical resting frequency, the famous alpha band. The most commonly used 2 Channel Sum training is probably 2 Channel Alpha-Theta training, which can therefore be considered paradigmatic for 2 Channel Sum training in general.

The EEG for the 1 Channel Alpha-Theta training, which was discussed above, is normally recorded at Pz, and excursions in alpha and theta amplitudes are rewarded. Increases of amplitudes in the reward bands correlate with locally synchronous activity in the reward band underneath the active electrode. In 2 Channel Alpha-Theta, normally one channel picks up the EEG at P3 and the other channel at the homotopic site P4 on the other hemisphere. This means that the training promotes synchrony in the reward frequency band simultaneously at two distal sites (P3 + P4). This results in an even greater degree of synchrony of neuronal network activity between the two hemispheres. In the work with clients it is advisable to start with 2 Channel midline (Fz + Pz) Alpha-Theta training to be sure that Synchrony training is tolerated by the client, especially in clients with instabilities. Then 2 Channel Sum training on the two hemispheres can be implemented as an alternative at (P3 + P4).

5.2.5 Synchrony Training in Classical Frequency Bands

There are special 2 Channel Neurofeedback applications available that not only reward the sum of signals in the reward band, but also explicitly reward synchrony, or phase correspondence, in the reward band at the two training sites. Compared to the traditional two-channel amplitude reward mode, people trained in this way sometimes report that they reach completely new and comfortable resting states faster and deeper than before.

Synchrony training can be seen as a further Neurofeedback training option. Whereas ILF awake state training promotes physiological self-regulation and Alpha-Theta training allows access to the resolution of unresolved trauma, Synchrony training is a training of calm mental states that has similar beneficial effects as mindfulness training.

In the past, the best experiences with Synchrony training were obtained with 10 Hz (Alpha) and 40 Hz (Gamma) training. The feedback options like fractals or natural environments support calm and peaceful states. In contrast to Alpha-Theta training, people are usually seated upright in Synchrony training and can also train with eyes open. The best starting positions are midline (Fz + Pz). Other useful sites are (P3 + P4) for Alpha (10 Hz) training and (Fp1 + Fp2) for Gamma (40 Hz) training. Alpha Synchrony training is often experienced as calming, especially for people with anxiety, tics, or agitation. Gamma Synchrony training can sometimes be too activating for those clients. For others, Gamma Synchrony often promotes an alert focused state, which is also true for anyone for whom Alpha is too sedating or dysregulating.

5.2.6 Synchrony Training in the ILF Range

Finding new Neurofeedback training modalities is always related to the questions where and how to train. The "where" relates to the electrode sites and the "how" to the training frequency, as well as to the training mode in signal processing. Therefore, the clinician needs at least basic knowledge in signal processing in order to use the right Neurofeedback software modules and electrode hook-up. In general, we train in differential mode in ILF HD awake state training for refined physiological regulation, including specific differentiated function, and we train in sum mode to promote synchrony of resting state rhythms. In the evolution of the ILF differential training over the years the midline electrode positions were skipped, because the training effects were not as impactful as the other intra- and inter-hemispheric basic sites on the multi modal association areas. As already described in Chapters 2 and 3, it is reasonable to assume that the ILF training targets the regulation of the Default Mode Network. The empirically derived electrode placements match up with the key nodes of the Default Mode Network. Nevertheless, there are still some important nodes of the Default Mode Network that are critically involved in self-reflection[10] and social cognition[11] that could not be addressed effectively with the ILF training so far, the so-called midline structures. The cortical midline structures seem to be the neurological basis of self-related processing.[12] The conventional Synchrony training showed beneficial effects for many people in terms of calming down the nervous system with 10 Hz and promoting alert focus with 40 Hz. Still, there was always the challenge to find the right frequency (10 Hz or 40 Hz) and the right training position ((Fz + Pz) or (P3 + P4) for Alpha or (Fp1 + Fp2) for Gamma). With all kinds of Synchrony training there is some risk of triggering instabilities. However, as midline (Fz + Pz) Synchrony training promotes synchrony between front and back, rather than across the two hemispheres, it minimizes the risk of triggering instabilities.

Clinical experience with the 10 Hz and 40 Hz midline Synchrony training did not lead to the expected changes that might be attributed to the above-described functions of the cortical midline structures. The state shifts achieved with 10 Hz and 40 Hz seem to be more related to a general resting state frequency than to the specific cortical midline structure. Taking into account that the Default Mode Network in general is oscillating at frequencies lower than 0.1 Hz, this might not be surprising. So, the question is how to address these important cortical midline structures if they do not react to the ILF HD differential training, nor to conventional Synchrony training at the classical frequency bands. Given the naturally low frequency oscillation of the Default Mode Network, the higher ILF range seems to be a good candidate for Synchrony training.

The Synchrony training modality at 0.05 Hz has been available since March 2018. Since then the clinical experiences with ILF Synchrony have been very promising. Clients get less bored or sleepy than with Synchrony training at the classical frequency bands. The effects of the training, of course, do depend on the initial clinical presentation but they have proven to be remarkably strong and distinct. The experiences are described as deep stillness and strong feelings of being in the body, feeling safe and settled, light and happy. Pain clients experience pain reduction in both body pain as well as headaches. Revisiting of core attachments is often described. Clients described themselves as more outgoing and friendlier, more at peace with themselves, with their emotions, and with others. So, one might conclude that the effects obtained from ILF Synchrony training seem to be more closely related to the above-described processing of self-relation and relation to others of the cortical midline structures of the Default Mode Network. The ILF Synchrony training is still a relatively new training option which needs further exploration. Already being used by some practitioners is the so-called "couple's Synchrony training," where two brains are hooked up with one system (active electrodes on Pz, linked reference at each person's ear lobe and shared ground). The expected result is the growth of harmony in the relations of the trained persons. Les Fehmi and Susan Shor Fehmi have, for years, conducted couples' workshops in Alpha Synchrony Training and have also published on their work.[13] While ILF-Synchrony for couples appears promising, it is considered to still be in an experimental stage.

For the combination of all these different and useful neurofeedback applications it is crucial to stick to a logical, sequential structure in the overall treatment plan. The foundation – and therefore always the beginning – is the ILF awake state training for physiological self-regulation of arousal, excitability, and autonomic balance as described above in Section 5.1. After achieving a certain level of physiological self-regulation, 0.05 Hz (ILF), Synchrony training (see Section 5.2.6) can be introduced for deeper calming, a stronger sense of self, and preparation for Alpha-Theta. For some clients Alpha Synchrony can be added for calming and Gamma for alert focus (Section 5.2.5), if needed and tolerated. Alpha-Theta training can be added for resolution of trauma (see Sections 5.2.1 to 5.2.4). For ILF Synchrony training with couples it is essential that both have an established ILF HD protocol and have tolerated ILF Synchrony training individually. For further training, the ILF and Sum training could be used, alternating from session to session or both done in one session, depending on available training time and the number of different electrode sites in the ILF protocol. The fact that EEG training is being done fruitfully with such a variety of immediate objectives, some of them even mutually inconsistent, compellingly demonstrates that the objective is not the attainment of specific states but rather the enhancement of the control of state. Alpha-Theta and Synchrony training complements this kind of training by using these same capabilities for experiential purposes that are clinically relevant and promote the fuller human experience.

5.3 Closing Remarks for Neurofeedback Clinicians

Clinicians should work respectfully with the client's brain and only use Neurofeedback methods in which they have been sufficiently trained! This chapter can only give a short overview to get an impression of the ILF Neurofeedback approach and how it can be combined effectively with older approaches to get the most beneficial effects for the clients. What is treated cursorily here cannot replace a training course with its practicum exercises, self-training experience with Neurofeedback under competent supervision, and live discussion of training results among the attendees.

Neurofeedback is a rapidly developing field due to more and more technically advanced and user-friendly, medically approved products. Neurofeedback is not a mechanical instrument that displaces traditional therapeutic work. It is a very effective tool that supports the therapeutic mission. To use this tool in the most beneficial way with clients, it needs to be emphasized that the paradigm of the symptom-guided ILF approach demands a high level of therapeutic skills, as well sensitive clinical decision making, and astute interpretation of training results in order to use this capability in the most beneficial way. Because of the complexity of this work, and because this method is still in its early stages of maturation, Neurofeedback practitioners using this method should be in contact with colleagues and mentors to refine their work, and always work respectfully within the scope of their professional expertise and support networks. In Neurofeedback we interact with a complex, self-organized system that is daunting in its complexity. We are still far from understanding it completely but at least we have learned to understand the reactions to the applied Neurofeedback training sufficiently in order to adapt the training accordingly.

Notes

1 Othmer S, Othmer SF, Kaiser DA, Putman J (2013) Endogenous neuromodulation at infra low frequency. *Semin Pediatr Neurol.* 20(4):246–257.
2 Othmer S (2019) *Protocol Guide for Neurofeedback Clinicians* 7th Edition. EEGInfoWoodland Hills, CA.
3 Broyd SJ, Demanuele C, Debener S, Helps SK, James CJ, Sonuga-Barke EJ (2009) Default-mode brain dysfunction in mental disorders: a systematic review. *Neurosci Biobehav Rev.* 33:279–296.
4 Menon V (2010) Large-scale brain network and psychopathology: a unifying triple network model. *Trend Cogn Sci.* 10:483–506.
5 Kamiya J (1968) Conscious control of brainwaves. *Psychology Today.* 1:56–60.
6 Green E, Green A (1977) *Beyond Biofeedback.* Published by arrangement with Dell Publlishing Co, Inc Seymon Lawrence Books/Delacorte Press, New York.
7 Fehmi L, Robbins J (2007) *The Open-Focus Brain.* Trumpeter, Boston and London.
8 Peniston E, Kulkosky P (1990) Alcoholic personality and alpha-theta brainwave training. *Medical Psychotherapy.* 3:37–55.
9 Scott WC, Kaiser DA, Othmer S, Sideroff SI (2005) Effects of an EEG biofeedback protocol on a mixed substance abusing population. *Am. J. Drug Alcohol Abuse.* 31:455–469.
10 Northoff G, Heinzel A, de Greck M, Bermpohl F, Dobrowolny H, Panksepp J (2006) Self-referential processing in our brain – a meta-analysis of imaging studies on the self. *Neuroimage.* 31(1):440–457.
11 Uddin LQ, Iacoboni M, Lange C, Keenan JP (2007) The self and social cognition: the role of cortical midline structures and mirror neurons. *Trends in Cognitive Sciences.* 11(4):153–157.
12 Qin P, Duncan N, Northoff G (2013) Why and how is the self-related to the brain midline regions? *Front. Hum. Neurosci.* 7:909
13 Fehmi LG (2007) Multichannel EEG phase synchrony training and verbally guided attention training for disorders of attention. In: *Handbook of Neurofeedback,* Evans JR editor, The Harworth Medical Press, New York: 301–320.

Chapter 6

Neurofeedback in an Integrative Medical Practice

Doreen McMahon

6.1 Introduction

Neurofeedback has been successfully applied to patients with a variety of mental health issues by professionals in the psychology and social work communities. However, neurofeedback is recognized by few practitioners in the allopathic (mainstream) medical community, even though it received the highest level of efficacy rating for the treatment of Attention Deficit Disorder by PracticeWise, a research service acting on behalf of the American Academy of Pediatrics (AAP).[1] This may be due to a paucity of published studies of neurofeedback in major medical journals and because neurofeedback is associated with treatment of non-medical issues.

However, numerous studies have been published that show the efficacy of neurofeedback in the treatment of sleep issues,[2] migraine headaches,[3, 4, 5] seizure disorders,[6,7,8,9,10] fibromyalgia,[11] chronic fatigue syndrome,[12] autistic spectrum disorder,[13] and traumatic brain injury.[14] Despite this evidence, many in the scientific community have difficulty accepting the efficacy of a treatment modality that does not lend itself to the supposed gold standard of a double-blind study. An experiment has not yet been designed in which it is not readily apparent to experimental subjects, as well as the personnel administering neurofeedback, when a sham neurofeedback treatment is being given.

Neurofeedback can be viewed as carefully applied brain fitness by exploiting latent brain plasticity.[15] Just as body fitness is desirable in maintaining good health and helping to overcome the symptoms of many health and mental health conditions, neurofeedback can similarly improve the functionality, both physical and psychologically, for "medical" issues.[16]

I was introduced to neurofeedback when I was exploring alternative techniques to help my then 10-year-old son with autistic spectrum disorder. Medications, behavioral therapy, speech therapy, occupational therapy, and social skills training provided little or only temporary relief from his symptoms. Electroencephalographic (EEG) neurofeedback slowly, but surely, enabled him to benefit from his therapies and be weaned from medications. He is now at college studying to become a psychologist.[17]

In this chapter, I am presenting recent case studies from my practice as a solo physician in a "neurointegrative" practice. In all cases, EEG neurofeedback, using the equipment and training protocols[18] of the EEG Institute of Woodland Hills, California, is the primary therapeutic modality, even as other treatments were integrated into patient care.

6.2 Assessment and Screening

The initial visit for a neurofeedback patient begins with a thorough history and physical examination. At a minimum, this should include a detailed description and history of the presenting issues, past medical and mental health histories, medications, non-prescription medications and dietary supplements, allergies and intolerances towards medications and foods, family health and mental health history, health habits (smoking, drinking, recreational drug use, caffeine use, exercise, and diet), and a review of major body systems. A physical exam should be performed with especial emphasis on areas of complaint, the nervous system, and brain function. Review of previous laboratory work and studies can be very helpful. The clinician should analyze these results and form a treatment plan.

As in regular medical practice, many patients presenting for neurofeedback have need for instruction and on-going coaching in basic health maintenance. Areas that frequently require attention include diet and nutrition, physical activity, sleep, and development of healthy brain behaviors.

6.2.1 Diet and Nutrition

A lack of basic vitamins, minerals, and other essential nutrients can adversely affect the function of many body systems, including the brain.[19] Therefore, patients' dietary practices are important in ensuring the effectiveness of neurofeedback. Underlying medical conditions that can cause nutritional deficiencies should be identified and adequately treated. Many patients have diets that are restricted in basic nutrients due to food flavors and/or textures, poor nutritional knowledge, unhealthy ingrained habits of eating, and neurological or gastrointestinal difficulties. Consultation and treatment by a dietician, nutritionist, or speech therapist may be an essential part of treatment for complicated or difficult patients. Many patients, however, can be treated with reminders to follow healthy dietary guidelines[20] with increased use of whole foods and decreased consumption of prepared, fatty, and sugary foods.[21]

There may be indications for special diets based on dietary history, specialized testing, and observation. These may include: Feingold diet,[22] Elimination/reintroduction diet,[23] Gluten-free/Casein-free diet,[24] Specific Carbohydrate Diet,[25] and GAPS diet.[26] Since patients may already utilize specific diet plans, clinicians should familiarize themselves with the basic guidelines of these diets even if they are not comfortable prescribing and helping patients adopt them.

Supplementation of commonly deficient nutrients is frequently indicated in patients receiving neurofeedback. Caution must be taken to carefully evaluate each patient who is receiving supplements for contraindications or complications from dietary supplements. A multivitamin is recommended for those who are unable to get adequate nutrition via a healthy diet.[27] While supplementation must be carefully individualized, omega-3 fatty acids, vitamin D3, and magnesium are commonly used in my neurofeedback practice.

Neurofeedback induces changes in the architecture of both grey and white matter in the brain.[28, 29] Essential fatty acids, in particular omega-3 fatty acids, are generally agreed to be vital to brain health, since they must be present to form the myelin sheathes that make up about 60% of brain volume.[30, 31] Omega-3 fatty acids via dietary and supplemental sources can ensure adequate molecular build-ing blocks for the brain remodeling process[32] induced by neurofeedback training. Omega-3 fatty acids are generally quite safe but they should not be mistaken for fish liver oil, which contains vitamin A that can be toxic at large doses.[33]

Vitamin D deficiency is estimated to be around 70% in white and 95% in Afri-can-American populations in the US.[34] Manifestations of vitamin D deficiency can include chronic fatigue, fibromyalgia, weakness, and mood disorders;[35] symptoms that are seen in many patients who present for neurofeedback. Vitamin D3 levels can be measured with blood work. Healthy serum concentrations are in the range of 50–125 nmol/L for almost all people.[36] However, daily supplementation of vitamin D3 of 1000–2000 IU is felt to be safe in those without obvious risk factors for over-supplementation.

Magnesium is another vital nutrient to nervous system function that is often deficient due to depleted farming soils and removal from municipal water supplies. Adequate levels of magnesium have been shown to treat depression, anxiety, head-aches, seizures, psychosis, and irritability. Magnesium supplements can interact with a number of medications including digoxin, oral anticoagulants, and quinolone and tet-racycline antibiotics. Kidney function should be normal. Magnesium doses of 200–350 mg. daily are usually well tolerated. For those who experience loose stools or cannot take oral supplements, Epsom salt baths (1–2 cups of Epsom salts and half a cup of baking soda in at least 6 inches of water) are an excellent and calming alternative.[37]

6.2.2 Brain–Gut Connection

The interconnected nature of the brain and the digestive system has been studied for over a century. Recent advances in functional brain imaging techniques have allowed scientific inquiry in central nervous system interactions with the human gut to flourish and shown that their relationship is far more intimate than previously supposed.[38] For example, the limbic system of the brain, which plays a central role in emotional regulation, is the area most concerned with gut control. Some neuro-transmitters have been demonstrated to be more plentiful in the gut than anywhere else in the body, including the brain.[39] The integrated nature of the function of these systems has been exhaustively demonstrated and may explain the emotional influ-ence on the body's control of insulin and blood pressure regulation.[40] Thus, ensuring the optimal function of both should be prioritized in a neurofeedback practice.

Eliciting good patient history data that goes beyond the usual review of systems is imperative. Dietary history should include information about patient intake and reactions to potentially neuroactive substances, such as coffee, tea, sodas, spices, and other foods and food additives. Functional history of chewing, swallowing, satiety, gastro-esophageal reflux, belching, nausea, vomiting, abdominal cramping, flatulence, bowel movements, and pain patterns may help guide treatment modalities in addi-tion to neurofeedback.

Of particular interest to practitioners of neurofeedback are the influences of food allergies and intolerances on brain function. Sensitivity to the wheat protein, gluten, and the milk protein, casein, in the form of elevated antibody levels have been clearly linked to neurological dysfunctions of unknown cause.[41, 42] National Institute of Allergy and Infectious Diseases (NIAID) Food Allergy Guidelines can steer investigation of food allergies.[43, 44]

Dysbiosis – abnormal microbial flora – can also contribute to immunological and physiological disruption of digestive and neurological function.[45, 46] A cycle of inflammation and abnormal function of intestinal and blood-brain barriers is thought to allow incompletely digested neuroactive substances such as casomorphins (from milk) and gluteomorphins (from wheat) to cause neurological symptoms.[47, 48, 49] Implications for treatment include removing offending foods from the diet, improving digestion function via enzyme supplements, and correcting dysbiosis.[50, 51, 52, 53]

6.2.3 Environmental Exposures

Avoidance of exposure to environmental toxins from physical and chemical agents is essential to good brain health. These include pesticides, toxic metals, solvents, and toxic gases. Many toxins are ubiquitous in everyday life, like food additives, household cleaners, nail polish and remover, automobile exhaust, building materials, and home furnishings.[54] Many people have concerns about exposure to electromagnetic fields such as those generated by household devices. Research to prove the safety of common devices, like cellular phones, is ongoing.[55]

6.2.4 Physical Exercise and the Brain

Lack of adequate physical activity is a frequent finding in the patient population presenting for neurofeedback. Regular aerobic exercise has been proven to increase physical and mental health.[56] Exercise, along with prudent dietary habits, promotes the activity of the brain derived neurotrophic factor (BDNF) system, which plays a critical role in the interface between metabolism and cognition.[57] Exercise has been shown to increase the effects of the BDNF system in conjunction with omega-3 fatty acids.[58] Treatment of anxiety and depression with exercise and yoga has been shown to be as efficacious as cognitive behavior therapy and medication.[59] Experiments have demonstrated that 5 hours a week of exercise at 80% of estimated aerobic capacity shows significant protective effects to neurotoxins in monkeys.[60] Exercise guidelines for children, adolescents, adults, and older adults are available at www.health.gov/paguidelines/guidelines.[61]

6.2.5 Sleep Management

Chronic lack of adequate sleep has been linked to many health and mental health issues that include obesity, poor dietary choices, heart disease, hypertension, elevated cholesterol levels, diabetes, cancer, Alzheimer's, depression, increase in inflammation, deterioration of performance of daily activities, substance abuse, and shorter life span.[62] Sleep disorders are estimated to be as prominent as 50% in children in the US and are felt to contribute to daytime sleepiness, irritability, behavioral problems, learning difficulties, poor academic performance, and in teenagers, to motor vehicle accidents.[63] The average American adult gets less than the recommended 7–9 hours a night.[64]

A thorough sleep history includes sleep initiation, sleep duration, arousals during the sleep period, ability to awaken, daytime sleepiness, bruxism, movements during sleep, dreaming patterns, snoring, apneic breathing patterns, enuresis, sleeping positions, sleep environment, and sleep timing.[65] Overnight polysomnography (sleep study) can be used to help identify sleep problems that are not readily distinguished by history. Neurofeedback can help with the management of many sleep issues in conjunction with specific therapies[66, 67] and pristine sleep hygiene.[68]

Even with effective neurofeedback and strict adherence to good sleep hygiene, sleep normalization can take weeks or months. Practitioner coaching and focusing on maximizing daytime functioning can help patients maintain patience while striving for the goal of satisfactory sleep.

6.2.6 Behavior Management

A psychological and physical environment that supports positive changes in behavior is vital to the success of neurofeedback. Even as neurofeedback therapy changes arousal levels of the brain and strengthens cortical neural pathways, the behaviors that allow improved function need to be strengthened. Just as sending an addict from a recovery program back to their "using" environment seems to correlate with relapse, having a neurofeedback patient stay in a setting that helped promote or did not prevent their symptoms can slow or confound progress towards wellness. History-taking during initial and follow-up encounters should be used to form impressions about psychosocial conditions that could be modified to encourage healthy functioning.

Among the environmental issues that can complicate neurofeedback treatment are poor or disrupted personal relationships. Mental health professionals and community resources can be utilized to guide patients and their significant others to

Table 6.1 Sleep Hygiene Rules

Keep the same wake time **7 days a week.**

- The bed should be used for sleep **only** (no TV, no radio, no reading, etc.).
- Sleep nowhere other than in bed.
- Leave the bedroom if you awaken and cannot get back to sleep within 15 minutes.
- Return to bed only when you are sleepy. Leave again if you cannot get to sleep within 15 minutes. Repeat as necessary.
- Do not time watch. Clocks should not be visible from the bed.
- Keep the sleeping area quiet, dark, and cool. Use earplugs, eyeshades, and other aids as necessary to accomplish this.
- Activity levels for 30–60 minutes prior to bedtime should be very leisurely and unimportant (not TV, especially news programs).
- Maintain a regular bedtime.
- Cut down on or eliminate caffeine.
- Cut down on or eliminate tobacco products.
- No alcohol consumption within 4 hours of bedtime.
- Don't go to bed hungry. No snacks with sugar or refined carbohydrates near bedtime.
- Use exposure to bright sunlight or artificial sunlight early in the day to awaken and reset light-reactive hormone cycles.
- School-aged children need a minimum of 8 hours, preferably at least 9 hours, of sleep/night.
- Adults need a minimum of 7 hours, preferably 8 hours of sleep/night.[69]

more useful modes of conduct and better cognitive states. Parent–child interaction problems can be especially troublesome since parenting skills are usually acquired "on the job" and reflect the parents' upbringing rather than the specific needs of an individual child. Parent–child relationships can get stuck in maladaptive ruts of unrealistic expectations and negative emotions. Carefully delineated behavioral incentive systems can foster improved behaviors, codify accountability between adults and children, and enable positive cognition.[70] Practitioner support in development, adaptation, and implementation of a behavioral system is often vital in making it a successful intervention.

The overuse of electronic media, including television, computers, and video games, is another concern for the general population as well as in patients receiving neurofeedback. The American Academy of Pediatrics has determined that the average child spends 7 hours using entertainment media, and recommends that children under the age of 2 use no media, with older children and teens using only 1–2 hours a day.[71] Media exposure is linked to drug use, alcohol use, low academic achievement, earlier initiation of risky sexual behaviors,[72] eating disorders, obesity, sleep disorders, and attention issues.[73] Functional MRI has shown that playing violent video games is directly connected with lasting changes in the brain regions associated with cognitive function and emotional control.[74, 75] A small percentage of child and teen video game players show multiple signs of behavioral addiction, including academic problems, increased lying, and inability to cut back on gaming.[76]

Practitioners need to be aware that it can be difficult to cut the electronic umbilical cords, since media is used as a safe and affordable distraction, as well as parents' modeling of heavy media use, i.e. the incorporation of media – especially TV – in household routines and a need to fill leisure time. Frank and frequent discussions with health care providers on ways to limit electronic media use to recommended levels may help households implement rules on media consumption. These should include paying attention to the amount of entertainment media utilized, not placing a television in a bedroom, eliminating background television, limiting television viewing (especially on "school days"), identifying non-screen, in-home activities that are pleasurable, and disconnecting television use from eating.[77]

6.2.7 Medications and Neurofeedback

Medications must be closely monitored and adjusted in someone receiving neurofeedback. As the brain becomes better self-regulated, symptoms may arise that look like medication overdose. For instance, a patient on a seizure medication may have an increase in lethargy and fatigue. This effect is not limited to medications that are generally considered to be brain specific. For example, blood pressure medications might become overly effective. Careful vigilance throughout the course of therapy is important. For many patients, decreasing or eliminating medications is a desirable goal of neurofeedback.

6.2.8 Medical Genomics

As the field of genetics advances, patients are eager to learn how their medical care can be individualized using their own genetic information.[78] This field is evolving rapidly and can have implications in recommending tailored health habits, such as specific dietary recommendations and nutritional supplementation.[79] However, most genetic interpretations have implications for lifestyle management and future planning given current technology.[80]

6.3 Case Presentations

6.3.1 Patient 1

38-year-old man presented with functional difficulties and constant, chronic pain from multilevel spinal injuries. Failed therapies included surgeries, implanted neural stimulator, and epidural medication. Therapies with limited effectiveness were acupuncture, chiropractic manipulation, massage, physical therapy, cranio-sacral therapy, meditation, TENS, antidepressant medication, neuromodulator medications, anti-inflammatory medications, muscle relaxers, and narcotic medications. He took Ultram, Flexeril, Dilaudid, Tylenol, and Advil on an as needed basis, which was usually multiple doses a day. Pain caused problems with sleep initiation and maintenance. Physical and mental stresses led to pain crises approximately weekly that confined him to bed for 2–4 days at a time. He was anxious about being able to provide for his family and his mood was depressed. He has heartburn 80% of the time. His ability to function at work and be available to his family was severely limited.

Treatment: Neurofeedback was started based on Othmer protocols at T4-P4 for physical calming and sensory integration. Reward was optimized at 0.1 mHz before gradually adding FP2-T4, T3-T4, and Fp1-T3 sites over ten sessions. Medication use was altered so that the patient took his most effective medications on a regular basis, and he used a set protocol at the onset of more significant discomfort. Education in sleep hygiene was undertaken and reinforced at each visit. Physical activity types and levels were reviewed. Regular low stress, better-tolerated exercise was initiated.

After approximately 25 sessions of neurofeedback, pain levels were reduced to manageable levels most days. Patient was aware of discomfort but felt like he was able to push it to the back of his mind and control it. Ultram was used on a daily basis. Dilaudid and Flexeril were needed for moderate pain flares every 7–10 days. Heartburn was resolved. He rarely missed work due to back issues. Sleep was longer and restful even though compliance with sleep rules is loose. Energy levels were significantly increased and mood was vastly improved. Activity tolerance was up. The patient felt much more involved with family activities. He saw his chiropractor infrequently. Over 50 sessions of neurofeedback were completed and the patient comes back for a "recalibration" session every few months.

6.3.2 Patient 2

56-year-old woman who was recently retired on disability for fibromyalgia. Her physical activity was severely limited due to pain and stiffness every day. Pain and restless legs disrupted sleep initiation and maintenance. She never felt rested and had problems with focus and memory. She had been diagnosed with ADD in the past. Mood was depressed and she was anxious about dealing with and providing for her teenage son as a single mother. Her house and yard were "a mess" because she had neither the energy nor the strength to organize or clean. Past medical history was significant for psoriasis with arthritis and osteoporosis. Medications were numerous and included Concerta, Cymbalta, Lamotrigine, Voltaren, Etodolac, Seroquel, and medications specific for psoriasis. Dietary supplements included multivitamin, CoQ10, curcumin, S-adenosyl methionine (SAM-e), vitamin D3, zinc, and krill oil. Family history revealed attention disorders and alcoholism. The patient was a non-smoker and non-drinker who avoided caffeine because it made her "jittery." She saw a mental health counselor on a twice a week basis. Physical exam was significant for sad affect with occasional crying. Patient moved slowly and with obvious discomfort. TOVA (Test of Variables of Attention) showed a significantly dysfunctional score of −7.43.

Treatment: The patient was started on a course of neurofeedback per Othmer protocols at T4-P4 for the calming of physical sensations and anxiety. Reward frequency was optimized to 0.1 mHz before gradually adding Fp2-T4, T3-T4, and Fp1-T3 sites over 12 sessions. Discussions about establishing daily routines and good sleep hygiene were initiated at each therapy session. By her tenth session she was experiencing better moods and increased energy to the point that she started swimming laps at the local pool 3–4 days/week. She was starting to tackle household chores for an hour or two a day. Episodes of depression, low energy, and physical discomfort still occurred every few days. By session 40, TOVA had normalized to +0.57. Weaning patient from Concerta, Cymbalta, Lamotrigine, and Seroquel was initiated. By session 50 she was no longer taking any of these medications. As long as she was following good sleep hygiene and swimming 4–5 days a week, energy levels and moods were good, even though her teenage son was having behavioral issues and she was caring for her terminally ill mother. A behavioral incentive program was set up for son. Counseling about realistic expectations for dealing with the dying process of her mother was included in each session, and the patient coped well when her mother died.

Patient found that she rarely experienced any inappropriate physical discomfort or mood problems as long as she had a neurofeedback session every 1–2 months. As long as she practiced good sleep hygiene, her energy levels were appropriate. She had a reasonably organized household including a normal relationship with her teenage son. She volunteered several days a week at an animal shelter where she tolerated mild to moderate physical effort. Friends and family told her that she was a "new person."

In her most recent "tune-up" sessions, the patient has re-optimized to 0.009 mHz. She is also using the Synchrony program at 0.05 mHz. She feels like the results are even stronger.

6.3.3 Patient 3

9-year-old girl had a history of traumatic head injury in the left fronto-temporal head areas resulting in seizure disorder. Multiple left-sided seizure foci were observed with EEG studies. Three different types of seizures have been diagnosed including absence seizures, myoclonic seizures, and rare generalized tonic-clonic seizures. Mother noted multiple daily episodes of unresponsiveness followed by decreased alertness, focus problems, and an inability to learn academic material. During the night, the child had 1–3 episodes of limb and body jerking associated with enuresis. She complained of almost constant feelings of "electricity" in her legs and sometimes in her arms. Her personality had gone from outgoing to intro- verted and fearful. She was unable to attend school because of seizures. She was home-schooled but was behind grade level due to inability to retain knowledge. Social interactions were fairly normal within her family but severely compromised by her social isolation and her worries of having seizures in front of peers. She had been minimally responsive to multiple trials of anti-epileptics including Lamictal, Topiramate, and Vimpat. Current medications were Lamictal, Topiramate, Pulmicort inhaler, Albuterol inhaler, Singular, and vitamin B12 injections.

Medical history was significant for recurrent ear and sinus infections until ton- sillectomy and adenoidectomy at age 3, pernicious anemia due to intrinsic factor antibodies, and celiac disease. Asthma was poorly controlled with frequent daily use of rescue inhalers. Known allergies were to penicillin, pollen, animal dander, and dust mites. Bowel function tended toward constipation with some complaints of bloating. Her diet was gluten- and sugar-free with an emphasis on vegetable and fruit consumption with healthy fats and complex carbohydrates. She participated in a number of physical activities including Tae Kwan Do and supervised swimming. Sleep routines were well enforced for a total of 11–12 hours of sleep/day. However, bedtime was compromised by patient anxiety, and sleep maintenance was always interrupted by seizures and bedwetting. She slept with her mother for comfort and supervision of seizures. Mother had a history of thyroiditis and environmental aller- gies. The patient saw a counselor, a speech therapist, and an occupational therapist.

Physical exam showed swollen, pale nasal turbinates with copious clear nasal discharge. Lungs were clear. Abdomen showed increased tympani to percussion with minimal generalized tenderness. Mild weakness was noted in muscles of right arm and leg. Patient walked with a mild limp. She could not cooperate to test deep tendon reflexes. Several episodes of staring, mouth movements with speech-like sounds, and random, small movements of arms and legs, lasting 10–20 seconds, were observed. Patient appeared unfocused, fidgeted, and had little spontaneous speech.

Treatment: Neurofeedback using Othmer protocols was started at T3-T4 to sta- bilize the seizures. Reward was optimized to 0.1 mHz. After eight sessions, additional sites were added after tolerance for each new site was established over three to four sessions: T4-P4 for control of physical sensations, Fp2-T4 for emotional trauma, and Fp1-T3 for attention issues. By session 30, patient was having fewer obvious daytime seizures. Nocturnal seizure activity decreased to none at all or once nightly, except for an increase that obviously correlated with the patient visiting a relative who exercised no dietary restrictions. Because of patient's strong history of atopy, food allergy testing was undertaken and multiple strong positive reactions were noted. Testing for casein sensitivity showed significant levels of casomorphins. Nutri- tionist consultation was obtained to design and institute a diet that accommodated the patient's medical conditions and sensitivities. Sleep hygiene and daily routines were modified as patient's functionality improved. Melatonin seemed to help patient fall asleep. Counselor and speech therapist emphasized social skill training.

When lower training frequencies became available, the patient re-optimized to 0.001 mHz, and Synchrony at 0.05 mHz was added. She has completed over 150 sessions of neurofeedback. She has had no generalized tonic-clinic seizures and absence seizures are rare. Nocturnal myoclonic seizures occurred only when there was dietary non-compliance or other major stressors such as getting off routines. She was on a single anti-convulsant. Her asthma was under excellent control with no need for any medication other than her prophylactic ones. Her anxiety decreased to appropriate levels, and the patient was thriving in school with an IEP geared to specific residual learning disabilities from her head trauma. She has many friends and participates fully, enjoying many social activities with groups of peers.

6.3.4 Patient 4

6-year-old girl with high functioning autistic spectrum disorder was having violent meltdowns with such frequency that her specialty school for children with developmental disorders wanted to expel her. She had already been asked to leave two previous preschools. There were problems getting her to focus unless she was interested in something, and then it was difficult to get her to break away. She was described as "wiggly" and impulsive. Extreme anxiety was causing issues with getting her to bed at night. Her pediatrician put her on omega-3 fatty acids and Metadate. Her anxiety and expressions of frustration seemed to increase, so she was switched to Vyvanse with no obvious changes in behavior.

Patient was born at 36 weeks' gestation and had been diagnosed with cholestasis. However, early milestones were generally within the normal range. She disliked loud sounds and noisy crowds. Daily bowel movements were described as hard and chunky. She had an unusually high pain tolerance with little or no crying after injuries, yet would not wear shoes until her socks were arranged to her satisfaction. She was a good consumer of a nutritious diet and exercised for hours a day in her school program that emphasized physical activity. She used media entertainment for 3 hours a day watching PBS children's shows and playing "Cool Math" and "Fun Brain" video games. Patient saw a child counselor weekly and seemed to have a good rapport with her. Physical exam was significant for child's unwillingness to speak in front of the examiner.

Treatment: Parents were willing to institute good sleep hygiene measures with emphasis on a quiet, calm bedtime routine that included Epsom salt baths. There was little interest in laboratory testing, resuming omega-3 fatty acids, or cutting down on media exposure. Neurofeedback treatment per Othmer protocols was initiated at T4-P4 for calming of anxiety and sensory integration issues. T4-T6 for social integration and Fp2-T4 for emotional regulation were added after several sessions. By session 12, the patient was consistently getting to bed with minimal drama and sleeping well through the night. She was able to show acceptable behaviors at school for at least 3–4 hours. The patient was consistently comfortable and talkative with the clinician. Pediatrician stopped Vyvanse and started Intuniv. Within 1 week, patient experienced volatile emotions, fatigue, and decreased appetite. Pediatrician added Prozac with possible decrease in behavioral issues. Parents insisted on continuing medications but agreed to get organic acid testing as well as an assessment of casein and gluten sensitivity.

Laboratory tests showed sensitivity to both casein and gluten. She also had elevated markers for gut dysbiosis of both yeast and bacteria. After a 10-day course of antifungal medication (Nystatin) she was started on a casein-free, gluten-free, anti-yeast diet with daily probiotics. The patient had a dramatic reduction in her symptoms over the next month. She was now considered to be the best-behaved and most promising student in her school and plans were underway to transfer her to a school with normal curriculum. Parents continued to insist that she take psychiatric medications. Follow up 5 months after finishing neurofeedback showed persistent positive behaviors and development.

6.3.5 Patient 5

18-year-old woman with Type 1 diabetes and hypertrophic cardiomyopathy suffered a cardiac arrest at age 16 in front of her father and a nurse. Resuscitation efforts were begun immediately. Subsequent events are uncertain due to misunderstandings between health care providers and the patient's family, who originate from a foreign culture and were legally excluded from her care. However, she suffered an anoxic brain injury and was in a coma for several months. She was in hospital and residential rehabilitation for over a year, but had stopped making any progress for over 6 months. She was discharged from further formal health care to her family. Speech was unintelligible except to some family members. She could not chew food. She was wheelchair bound because of spastic arms, legs, and body. Balance was poor and her mood was anxious and depressed. She felt trapped in an uncooperative body and upset that she was totally dependent on her family for everything, including activities of daily living. Feelings of social isolation were prominent. Her premorbid condition was that of a high achieving, well focused, musical, and social high-school student.

Type 1 diabetes mellitus was diagnosed at age 3 and was reasonably well controlled on insulin injections until her cardiac arrest. An automatic implantable cardioverter defibrillator had been surgically placed after her cardiac arrest. Medications included insulin, birth control pills for menstrual management, and clonazepam as needed for anxiety. She was sensitive to sodium benzoate, soy, and food dyes. She slept well for 8–9 hours/night. She rarely consumed caffeine. Bowel function tended towards constipation. Her diet was a high fiber, diabetic diet. Mouth articulation problems made eating difficult and patient was underweight.

Physical exam was commensurate with described handicaps. Neurological exam showed slow, unintelligible speech, spasticity in both legs and right arm, profound weakness in left arm, and a lack of intentional movement. She could balance for a couple of seconds on her feet when pulled up to a standing position but could not move her legs or feet in any meaningful way.

Treatment: A course of neurofeedback per Othmer protocols was initiated at T3-T4 and optimized to a reward of 0.1 mHz. The patient and her family were unwilling to see speech, occupational, or physical therapists because of previous adverse encounters during residential rehabilitation. However, the family was willing to implement any measures thought necessary at home. Detailed instruction for home therapy was given at each neurofeedback session. Bowel care measures were implemented.

Improvements in patient's function were rapid and dramatic over three to four sessions at T3-T4. Neurofeedback sites were added at T4-P4 for body awareness, Fp2-T4 for emotional stability, and Fp1-T3 for focus. Within 3 months, patient's speech was intelligible, eating was easier, and body weight had risen to more appropriate levels. Diabetes control was more consistent. Bowel function normalized. She was able to use a computer keyboard and write slowly. She could get to sitting and standing positions with minimal help. She could ambulate with a walker. Frustrations with physical limitations contributed to ongoing feelings of depression and anxiety, however, the patient successfully applied, was admitted, and went to a pre-medical university program where she received straight As.

6.3.6 Patient 6

20-year-old woman presented with 5-month history of nausea and vomiting spells that occurred at least daily. Associated symptoms included chronic fatigue, palpitations, flushing, diaphoresis, urgent need to defecate, syncope or near-syncope, anorexia, and 20 lb. weight loss. Medical work up included normal pelvic ultrasound, normal head and abdominal CT scans, normal colonoscopy, and unremarkable stool analysis. Upper endoscopy showed "reactive gastropathy." Gastric emptying test was significant for markedly prolonged gastric emptying time and established a diagnosis of gastroparesis. Dynamic defecography demonstrated pelvic floor laxity with cystocele and rectocele. Blood work confirmed mild malnutrition with low albumin and vitamin D levels but had no signs of inflammation, hormonal dysfunction, or liver problems.

Past medical history was significant for chronic yeast infections, eczema, and food intolerances controlled with avoidance of milk products, wheat, and sugar. A history of abdominal bloating, constipation, and encopresis dated to toddlerhood. Medications included Prozac, Xanax, Promethazine, and Zofran. She considered Xanax to be most effective for treating her symptoms. Dietary supplements consisted of vitamin D and probiotics. She was a non-smoker who avoided caffeine and recreational drugs. She drank occasionally to "numb" her stomach but would later get nauseated. She described herself as needing at least 10 hours of sleep to feel rested and felt dependent on Xanax to initiate sleep. History of hypersensitivity to sounds, touch, smell, and taste was elicited. Anxiety and depressed moods were prominent. She was unable to exercise or go to school. Family history was significant for anxiety, depression, and syncope due to "hypotension."

The physical exam was significant for increased heart rate of 93, with an otherwise normal cardiac examination. Her abdomen demonstrated generalized tenderness with no other findings. Skin showed livedo reticularis.

Treatment: A course of neurofeedback per Othmer protocols was initiated at T4-P4 for physiological and psychological calming. Reward was optimized to 0.1 mHz. Several additional sites were added one at a time over the next several sessions: Fp2-T4 for anxiety control, T3-T4 for physiological stabilization, and Fp1-T3 for depressed mood. The patient was overwhelmed with medical recommendations and wanted to avoid any further consultations, testing, or therapies. By her fifth session of neurofeedback she was having some symptom-free days, and was starting to increase the quality and quantity of her food. A schedule to taper bedtime Xanax was established, with melatonin to be used instead. Patient was willing to use stool softeners for constipation. Energy levels were increasing. By session

15, patient was contemplating re-enrolling in college. Reviewing the practical and cognitive issues with symptom management at school was incorporated into each session. Her moods improved and anxiety decreased as she met with success in her classes. A Prozac taper was initiated and well tolerated. By session 30, further increases in food amounts and diversity, including eating in restaurants, was noted. Omega-3 fatty acid and vitamin D supplements were added. By session 40, she was feeling well enough that she was testing her tolerances for food types and quantities. She was also breaking sleep routines and mild recurrences of symptoms were associated with these. Neurotherapy sessions were gradually tapered. At last check-up she was able to eat a carefully selected diet and regained all the weight she had lost. She was able to eliminate all medicines and was at college fulltime, exercising regularly, socializing, and thriving.

6.3.7 Patient 7

16-year-old boy with Tourette's Syndrome, ADD, and social anxiety presented with constant, debilitating nausea and exacerbation of his tics that began 5 months prior during a stressful time at school. He had a multi-year history of anxiety about going to school that would crescendo at the end of a weekend and thus had a record of poor school attendance. On one Sunday evening he had an episode of extreme agitation and violence in which he physically tore apart portions of the house. He was hospitalized and medicated with Haldol for a "psychotic" episode. He had not attended school since that time. He spent all his time either in bed or in front of electronic media. He rarely left the house unless physically forced. Nausea is moderate and vaguely located in the abdomen. He vomited twice since symptoms began. Appetite was rarely compromised, and patient had gained about 40 lbs. Bowel movements were formed and occurred daily to every other day. Anti-nausea medications had been ineffective, including Zofran. At presentation his only medicine was Prilosec (40 mg. daily). Tourette's syndrome had been diagnosed at 4 years of age. The patient expressed much embarrassment and distress about his tic disorder: "on a scale of 1 to 10, it is a 13."

Patient had undergone exhaustive medical workup. Upper endoscopy showed only minimal esophagitis and negative testing for *Helicobacter pylori*. Food allergy testing revealed multiple mild reactions to foods that patient was unwilling to forego. Blood analyses showed borderline low vitamin D, high triglycerides, low high density lipoprotein (HDL) cholesterol, normal metabolic profile, normal blood counts, normal thyroid functions, normal adrenal function, normal androgens, normal inflammatory parameters, negative Epstein-Barr virus profile, negative Lyme disease profile, and negative *Babesia microti* and *Ehrlichia chaffeensis* testing. Brain magnetic resonance imaging (MRI), electrocardiogram (EKG), sleep-deprived EEG, and overnight polysomnogram were normal. Two neuropsychological workups had been performed. One concluded that the patient had encephalopathy, tic disorder, learning disabilities, sleep disorder, and mood disturbance; the other found autistic spectrum disorder, high-functioning cognitive disorder, learning disorders, mood disorder, bipolar type, and Tourette's syndrome. The patient was tried on multiple treatments, including Vyvanse, Strattera, clonidine, Topamax, Risperdal, Seroquel,

Haldol, Xanax, Ativan, Zoloft, Effexor, chlorpromazine, omeprazole, omega-3 fatty acids, vitamin D, and probiotics. For a couple of months prior to consultation for neurofeedback, he refused to take any further medications.

The past medical history was significant for neuropsychological issues going back to 4 years of age. A recurring theme involved altercations with his father who had bipolar disorder with a predominantly hypomanic affect, and disengagement of his ADD-diagnosed mother. Patient reported nearly daily headaches consisting of intense pressure in random locations around his head that would last up to a day. However, he "ignored most pain." His sleep schedule was chaotic, with the patient sleeping any time of the day or night. His diet included few vegetables and fruits. He did not exercise. Family history was significant for father with bipolar disorder, mother with ADD and obsessive-compulsive disorder (OCD), and paternal relatives with bipolar disorder and addiction problems.

The physical exam showed a shoddily dressed, overweight, poorly groomed, slouching teenage boy with moderate acne and acne scars on his face. Tics were observed in the face, especially the forehead, with variable occurrence from constant to up to 10 minutes tic free. He argued repeatedly with his father who was emotionally volatile and provocative.

Treatment: A course of Othmer protocol neurofeedback was started at T4-P4 electrode placement that was optimized to a reward of 0.1 mHz to initiate physical calming. Every couple of sessions, additional sites were added: Fp2-T4, T3-T4, and Fp1-T3. Much of each session was spent establishing a rapport with the therapist as a reliable adult who would advocate for his best interests. He also started sessions with a psychiatrist who specialized in adolescents with somatic disorders. Parenting skills training was undertaken with inconsistent effect. Further medical consultations were discouraged to break the constant distraction of multiple appointments, the psychological trauma of looking for something "wrong" with the patient, and the physical disruption of testing and invasive treatment. As patient calmed, sleep hygiene was introduced with melatonin use to help regulate sleep onset. A personal trainer came to the home every morning to help the patient get out of bed at a regular time and then do aerobic and strengthening exercise. Patient started and did well with a remote curriculum from his high school. Patient was successfully weaned from excessive entertainment media. By session 20, nausea-free periods lasted for a day or two at a time. Patient was able to consume a healthier diet. By session 30, sleep routines were well established and fatigue abated. Tics and nausea were well controlled, except for confrontations with parents and the prospect of returning to school classrooms. By session 40, the patient had lost 40 lbs. and completely altered his physical appearance with improved posture, good personal hygiene, and appropriate clothing.

After consultation with his psychiatrist, it was felt that the patient would be able to move on in his personal growth in a setting that emphasized stability and routine with consistent positive behavioral reinforcement. Parents were unable to provide this in their home, even with extensive family therapy, so the patient was enrolled in and attended a boarding school with a reputation for providing a constructive environment for special needs students. He was a top student at this school, and he coped well with visits and vacations with his family. Parents were more relaxed and positive with their interactions with him. Tics were rare events and somatic symptoms were resolved. He was off all medicines.

After graduating from high school the patient moved back into the family home before continuing his education at a local university. His parents insisted that he enroll in engineering courses that he did not care for. He stopped going to classes and so failed most of them. He returned for neurofeedback. He re-optimized to a training frequency of 0.005 mHz at T4-P4, Fp2-T4, T3-T4, and Fp1-T3. He enjoyed working at a part time job until returning to school to successfully take courses in fields that he enjoyed.

6.3.8 Patient 8

9-year-old boy presented with a 2-year history of generalized tonic-clonic seizures and nocturnal Rolandic seizures that occur at least weekly while on medications. EEG showed multifocal sharp-wave discharges in multiple brain areas, including mid-central, mid-parietal, right temporal, and left parietal regions. MRI showed right hippocampal sclerosis. For religious reasons, the patient's family wanted to have him off medications, but they agreed to start medicine after an episode of status epilepticus that resulted in hospitalization about 6 months prior to presentation for neurofeedback treatment. Mother observed that medications (Trileptal and Lamictal) have caused side effects of slurred speech, tremors, poor motor coordination, decreased processing speed, and fatigue.

Past medical history was significant for prolonged labor and fetal distress during the birth process. As a baby, he was diagnosed with reflux. As he matured, he continued to have daily upper abdominal discomfort with belching and regurgitation. As a toddler he met most developmental milestones except for issues of low neurological tone, causing some delay in gross motor skills. Iron supplements were prescribed for mild anemia. Mother noted ongoing issues with anxiety and obsessive thoughts about bad things happening to him or his family. He was worried about various body sensations representing significant disease. He was prone to getting generalized tightness around his head for an hour or so after using electronic media. He was under the care of a naturopath and receiving a large number of supplements, including Vitamin B complex, magnesium, zinc, vitamin A, vitamin C, vitamin D, taurine, probiotics, and digestive enzymes.

The patient was on a diet that was based on the GAPS plan. He consumed no caffeine and took part in daily exercise routines that included running, cycling, and bouncing on a trampoline. He was home-schooled because of seizures and fatigue. He was at grade level even though he worked very slowly and had trouble with focus. Screen time was strictly limited to academic purposes. Days were very scheduled with predictable routines, including sleep. Bedtime was 8 PM, but patient was often awake for hours with physical restlessness and obsessive thoughts. He usually slept through his nocturnal seizures and was sluggish and slow to arise around 7 AM. A year-old overnight sleep study showed mild apnea and restless sleep.

The physical exam was significant for a pale and very slender boy with speech that was so slurred that it was often unintelligible. Muscular tone and strength were generally decreased. A mild tremor of the hands was observed. He was unable to balance on one foot. The patient brought up his anxieties about his physical well-being frequently and at length.

Treatment: A course of neurofeedback using Othmer protocols was undertaken, beginning at T3-T4 for seizure stabilization. Reward was optimized to 0.1 mHz. T4-P4 for calming of somatization, Fp2-T4 for anxiety, and Fp1T3 for OCD and focus were gradually added over ten sessions. The patient was slowly weaned off medications over 11 months and 50 neurofeedback sessions. His seizures decreased in frequency to one every 1–2 months. All seizures were about 30 seconds or less and occurred around waking time. Seizures did not interfere with getting up promptly, being alert, and having a productive day. Speech intelligibility issues cleared up completely. Some mild tiredness during the daytime persisted but tremors and balance issues resolved. Melatonin and Epsom salt baths were used successfully to decrease sleep onset time. School achievement rose to above grade level, except for math and physical sciences which remained at grade level. Cognitive counseling techniques were used at each session to allow correct interpretation of body sensations. Expressions of anxiety and obsessive worries normalized. Headaches and gastric reflux symptoms were rare.

6.3.9 Patient 9

63-year-old woman with lifelong history of headaches presented with crescendo, complex migraines. She was hospitalized twice in 2 months to rule out cerebrovascular accident (CVA) when she presented with left facial droop, confusion, and left arm weakness and paresthesias, in addition to left-sided throbbing headache. Headaches were preceded with auras of huge blue and yellow splatters in all visual fields for about 20 minutes. MRI showed supratentorial bright spots that were thought to be commensurate with history of migraines. Other testing was negative for CVA. She also had a history of chronic daily headaches that involve discomfort in the left side of her head and heaviness in her left eye that prevented her from opening it fully. Her headaches caused difficulties with memory, reasoning, and organization. She typically tried treating her migraines with caffeine as a first step. If caffeine did not help, she took Tylenol #3, which did not help with the recent, more severe headaches. Amitriptyline prophylaxis had been unsuccessful.

The past medical history was significant for decreased renal function secondary to childhood streptococcal infection, generalized osteoarthritis, hiatal hernia with Nissen repair, environmental allergies, and lifelong chronic depression and anxiety. In the past, the patient tried a number of antidepressant and anxiolytic medicines and had side effects including decreased alertness, palpitations, tremors, and flushing. Taking Adderall on an as needed basis was considered effective and reasonably comfortable. Feeling of sadness increased in the fall and winter, but improved in the spring when she could resume gardening. Medications include Tylenol #3, Excedrin, Adderall, and nasal corticosteroids. Glucosamine was the sole dietary supplement. Family history was significant for a "seven generation" history of migraines. She was a non-smoker who had about one alcoholic drink a week and up to a liter of Diet Coke daily. Sleep time was scheduled for 6 hours per night. Patient fell asleep quickly because of exhaustion, but then awoke every couple of hours. She felt minimally refreshed in the morning and experienced chronic fatigue. Her diet was nutritious with an emphasis on green vegetables, but she had recent carbohydrate cravings that she indulged. She worked long hours as a nurse treating brittle diabetic patients. Her husband was retired and had recently been diagnosed with a blood dyscrasia. He and a mildly disabled adult son living at home were completely dependent on her for all household chores. The house was disorganized and filled with clutter. She repeatedly expressed anxiety, anger, and frustration about her work and family situations.

The physical exam was significant for left eyelid drooping. She cried easily and had problems with word retrieval when she was emotional.

Treatment: A course of neurofeedback was started per Othmer protocols with an initial site of T3-T4 for headache stabilization at an optimal reward of 0.1 mHz. Good sleep hygiene was reviewed and begun. Omega-3 fatty acids and vitamin D3 2000 International Units (IU) per day were started. 5-hydroxytryptophan (5-HTP) supplements, full spectrum lights in the morning, and the need for ongoing mental health counseling were discussed, but patient did not "get around" to trying them. A household chore chart was concocted for patient's husband and son. Severe headaches abated within 10 sessions of neurofeedback. Facial droop cleared except for times of extreme stress. Additional neurofeedback sites included T4-P4 for physical and emotional calming, Fp2-T4 for anxiety, and Fp1-T3 for focus issues. By 30 sessions, chronic daily headaches were resolved and the patient had only mild headaches every week or two. Fatigue was still an issue at the end of a long working day, but the patient rarely used Adderall to get through the day. The patient continued to be unhappy about aspects of her home and work life but felt like things were considerably less stressful.

6.3.10 Patient 10

18-month-old boy presented with developmental delay, lack of speech, poor balance and coordination (including inability to walk), seizures once or twice a week for 4 months, difficulties with sleep onset and maintenance, and hyperactivity. He had been recently diagnosed with Angelman's Syndrome, a defect in the UBE3A gene which regulates protein synthesis and degradation in the brain. His seizures were relatively well controlled on levetiracetam (Keppra) and clonazepam, but parents were concerned that he was over-sedated. It was difficult to get the child to sleep. He often awoke in the middle of the night and made enough commotion to arouse the rest of his family.

The past medical history was significant for a normal pregnancy and delivery. He was hospitalized for respiratory syncytial virus (RSV) at age 7 months and work up of seizures at 15 and 16 months. His diet consisted of little processed food with lots of vegetables and fruit. Sugar intake was strictly limited. Dietary supplements included multivitamins, vitamins C and D, and probiotics. He was an active crawler and enjoyed physical activity with his older siblings. Family history was significant for a brother with a congenital heart defect that was corrected with surgery.

Physical exam showed a smiling, very fair haired and skinned child. He drooled almost constantly as he sucked on chew toys. Muscle tone was decreased. Movements were ataxic (poorly coordinated), including poor neck control. He could sit and stand with support and could throw a toy. He was able to make eye contact for a short while but gaze and attention was fleeting. He did not vocalize.

Treatment: A course of Othmer protocol neurofeedback with sessions twice a week was initiated at T3-T4 for stabilization of seizures. The training frequency was rapidly titrated to 0.01 mHz (the lowest frequency available at that time). Mother was supported in changing the child's diet to a modified ketogenic diet to decrease excitability of seizure foci. The child was seizure-free until he contracted an upper respiratory infection 3 weeks later. Mother felt that he recovered much more quickly than usual from several minor seizures while he was ill. At session 8, he began to walk independently. At session 13, a software update allowed further titration of the training frequency to 0.005 mHz. Patient remained seizure-free until he grabbed and ate several cookies when he was temporarily unsupervised by an adult. He had a couple of small seizures a few hours later.

The child's family was so pleased with his progress in gross motor skills that they inquired about trying to stimulate verbalizations. F7-F8 was added to his treatment at session 24. A week later he began to vocalize spontaneously. By session 35, child began to have crying spells when he was placed in his crib to go to bed. T4-P4 was added to help with sleep induction and physical calming and coordination. Bedtimes normalized within a few days. Parents inquired about stimulating more verbal behaviors because his progress in speech therapy had stalled. So F7-F8 was eliminated and F7-T3 was initiated. Within a week, his speech therapist felt that he had progressed enough that he was started on an assisted language device.

At session 42, increased Cygnet software capability allowed for lower training frequencies. Child's training frequency was re-optimized to 0.001 mHz at all sites. EEG neurofeedback sessions were tapered to weekly. By session 46, child, now 27 months old, was reliably toilet trained during the day. He began special education preschool.

Patient had been seizure-free for months, so his neurologist approved tapering of medications. The child was weaned off all medications. Since then, he has had only mild seizures when he has had a fever from which he recovers very quickly. When he was just 3 years old, he attended a conference for families with children who have Angelman's Syndrome. His parents felt that he was clearly one of the most capable children there with skills exceeding those of much older children, including teenagers. He continues to receive neurofeedback every week or so.

6.4 Conclusion

Neurofeedback is a vital tool in an integrative medical practice that emphasizes good brain regulation and fitness as the basis for improved function in patients with a wide variety of presenting complaints and symptoms. Even medical conditions, like asthma, diabetes, and gastrointestinal problems, which are not normally considered to be brain based, can be better controlled. Potentially harmful or poorly effective treatments can be scaled back or eliminated. Twice-weekly neurofeedback sessions give the practitioner a platform to communicate frequently with patients. This enables rapport that can be used to educate patients and help them implement better lifestyle habits and management of health conditions.

Notes

1 PracticeWise. 2010. Evidence based child and adolescent psychosocial intervention. http://pediatrics.aappublicationslorg/content/125/Supplement_3/S128.full.pdf+html.

2 Hauri PJ, Percy L, Hellekson C, Hartmann E, Russ D. 1982. The treatment of psychophysiologic insomnia with biofeedback: a replication study. *Biofeedback Self Regul* 7(2): 223–235.

3 Stokes DA, Lappin MS. 2010. Neurofeedback and biofeedback with 37 migraineurs: a clinical outcome study. *Behav Brain Funct* 6: 9.

4 Walker J. 2011. QEEG-guided neurofeedback for recurrent migraine headaches. *Clin EEG and Neurosci* 42(1): 59–61.

5 Siniatchkin M, Hierundar A, Kropp P, Kuhnert R, Gerber WD, Stephani U. 2000. Self-regulation of slow cortical potentials in children with migraine: an exploratory study. *Appl Psychophysiol Biofeedback* 25(1): 13–32.

6 Sterman MB, Macdonald LR. 1978. Effects of central cortical EEG feedback training on incidence of poorly controlled seizures. *Epilepsia Jun* 19(3): 207–222.

7 Kuhlman W. N. 1978. EEG feedback training of epileptic patients: clinical and electroencephalographic analysis. *Electroencephalogr Clin Neurophysiol* 45(6): 699–710.

8 Tozzo CA, Elfner LF, May JG Jr. 1988. EEG biofeedback and relaxation training in the control of epileptic seizures. *Int J Psychophysiol* 6(3): 185–194.

9 Walker JE, Kozlowski GP. 2005. Neurofeedback treatment of epilepsy. *Child Adolesc Psychiatr Clin N Am* 14(1): 163–176.

10 Legarda SB, McMahon D, Othmer S, Othmer S. 2011. Clinical neurofeedback: case studies, proposed mechanism, and implications for pediatric neurology practice. *J Child Neurol* 26(8): 1045–1051.

11 Kayiran S, Dursun E, Dursun N, Ermutlu N, Karamursel S. 2010. Neurofeedback intervention in fibromyalgia syndrome; a randomized, controlled, rater blind clinical trial. *Appl Psychophysiol Biofeedback* 35: 293–302.

12 James LC, Folen R. A. 1996. EEG biofeedback as a treatment for chronic fatigue syndrome: a controlled case report. *Behav Med* 22(2): 77–81.

13 Coben R, Padolsky I. 2007. Assessment-guided neurofeedback for autistic spectrum disorder. *J Neurotherapy* 11(1): 5–23.

14 Nelson DV, Esty ML. 2012. Neurotherapy of traumatic brain injury/posttraumatic stress symptoms in OEF/OIF veterans. *J Neuropsychiatry Clin Neurosci* 24(2): 237–240.

15 Othmer S, Othmer S, Kaiser DA, Putman J. 2013. Endogenous neuromodulation at infralow frequencies. *Semin Pediatr Neurol* 20(4): 246–257.

16 McMahon D. 2013. Notes from clinical practice: an MD's perspective on 9 years of neurofeedback practice. *Semin Pediatr Neurol* 20(4): 258–260.

17 McMahon D. 2013. My road to neurofeedback and integrative medicine. *Novaneurotherapy.com Blog*.

18 Othmer S. 2017. Optimizing assessment and training with infra-low frequency HD and alpha-theta neurofeedback. *The Neurofeedback Clinicians' Protocol Guide: Optimizing assessment and training with Infra-low frequency HD, Alpha-Theta and Synchrony neurofeedback* (6th edition). Woodland Hills, CA: EEG Institute.

19 Gomez-Pinilla F. 2008. Brain foods: the effects of nutrients on brain function. *Nat Rev Neurosci* 9(7): 568–578.
20 Office of Disease prevention and Health Promotion. 2015. Dietary guidelines for Americans. www.health.gov/dietaryguidelines/2015.
21 Gomez-Pinilla F. 2008. Brain foods: the effects of nutrients on brain function. *Nat Rev Neurosci* 9(7): 568–578.
22 Feingold Association of the United States. What is the Feingold Diet Program? www.feingold.org.
23 Matthews J. 2008. Nourishing hope for autism. 193.
24 The GFCF Diet Support Group. The GFCF Diet Intervention Autism Diet. www.gfcfdiet.com.
25 Gottschall E. Breaking the vicious cycle. www.breakingtheviciouscycle.info.
26 Campbell-McBride N. The GAPS diet. www.gapsdiet.com.
27 Office of Dietary Supplements, National Institutes of Health, US Department of Health & Human Services. 2015. https://ods.od.nih.gov/factsheets/MVMS-HealthProfessional/.
28 Lubar J. F. 1997. Neocortical dynamics: implications for understanding the role of neurofeedback and related techniques for the enhancement of attention. *Appl Psychophysiol and Biofeedback* 22(2): 111–126.
29 Chang CY, Ke DS, Chen J. Y. 2009. Essential fatty acids and human brain. *Acta Neurol Taiwan* 18(4): 231–241.
30 Robinson JG, Ijioma N, Harris W. 2010. Omega-3 fatty acids and cognitive function in women. *Womens Health* 6(1): 119–134.
31 Wu A, Ying Z, Gomez-Pinilla F. 2008. Decosahexaenoic acid dietary supplementation enhances the effects of exercise on synaptic plasticity and cognition. *Neuroscience* 155(3): 751–759.
32 National Center for Complementary and Integrative Health, National Institutes of Health, US Department of Health & Human Services. 2018. Omega-3 supplements: in depth. nccih.nih.gov/health/omeg3/introduction.htm.
33 Kennel KA, Drake MT, Hurley DL. 2010. Vitamin D deficiency in adults: when to test and how to treat. *Mayo Clin Proc* 85(8): 752–758.
34 Holick MF, Chen TC. 2008. Vitamin D deficiency: a worldwide problem with health consequences. *Am J Clin Nutr* 87(suppl 4): 1080S–1086S.
35 Deans E. 2011. Magnesium and the brain: the original chill pill. *Evol Psychiatry* http://evolutionarypsychiatry@blogspot.com.
36 Deans E. 2011. Magnesium and the brain: the original chill pill. *Evol Psychiatry* http://evolutionarypsychiatry@blogspot.com.
37 Ibid.
38 Aziz Q, Thompson DG. 1998. Brain-gut axis in health and disease. *Gastroenterology* 114: 559–578.
39 Brown H. 2005. The other brain also deals with many woes. *The New York Times*, August 23.
40 Jones MP, Dilley JB, Drossman D, Crowell M. D. 2006. Brain-gut connections in functional GI disorders: anatomic and physiologic relationships.
41 Whitford T. 2000. The underlying mechanisms of brain allergies. *J Orthomolecular Med* 15(1): 5–14.

42 Hadjivassiliou M, Gibson A, Davies-Jones GAB, Lobo AJ, Stephenson TJ, Mitford-Ward A. 1996. Does cryptic gluten sensitivity play a part in neurological illness? *Lancet* 347(8998): 369–371.

43 Vojdani A, Kharrazian D, Mukherjee P. S. 2014. The prevalence of antibodies against wheat and milk proteins in blood donors and their contribution to neuroimmune reactivities. *Nutrients* 6(1): 15–36.

44 Yawn BP, Fenton MJ. 2012. Summary of the NIAID-sponsored food allergy guidelines. *Am Fam Physician* 86(1): 43–50.

45 National Institute of Allergy and Infectious Diseases, US National Institutes of Health. 2017. Guidelines for clinicians and patients for diagnosis and management of food allergy in the United States. www.niaid.nih.gov/diseases-conditions/guidelines-clinicians-and-patients-food-allergy.

46 Fedorak RN, Madsen KL. 2004. Probiotics and the management of inflammatory bowel disease. *Inflamm Bowel Dis* 10(3): 286–299.

47 Theoharides TC, Zhang B. 2011. Neuro-inflammation, blood-brain barrier, seizures and autism. *J Neuroinflammation* 8(168): 1–6.

48 Zioudrou C, Streaty RA, Klee W. A. 1979. Opioid peptides derived from food proteins. *J Biol Chem* 254(7): 2448–2449.

49 Reichelt KL, Knivsberg AM. 2003. Research: can the pathophysiology of autism be explained by the nature of the discovered urine peptides? *Nutr Neurosci* 6(1): 19–28.

50 Sienkiewicz-Szlapka E, Jarmolowska B, Krawczuk S, Kostyra E, Kostyra H, Bielikowicz K. 2009. Transport of bovine milk-derived opioid peptides across a caco-2 monolayer. *Internat Dairy J* 19(4): 252–257.

51 Rhee SH, Pothoulakis C, Mayer E. A. 2009. Principles and clinical implications of the brain-gut-enteric microbiota axis. *Nat Rev Gastroenterol Hepatol* 6: 306–314.

52 Pennesi CM, Klein LC. 2012. Effectiveness of the gluten-free, casein-free diet for children diagnosed with autism spectrum disorder: based on parental report. *Nutr Neurosci* 15(2): 85–91.

53 Champeau R. 2013. Changing gut bacteria through diet affects brain function, UCLA study shows. http://newsroom.ucla.edu/releases/changing-gut-bacteria-through–245617.

54 Collaborative on Health and the Environment. 2008. Mental health and environmental exposures. www.healthandenvironment.org/uploads-old/MentalHealthFactSheet.pdf.

55 National Institute of Environmental Health Sciences, National Institutes of Health. 2018. Electric and magnetic fields. www.niehs.nih.gov/health/topics/agents/emf/index.cfm.

56 Hillman CH, Erickson KI, Kramer AF. 2008. Be smart, exercise your heart: exercise effects on brain and cognition. *Nat Rev Neurosci* 9(1): 58–65.

57 Vaynman S, Gomez-Pinella F. 2006. Revenge of the "sit": how lifestyle impacts neuronal and cognitive health through molecular systems that interface energy metabolism with neuronal plasticity. *J Neurosci Res* 84(4): 699–715.

58 Wu A, Ying Z, Gomez-Pinilla F. 2008. Decosahexaenoic acid dietary supplementation enhances the effects of exercise on synaptic plasticity and cognition. *Neuroscience* 155(3): 751–759.

59 Safeed SA, Antonacci DJ, Bloch R. M. 2010. Exercise, yoga, and meditation for depressive and anxiety disorders. *Am Fam Physician* 81(8): 981–986.

60 Sanders L. 2009. Exercise helps brain rebound. *Science News* 176(11): 8.
61 Office of Disease Prevention and Health Promotion, US Department of Health and Human Services. 2008. *Physical activity guidelines for Americans*. https://health.gov/paguidelines/guidelines/.
62 Saey T. H. 2009. Dying to sleep. *Science News* 176(9): 28–32.
63 Carter KA, Hathaway NE, Lettieri C. F. 2014. Common sleep disorders in children. *Am Fam Physician* 89(5): 368–377.
64 Ramar K, Olson EJ. 2013. Management of common sleep disorders. *Am Fam Physician* 88(4): 231–238.
65 Carter KA, Hathaway NE, Lettieri C. F. 2014. Common sleep disorders in children. *Am Fam Physician* 89(5): 368–377.
66 Carter KA, Hathaway NE, Lettieri C. F. 2014. Common sleep disorders in children. *Am Fam Physician* 89(5): 368–377.
67 Ramar K, Olson EJ. 2013. Management of common sleep disorders. *Am Fam Physician* 88(4): 231–238.
68 Harsora P, Kessman J. 2009. Nonpharmacologic management of chronic insomnia. *Am Fam Physician* 79(2): 125–130.
69 Jordan AB, Hersey JC, McDivitt JA, Heitzler CD. 2006. Reducing children's television-viewing time: a qualitative study of parents and their children. *Pediatrics* 118(5): e1303–e1310.
70 Heininger JE, Weiss S. K. 2001. *From Chaos to Calm: Effective Parenting of Children with ADHD and Other Behavioral Problems*. New York: Perigee Books.
71 Council on Communications and Media, American Academy of Pediatrics. 2011. Policy statement: Media use by children younger than 2 years. *Pediatrics* 128: 1040–1045.
72 Ashby SL. 2006. Television viewing and risk of sexual initiation by young adolescents. *Arch Pediatr Adolesc Med* 160: 375–380.
73 Nunez-Smith M, Wolf E, Huang HM, et al. 2008. Media + Child and Adolescent Health. Common Sense Media (online service), http://ipsdweb.ipsd.org/uploads/IPPC/CSM%20Media%20Health%20Report.pdf.
74 Wang Y, Hummer T, Kronenberger W, Mosier K, Mathews V. P. 2011. Violent video games alter brain function in young men. *Science Daily* www.sciencedaily.com/releases/2011/11/111130095251.htm.
75 Mathews V, Wang Y, Kalnin A, Moster K, Dunn D, Kronenberger W. 2006. Short-term effects of violent video game playing: an fMRI study. Session: Neuroradiology/Head and Neck (Brain: Functional MR). RSNA 2006. rsna2006.rsna.org/rsna2006/V2006/conference/event_display.cfm?em_id=4433801.
76 Gentile D. 2009. Pathological video game use among youth 8 to 18: a national study. *Psychol Sci* 20(5): 594–602.
77 Jordan AB, Hersey JC, McDivitt JA, Heitzler C. D. 2006. Reducing children's television-viewing time: a qualitative study of parents and their children. *Pediatrics* 118(5): e1303–e1310.
78 National Human Genome Research Institute, US National Institutes of Health. 2018. What is Genomic Medicine? https://www.genome.gov/27552451/what-is-genomic-medicine//genomic-medicine/.
79 Lynch B. 2018. *Dirty Genes*. HarperOne.
80 David SP, Palaniappan L. 2018. Clinical and Personal Utility of Genetic Risk Testing. *Am Fam Physician* 97(9): 600–602.

Chapter 7

Neurofeedback in Combination with Psychotherapy

Keerthy Sunder

7.1 Overview

In psychiatry two conventional treatment modalities, pharmacotherapy and psychotherapy, have been consistently utilized in clinical settings. The clinical dichotomy that psychotherapy is reserved for "psychologically based disorders" and pharmacotherapy for "biologically based" disorders has fortunately been revisited with advances in brain-based understandings of mental processes.[1] Furthermore, during the time period of the Decade of the Brain the fields of neuroscience and neuroimaging made tremendous gains, which led to the rise of both scientific publications and public interest in the field of mental illness. (The Decade of the Brain was a designation given to the time period of 1990–1999 by U.S. president George H.W. Bush as part of a larger effort involving the Library of Congress and the National Institute of Mental Health of the National Institutes of Health "to enhance public awareness of the benefits to be derived from **brain** research.") Collectively, these developments helped to decrease the stigma surrounding mental illnesses and paved the way for empirically driven, brain-centered approaches to treatment interventions.[2]

Pharmacological treatment aims at reducing psychiatric symptoms using psychotropic medications. Pharmacotherapy has shown considerable benefits for the acute and chronic treatment of the major mood syndromes, namely major depressive disorder, dysthymic disorder, and bipolar disorder, as well as other psychiatric disorders. There is some evidence that medications can assist in normalizing decreased brain volumes in the brain regions of the amygdala, hippocampus, and subgenual prefrontal cortex, which are implicated in the impairment of emotional regulation in patients with bipolar disorder.[3, 4, 5]

However, even with treatment, the relapse rates in patients with bipolar disorder remain high. About 37% of patients relapse into mania or depression within one year and 60% relapse within two years.[6]

The longitudinal course of bipolar disorder is primarily depressive rather than manic, with fluctuating levels of severity. It does not necessarily respond to medications and therapy alone. Additionally, despite pharmacotherapy and psychotherapy interventions, residual depressive symptoms may persist in patients with bipolar disorder for about a third of their lives.[7]

Antidepressant medications, when used as a monotherapy in placebo-controlled registration trials, typically result in 30–35% remission rates.[8] Antidepressant medications work for many patients but some build tolerance, or intolerance, to medications. Other patients do not respond to medications, refuse to take them, or, in many parts of the world, do not have access to them or simply cannot afford them.

Moreover, pharmacological treatment methods lack specificity for target areas in the brain and can lead to unwanted side effects and/or unpleasant outcomes, such as dry mouth, headache, nausea, constipation, and sexual dysfunction, adversely affecting the patients' quality of life.[9]

A significant proportion of medication responders experience residual symptoms that predispose them to recurrence or relapse of their mood disorders. For all of these patients, and those who partially respond to medications, psychotherapy interventions offer a possibility for augmentation towards both symptom remission and relapse prevention.

Psychotherapy modalities include psychodynamic psychotherapy, cognitive behavioral therapy, dialectical behavior therapy, and interpersonal psychotherapy. According to Lynch et al., the effect of cognitive behavioral therapy was found to be similar to that of pharmacotherapy in depressive disorders.[10] Available literature informs us that combining psychotherapy with pharmacotherapy appears to be at least as effective as psychotherapy or pharmacotherapy alone for depressive disorders.[11]

Structured psychotherapy in the hands of a good clinician results in favorable changes in the brain, as demonstrated in neuroimaging studies. Functional MRI data confirms less limbic activity (decrease in emotionality) and increased dorsolateral frontal activity (increase in thoughtfulness) following the administration of cognitive behavioral therapy in depressed patients.[12]

It is clear that within the conventional modalities of treatment we are able to modulate the neurochemical and structural domains of the brain with varying degrees of success. However, incomplete remission of symptoms is common and seldom responds to increasing doses of psychotherapy or pharmacotherapy. In our clinical practice setting, I was continuously challenged with suboptimal responses to traditional interventions and recognized the need for augmentation therapies to improve response and promote remission for psychiatric disorders.

This challenge prompted us to examine therapies that addressed the neuroelectrical domain of brain functioning. Although overshadowed by the dominance of pharmacological treatment for the past 60 years, the neuroelectrical domain of treatment has had a long tradition going back to Electroconvulsive therapy (ECT). However, ECT was not only intrusive but largely restricted to institutional settings where it suffered from a lack of financial support for longitudinal systematic research.[13]

Neuromodulation with ECT and Transcranial Magnetic Stimulation (TMS) are both established brain stimulation therapies that target the neuroelectrical domain. However, they are both limited to a few indications and are not universally available for application. An additional sophisticated and well-studied method in the neuroelectrical domain, available to enhance treatment effectiveness and address the limitations of conventional methods, is neurofeedback.

Neurofeedback has successfully addressed this suboptimal clinical response gap by producing global brain effects and harnessing the interconnectivity between different functional networks.

Neurofeedback is an active training program in which the individual can restore the regulation of the brain network spontaneously.[14] Just as the ballerina benefits from practice in the mirror to correct imperfect movements, so does the brain from witnessing its own dysregulation via the captured EEG signals on a computer screen that functions like a mirror, enabling the brain to observe its own activity and self-regulate.

Since 1960, neurofeedback has been verified to be effective in epilepsy and applied to various fields. In psychiatry, neurofeedback has been used in the treatment of attention deficit hyperactivity disorder,[15] depressive disorders, anxiety disorders,[16] sleep disorders,[17, 18] substance abuse,[19] and the cognitive rehabilitation of patients with head trauma or cerebrovascular disorders.[20, 21] In addition, it has been used to improve performance (peak performance) in normal individuals.[22] The application of neurofeedback to most of these issues is covered in greater detail in other chapters.

The use of Infra-Low Frequency (ILF) Neurofeedback has helped our clinical practice in addressing mood, anxiety, and trauma-related dysregulation among refractory patients differentially responsive to pharmacotherapy or psychotherapy. Similarly, the subset of patients who experience mood oscillations due to neuroendocrine disruptions in pregnancy, postpartum, and lactational periods are excellent candidates for the calming effects that can be obtained with neurofeedback. With ILF Neurofeedback, we now have a powerful and sophisticated tool to augment our treatments along an additional domain, namely neuroelectrical, that has thus far been neglected. Neurofeedback helps the brain to observe itself in a clinical setting, if and when it is ready, and on its own terms, to promote self-regulation. Thus, we are able to seamlessly facilitate the introduction of medications and psychotherapy by breaking down defenses easily, without needing to work extensively with the inevitable psychological resistance among conventional treatment refractory patients. Our ability to modulate the signal-noise ratio so as to decrease the noise of unhelpful thoughts and feelings that impair functional progress has improved significantly with the introduction of ILF Neurofeedback. This, in turn, has facilitated successful resolution of symptoms in the treatment of refractory patients, without the need for escalating doses of psychotherapy or medications fraught with the risk of systemic adverse effects. Additionally, neurofeedback often allows for a decrease or discontinuance of medications in a subset of patients under careful supervision.

What follows is two recent case studies from our integrated psychiatry practice that illustrate augmentation strategies and the effects of neurofeedback on adult psychiatric patients in a naturalistic setting. In both cases, EEG ILF Neurofeedback, using the training protocols of the EEG Institute of Woodland Hills, California, was the primary neurofeedback therapeutic modality at our clinical practice.[23]

7.2 Case Study #1: Bipolar I Disorder, Postpartum Mixed Episode

Jane is a 35-year-old woman who had previously been diagnosed with bipolar I disorder as a teenager. She presented to us at six weeks postpartum following the birth of her first child with anxiety attacks, mood swings, feelings of guilt, and insomnia. A thorough medical history and physical examination, including baseline laboratory evaluation, were completed at her initial visit. The findings were unremarkable.

Jane reported a history of inpatient psychiatric hospitalization as a teenager following a severe manic episode. She was prescribed mood stabilizing medications that included Oxcarbazepine (Trileptal). Although the treatment had been successful, she described her experience on the ward during the mania as psychologically traumatic. She continued under the care of her psychiatrist without major symptom exacerbations, hospitalizations, or any changes in her medication regimen. Following her marriage in her twenties, Jane elected to defer pregnancy in favor of pursuing higher education and a full time job, whilst continuing on her medication. She worked in a health care setting providing supportive counseling, and found tremendous satisfaction in helping the lives of others improve over time. She worked full time and was able to carry a full caseload without any difficulties. Now in her thirties, feeling ready to begin a family, the couple elected to discontinue contraception and she conceived shortly after. After a risk–benefit decision analysis with her psychiatrist regarding continuing with medication versus no medication during pregnancy, she elected to discontinue her use of medication during her pregnancy. The course of her pregnancy was uneventful and she continued to work full time, with a plan to take time off after childbirth. Despite being advised about the risks of postpartum mania, depression, and psychosis in women with a history of bipolar disorder and the need for prophylactic medication, she decided not to re-commence her medication. Jane felt compelled to protect her baby from exposure to medications during breastfeeding. Unfortunately, the disruption in sleep–wake cycles, loss of role identity from being unable to work, and the role transition to motherhood were sufficient stressors to create instability in her brain. She developed a postpartum mixed manic and depressive episode at four weeks following delivery, that led to an involuntary psychiatric hospitalization to stabilize her symptoms. Following a week of rest and recuperation in the hospital, which included the initiation of medications such as Oxcarbazepine (Trileptal) and Quetiapine (Seroquel), she was discharged. It was at this point that Jane touched base with us, having heard about neurofeedback at a postpartum support meeting. She wanted to explore neurofeedback as a possible intervention for her symptoms, without the side effects she had been experiencing from her medications. She was distraught from her experience in the hospital and her brief separation from her baby. Additionally, she was distressed by her decision to stop breastfeeding due to the need to reinstate her medication regimen. During her internment, her husband and mother had taken over the care of her baby and the infant was being bottle fed. Jane was experiencing moderate sedation, racing thoughts with recurrent feelings of shame, guilt, regret, anxiety, and sadness during the day. She said she felt "flat and robotic." She was not able to sleep well and felt exhausted during the day.

A course of neurofeedback was initiated at T4-P4 for physiological and psychological calming. An additional site at T3-T4 was added for stabilization, and to maintain the left/right balance necessary for instabilities related to bipolar disorder. We tracked the changes in physiological arousal to find the optimal training frequency that would be sufficiently calming but not sedating. Reward was optimized at 0.01 mHz. By her fourth session of neurofeedback Jane was sleeping better and she reported her thoughts as more organized. She was looking and feeling less anxious. After one week of sessions, we carefully down-titrated her daytime Seroquel dosage to minimize sedation and optimize her function. She gradually regained her sense of self in relation to her newborn child and her husband. At this point, we collaborated with her therapist to introduce the principles of interpersonal social rhythm therapy (IPSRT) that is supported by clinical research to help with relapse prevention in patients with bipolar disorder. Her husband was also included in couple therapy sessions to address any ongoing relational conflicts that could become potential triggers for mood episodes.

By session 20, Jane was looking forward to getting back to part-time work and was decreasing the frequency of her neurofeedback sessions. She was no longer preoccupied with her feelings of guilt related to her cessation of breastfeeding and not yet being back at work full-time. She had consolidated her new role identity and had made peace with her role transition. By session 30, Jane had returned to work full-time and was on a maintenance low dose of her medication. She continued to receive weekly therapy sessions and chose to discontinue neurofeedback follow up. She felt the treatments had helped her down-titrate the medication dosage over time, re-capture her motherhood, and get back to her job. Her husband reported their relationship had returned to normal.

7.2.1 Discussion

Bipolar disorder is a chronic relapsing and remitting disorder with progressive disability across the lifespan. The depressed state is characterized by sad or hopeless feelings, anger and frustration, as well as irritability in varying degrees of severity. There is also a noticeable change in sleep and appetite, tiredness, feelings of worthlessness, and loss of interest in pleasurable endeavors. The hypomanic phase involves an increase in grandiose thinking, talkativeness, decreased need for sleep, distractibility, and excessive need to indulge in activities that are likely to produce painful consequences. The manic phase is more severe and causes a marked impairment in functioning, and patients may require hospitalization. These individuals suffer from the loss of functional lives due to constant mood swings and disrupted personal relationships. Often, hospitalizations and re-hospitalizations are necessary and provide temporary relief of the symptoms.

The treatment of bipolar disorder typically involves acute stabilization with the goal of bringing a patient with mania or depression back to a stable mood. However, the treatments that alleviate each pole of the disorder can inadvertently result in rebound episodes. Consequently, patients often experience mixed symptoms or subthreshold symptoms, despite overt reports of stabilization. Patients with bipolar disorder struggle with medication compliance and tend to self-medicate with alcohol and other substances. Most of them tend to seek help when they are in the throes of depression but, because they miss their manias, a significant number discontinue anti-depressant medications. In neurofeedback terms, the brain experiences state instabilities that manifest as mood swings. Such shifts of arousal and excitability are eminently addressed with inter-hemispheric and right-sided calming protocols. The brain is guided to regulate itself in both states of hyper-arousal (hypomania or mania) or under-arousal (depression). Neurofeedback facilitates the taming of a kindling, reactive, chaotic nervous system. One of the main advantages of neurofeedback is that it breaks the craving for disregulated manias while also addressing the issue of addictions. Additionally, we prepare the brain to receive the insights from psychotherapy sessions, thus minimizing the frequency, intensity, and duration of mood swings.

In Jane's case, we utilized the principles of interpersonal therapy (IPT) and social rhythm therapy (IPSRT) to target both her postpartum depressive symptoms and her symptoms of bipolar disorder. IPT is based on the so-called common factors of psychotherapy; a treatment alliance in which the therapist empathically engages the patient, helps the patient to feel understood, arouses affect, presents a clear rationale and treatment ritual, and yields successful experiences.[24] On this foundation IPT builds on two major principles. First, that depression is a medical illness rather than the patient's fault or personal defect; moreover, it is a treatable condition. This definition has the effect of defining the problem and excusing the patient from symptomatic self-blame. Second, is that mood and life situations are related. Building on interpersonal theory and psychosocial research on depression,[25] IPT makes a practical link between the patient's mood and disturbing life events that either trigger or follow from the onset of the mood disorder. In turn, these benefits translate to a return to normal functions at home, work, or school.

Neurofeedback augments conventional treatments without adding to the burden of side effects. After beginning neurofeedback, patients feel that they can trust their brain a lot more, and often report less susceptibility to mood swings, an increased ability to focus, and reduced anger. Their ability to function may increase as they find themselves less reactive and increasingly able to respond and act appropriately in situations that would have triggered mood episodes in the past.

7.3 Case Study #2: Severe Generalized Anxiety Disorder with Severe Alcohol Use Disorder

Mary is a 22-year-old woman who presented with a five-year history of progressive use of alcohol to self-medicate her symptoms of anxiety and panic attacks. A thorough medical history, physical examination, and baseline lab evaluation was completed at her initial visit. Her lab results were significant for borderline elevation of liver enzymes due to alcohol use disorder. Her past history was significant for an episode of sexual abuse perpetrated by a neighbor during her childhood. She had attended counseling sessions but was reluctant to relay her experiences of sexual abuse and did not confirm whether or not the counseling sessions had helped her resolve the experience. She felt as though she was "stuck in the past." She endorsed chronic feelings of low self-esteem, worthlessness, intrusive negative thoughts, and feeling "dirty" most of the time with episodic panic attacks. She said she felt a low level of sadness most of the time with a high level of anxiety all the time.

She had experienced high anxiety symptoms throughout her teenage years and had struggled to complete her secondary education. She reported a significant relief in her anxiety symptoms following her first exposure to alcohol in high school. She quit studying after high school because her high levels of anxiety impeded her ability to focus on her studies. She then began to work as a bartender, giving her easy access to her medication of choice for her symptoms. Following two emotionally and sexually abusive relationships with boyfriends, whom she met at her work place, her alcohol use escalated to the point that she was needing a daily eye opener just to get out of bed. At this point, she was urged by her concerned parents to seek help from her primary care physician and was prescribed a benzodiazepine (Xanax) to ease her symptoms. She began to abuse the prescription medication and continued using alcohol. This resulted in tardiness at work, dependence on substances to get her through the day, and a failed attempt at alleviation of symptoms. She declined helpful interventions from her employer and abruptly stopped going to work. After a more successful intervention from her parents, she touched base with us at the urging of her family to explore options for treatment. She did not want to become dependent on psychotropic medications, but at the same time wanted lasting relief from her unrelenting symptoms of anxiety. At this stage, she was still unwilling to talk about her previous history of sexual abuse.

Following a risk–benefit decision analysis at intake assessment regarding the various treatment options, she elected to proceed with outpatient medical detoxification for alcohol withdrawal symptoms. We addressed her symptoms with a standard ASAM (American Society of Addiction Medicine) benzodiazepine taper protocol that lasted five days. She agreed to commence a low dose of sertraline (Zoloft) for her anxiety symptoms. To augment her treatment and promote recovery, a course of neurofeedback was started at T4-P4 and optimized to a reward of 0.01mHz. Mary tolerated the sessions very well and reported a modest decrease in her anxiety symptoms following the first session. She went in feeling skeptical about the intervention but after an hour of neurofeedback she felt more confident and willing to pursue this course of treatment.

T4-P4 sessions were continued for 10 twice-weekly sessions to stabilize her brain and early trauma-related dysregulation with good effect. T4-P4 protocols remained the baseline whilst other sites were added to address more specific symptoms such as panic attacks and impulse control. Neurofeedback sites were added at T3-T4 for panic attacks, T4-FP2 for emotional stability, and T3-FP1 for impulse control and cravings. Significant improvements were noted as she completed her detox protocol and continued low dose sertraline over the next two weeks. She reported better sleep, resolution of panic symptoms, and decreased cravings. By session 30, over a 15-week period, she was no longer experiencing cravings for alcohol or xanax and was keen to get back to work. Mary commenced motivational interviewing and cognitive behavior therapy sessions soon after session 20. She also elected to continue with a low dose of sertraline. At the six-month follow up she was sober, working her twelve steps, and went back to work as a customer service representative. She elected to consolidate her gains with monthly maintenance neurofeedback sessions.

7.3.1 Discussion

Abuse and maltreatment during childhood are major risk factors for internalizing disorders, such as depression and anxiety, which can lead to significant disability.[26]

Altered connectivity of the brain's fear circuitry represents an important candidate mechanism linking maltreatment and internalizing symptoms such as anxiety, low self-esteem, feelings of worthlessness, and low levels of depression. In a study using resting-state functional brain connectivity in adolescents, it was shown that maltreatment predicts lower prefrontal–hippocampal connectivity in females and males, but lower prefrontal–amygdala connectivity only in females. These results indicate the importance of fronto–hippocampal connectivity for both sexes in internalizing symptoms following maltreatment. In females, the finding of fronto–amygdala connectivity may help explain their higher risk for anxiety and depression.[27]

Benzodiazepines represent a popular class of drugs that have shown efficacy in the treatment of anxiety disorders, but they suffer from the potentiality of producing dependence with chronic use.[28, 29] Abrupt discontinuation of benzodiazepines after more than a couple of weeks use can lead to insomnia and anxiety.[30] More recently, newer antidepressants, selective serotonin reuptake inhibitors (SSRIs), have shown efficacy in anxiety disorders without raising the same concerns regarding dependence.[31, 32] These medication, however, do have their own side effects, which may influence the ability of patients to adhere to therapy.[33]

A recent 2018 study found what was referred to as "worrying results" implicating benzodiazepine use to dementia risk. The study results concluded that benzodiazepine and related drug use in general were associated with a modestly increased Alzheimer's disease risk, with no major differences between benzodiazepine and other related drug subcategories. The study authors recommended that benzodiazepine and related drug subcategories should be avoided when possible and that the threshold for prescribing should be high due to their overall adverse effect profile.[34]

With the introduction of the SSRIs in the 1980s, and their effectiveness in the treatment of depression and anxiety, they have become the most widely and frequently prescribed drugs in the world. Patients need to be closely monitored during initiation of SSRI therapy due to the reported risks of increased suicidal ideation. This has led to considerable controversy regarding their overall efficacy and safety in the treatment of major depressive disorders.[35, 36, 37] SSRIs include fluoxetine, fluvoxamine, sertraline, citalopram, paroxetine, and the mixed serotonin and norepinephrine reuptake inhibitor venlafaxine. These drugs are now used in both pediatric and adult populations for many anxiety and depressive disorders. They have not been reported to cause dependence or abuse, though a withdrawal discontinuation syndrome has been reported.[38, 39] One major drawback to their use, however, has been the lag between treatment initiation and the onset of therapeutic response. Typically, the response may be seen only after 3–4 weeks of initiation. Hence, they are not useful for the treatment of acute anxiety or depression. Additional limitations to their routine use include various side effects and their tolerability.[40] These side effects include, but are not limited, to sexual dysfunction, weight gain, initial insomnia, restlessness, and agitation.

Some researchers have suggested that there may be a genetic link influencing a person's anxiety level and their alcohol consumption.[41] These biological theories suggest that a brain mechanism is responsible for both anxiety symptoms and drinking behaviors. Other researchers proposed an expectancy component in alcohol consumption and anxiety symptoms. This means a person would expect to experience relief from their anxiety symptoms after consuming alcohol due to its calming effect on the central nervous system. Drinking behaviors are based on the person's level of anxiety and the expected relief alcohol will provide. Thus, based on this theory, one would expect higher anxiety levels to be eased with a greater consumption of alcohol.

People with anxiety disorders are up to three times more likely to suffer an alcohol or other substance abuse disorder than those without an anxiety disorder. Studies have shown that problem drinking is more prevalent in patients with anxiety disorders. Because the suffering with these disorders is substantial, anxiety disorders should not go untreated. An additional problem is that long-term alcohol abuse usually means building a tolerance to its effects. This results in increased alcohol consumption to get the desired result. Therefore, what begins as a way to cope with anxiety can quickly have the opposite effect of increasing anxiety. Problem drinking leads to alcohol withdrawal, known as a "hangover." The symptoms of alcohol withdrawal include anxiety and panic attacks, besides other possible symptoms such as agitation, nausea, vomiting, elevated blood pressure, elevated heart rate, and increased body temperature. These symptoms tend to create a cycle of heightened anxiety and increased problem drinking.[42, 43, 44]

Addiction is characterized by improper engagement of neurobiological systems involved in adaptive decision making. The prevalence of relapse among addiction patients may be explained by the persistence of maladaptive patterns of synaptic connectivity. An effective approach to addiction treatment and relapse prevention may thus rely on enhancing the brain's capacity for neuroplasticity and self-regulation.

In a review paper published by Sunder et al., the authors found that altered functional connectivity has been postulated to be a key failure mechanism in addiction psychopathology. Addiction patients who underwent neurofeedback training reported experiencing dysphoria when they used a substance following the treatment, indicating that the intervention may have rewired the brain's response to substance use. Neurofeedback training may thus operate by promoting neuroplasticity, facilitating adjustments in neuronal activity that support optimum functioning. More specifically, as stated in Chapter 4, neurofeedback has been proven to activate astrocytic mechanisms that facilitate synaptogenesis and manage network excitability through capillary blood flow.[45] These promising findings indicate that it is possible to rewire the brain for optimal functioning via the use of neurofeedback.

7.4 Conclusion

Treatment modalities such as neurofeedback offer the possibility of a wider spectrum of efficacy without the concerns of pharmacological dependence or their associated side effects. It is hoped that neurofeedback training will allow many more clinicians to confidently treat patients with psychiatric disorders, without the need to prescribe medications known to have potentially adverse effects, abuse, or dependency. Neurofeedback has proven to be an outstanding tool within a psychiatric practice setting. By calming the brain, neurofeedback cuts down or eliminates any resistance to psychotherapy that the patient might already have, or experience in ongoing therapy sessions. Thus, after neurofeedback, they are more open to choose effective psychotherapy treatment, possibly in combination with low dose pharmacotherapy. Neurofeedback may decrease the need for medication or eliminate the need altogether.

Neurofeedback has taught me, as an integrative psychiatrist, to be more discerning and reflective about when to talk, when to medicate, and when to train the brain.

Notes

1 Kandell ER. A new intellectual framework for psychiatry. *Am J Psychiatry.* 1998;1998(155):457–469.
2 Goldstein M. Decade of the brain-an agenda for the nineties, in neurology – from basics to bedside (special issue). *West J Med.* 1994;1994(161):239–241.
3 Baloch HA, Hatch JP, Olvera RL, Nicoletti M, Caetano SC, Zunta-Soares GB, Soares Jair C. Morphology of the subgenual prefrontal cortex in pediatric bipolar disorder. *J Psychiat Res.* 2010;44(15):1106–1110.
4 Baykara B, Inal-Emiroglu N, Karabay N, Çakmakçı H, Cevher N, Pilan BS, Alşen S. Increased hippocampal volumes in lithium treated adolescents with bipolar disorders: A structural MRI study. *J. Affective Disorders.* 2012;138(3):433–439.
5 Chang K, Karchemskiy A, Barnea-Goraly N, Garrett A, Simeonova DI, Reiss A. Reduced amygdala gray matter volume in familial pediatric bipolar disorder. *J Am Acad Child Adolescent Psych.* 2005;44(6):565–573.
6 Gitlin MJ, Swendsen J, Heller TL, Hammen C. Relapse and impairment in bipolar disorder. *Am J Psychiatry.* 1995;152(11):1635–1640.
7 Judd LL, Akiskal HS, Schettler P. J., et al. The long-term natural history of the weekly symptomatic status of bipolar I disorder. *Arch Gen Psychiatry.* 2002;59:530–537.
8 Rush AJ, Trivedi MH, Stewart J. W., et al. Combining medications to enhance depression outcomes (CO-MED): acute and long-term outcomes of a single-blind randomized study. *Am. J. Psychiatry.* 2011;168:689–701.
9 Lam RW, Kennedy SH, Grigoriadis S, McIntyre RS, Milev R, Ramasubbu R., et al. Canadian Network for Mood and Anxiety Treatments (CANMAT) clinical guidelines for the management of major depressive disorder in adults. *J. Affective Disorders.* 2009;117:S26–2S4.
10 Lynch D, Tamburrino M, Nagel R, Smith MK. Telephone-based treatment for family practice patients with mild depression. *Psychological Reports.* 2004;94:785–792.
11 Manning D, Markowitz J, Frances A. A review of combined psychotherapy and pharmacotherapy in the treatment of depression. *J Psych Pract Res.* 1992;1(2):103–116.
12 Clark DA, Beck AT. Cognitive theory and therapy of anxiety and depression: convergence with neurobiological findings. *Trends Cogn Sci.* 2010;14:418–424. 10.1016/j.concog.2011.03.024.

13 Versiani M, Cheniaux E, Landeira-Fernandez J. Efficacy and safety of electroconvulsive therapy in the treatment of bipolar disorder: a systematic review. *J Ect.* 2011;June;27(2):153–164.

14 Johnston SJ, Boehm SG, Healy D, Goebel R, Linden DEJ. Neurofeedback: a promising tool for the self-regulation of emotion networks. *Neurolmage.* 2010;49(1):1066–1072.

15 Moriyama TS, Polanczyk G, Caye A, Banaschewski T, Brandeis D, Rohde LA. Evidence-based information on the clinical use of neurofeedback for ADHD. *Neurotherapeutics.* 2012;9(3):588–598.

16 Hammond DC. Neurofeedback with anxiety and affective disorders. *Child and Adolescent Psychiatric Clinics of North America.* 2005;14(1):105–123. Vii.

17 Arns M, Kenemans JL. Neurofeedback in ADHD and insomnia: vigilance stabilization through sleep spindles and circadian networks. *Neurosci Biobehavioral Rev.* 2014;44:183–194.

18 Cortoos A, Valck E, Arns M, Breteler MHM, Cluydts R. An exploratory study on the effects of tele-neurofeedback and tele-biofeedback on objective and subjective sleep in patients with primary insomnia. *Applied Psychophysiology and Biofeedback.* 2009;35(2):125–134.

19 Sokhadze TM, Cannon RL, Trudeau DL. EEG biofeedback as a treatment for substance use disorders: review, rating of efficacy, and recommendations for further research. *Appl Psychophysiol Biofeedback.* 2008;33(1):1–28.

20 Angelakis E, Stathopoulou S, Frymiare JL, Green DL, Lubar JF, Kounios J. EEG neurofeedback: a brief overview and an example of peak alpha frequency training for cognitive enhancement in the elderly. *Clin Neuropsychologist.* 2007;21(1):110–129.

21 Thornton K. Improvement/rehabilitation of memory functioning with neurotherapy/QEEG biofeedback. *J Head Trauma Rehabil.* 2000;15(6):1285–1296.

22 Vernon DJ. Can neurofeedback training enhance performance? An evaluation of the evidence with implications for future research. *Appl Psychophysiol Biofeedback.* 2005;30(4):347–364.

23 Othmer S. *The Neurofeedback Clinicians' Protocol Guide.* 6th edition. Woodland Hlls, CA: EEG Institute, 2017.

24 Frank J. Therapeutic factors in psychotherapy. *Am J Psychother.* 1971;25:350–361.

25 Klerman GL, Weissman MM, Rounsaville B. J., et al. *Interpersonal psychotherapy of depression.* New York: Basic Books, 1984.

26 Herringa RJ, Phillips ML, Fournier JC, Kronhaus DM, Germain A. Childhood and adult trauma both correlate with dorsal anterior cingulate activation to threat in combat veterans. *Psychol Med.* 2013;43(7):1533–1542.

27 Herringa RJ, Birn RM, Ruttle PL, Burghy CA, Stodola DE, Davidson RJ, Essex M. J. Childhood maltreatment is associated with altered fear circuitry and increased internalizing symptoms by late adolescence. *Proc Nat Acad Sci USA.* 2013;110(47):19119–19124.

28 Möller H. J. Effectiveness and safety of benzodiazepines. *J Clin Psychopharrnacol.* 1999;19(Suppl 2):2S–11S.

29 Woods JH, Katz JL, Winger G. Benzodiazepines: use, abuse, and consequences. *Pharmacol Rev.* 1992;44:151–347.

30 Greenblatt DJ, Shader Rl, Abernethy DR. Drug therapy. Current status of benzodiazepines. *N Engl J Med*. 1983;309:354–358.

31 Ninan PT. New insights into the diagnosis and pharmacologic management of generalized anxiety disorder. *Psychopharrnacol Bull*. 2002;36:105–122.

32 Kasper S, Resinger E. Panic disorder: the place of benzodiazepines and selective serotonin reuptake inhibitors. *Eur Neuropsychopharmacol*. 2001;11:307–321.

33 Masand PS, Gupta S. Selective serotonin-reuptake inhibitors: an update. *Harv Rev Psychiat*. 1999;7:69–84.

34 Tapiainen V, Taipale H, Tanskanen A, Tiihonen J, Hartikainen S, Tolppanen AM. The risk of Alzheimer's disease associated with benzodiazepines and related drugs: a nested case–control study. *Acta Psychiatr Scand*. 2018;August;138(2):91–100.

35 Gorman JM. Treatment of generalized anxiety disorder. *J Clin Psychiatry*. 2002;63(Suppl 8):17–23.

36 Masand PS, Gupta S. Selective serotonin-reuptake inhibitors: an update. *Harv Rev Psychiatry*. 1999;7:69–84.

37 Barbey JT, Roose S. P. SSRI safety in overdose. *J Clin Psychiatry*. 1998;59(Suppl 15):42–48

38 Haddad PM. Antidepressant discontinuation syndromes. *Drug Safety*. 2001; 24:183–197.

39 Judge R, Parry MG, Quail D, Jacobson JG. Discontinuation symptoms: comparison of brief interruption in fluoxetine and paroxetine treatment. *Int Clin Psychopharrnacol*. 2002;17:217–225.

40 Masand PS, Gupta S. Selective serotonin-reuptake inhibitors: an update. *Harv Rev Psychiatry*. 1999;7:69–84.

41 Pandey SC, Zhang H, Roy A, Xu T. Deficits in amygdaloid cAMP-responsive element-binding protein signaling play a role in genetic predisposition to anxiety and alcoholism. *J Clin Invest*. 2006;December;116(12):3292.

42 Hasin DS, Stinson FS, Ogburn E, Grant B. F. Prevalence, correlates, disability, and comorbidity of DSM-IV alcohol abuse and dependence in the United States: results from the national epidemiologic survey on alcohol and related conditions. *Archives of General Psychiatry*. 2007;64:830–842.

43 Kessler RC, Nelson CB, McGonagle KA, Edlund MJ, Frank RG, Leaf PJ Am. The epidemiology of co-occurring addictive and mental disorders: implications for prevention and service utilization. *J Orthopsychiatry*. 1996;January;66(1):17–31.

44 Kushner MG, Krueger R, Frye B, Peterson J. Epidemiological perspectives on co-occurring anxiety disorder and substance use disorder. In: Stewart SH, Conrod P, editors. *Anxiety and Substance Use Disorders: The Vicious Cycle of Comorbidity*. New York: Springer, 2008, pp. 3–17.

45 Sunder KR, Bohnen J. L. The progression of neurofeedback: an evolving paradigm in addiction treatment and relapse prevention. *MOJ Addict Med Ther*. 2017;3(3):00037. DOI:10.15406/mojamt.2017.03.00037

Chapter 8

Remediating Brain Instabilities in a Neurology Practice

Stella B. Legarda

8.1 Introduction

This chapter acquaints the reader with a neurologist's experience using EEG-based neuromodulation and infra-low frequency (ILF) brain training[1,2] to manage significant neurological disorders. Let us dive into this subject matter by introducing actual patient profiles (using pseudonyms) and their responses to this form of neurotherapy.

8.2 Case Vignettes

8.2.1 Patient A

Mr. Robinson, a 74-year-old male is a new patient accompanied by his wife. He has uncontrollable shaking and requires a walker to walk long distances. His cane hangs on the side of the walker. I ask him why he needs the walking aids. He states that he woke up from surgery, couldn't walk, and that he was diagnosed with a foot drop. He has anger as a clear component of his presentation. "This all started after a failed surgery," he growls. He is involved in a lawsuit with the hospital. After 30 years of being in practice, I know the type. Having placed great faith in his doctors he feels cheated, disillusioned, and has become over-critical and distrustful. Angry. His anger and general disposition are wreaking havoc on his marriage; his wife is in psychiatric counseling, not coping well. This fact makes him even more furious. I look at his list of medications; there are twelve. Among them are these powerful medications: lithium, olanzapine, ziprasidone, valproate, primidone, and alprazolam – all at high doses. His exam is significant for marked motor dyscontrol, marked anxiety, and rage. As he sits, he continues with movements best described as resting shakes. The foot drop is unexplainable; he has intact reflexes, intact power of the isolated plantar flexion and extension ranges of motion, and no relative disuse foot atrophy. He is informed that his central nervous system is dysregulated. "Well of course it is! Is there anything to fix it? I'm on all these drugs and nothing works," he yells. I venture to say there is a novel intervention he has not yet tried. No, it is not another drug. It is a form of EEG-based neuromodulation to re-regulate his markedly dysregulated state and I offer him a brain training session right there and then – no promises, but what does he have to lose? "Nothing else has worked." Should he not experience immediate benefit after this one session then I would attempt to optimize his medical regimen. Defensive in his stance, he acts helpless all the same. He agrees, his interest is piqued. After the tailored brain training session immediate benefits are evident and felt by the patient: the uncontrollable shaking stops, the anger is reduced, he states he has not felt this calm for a very long time (the surgery was three months ago), and he walks out of the office carrying his walker, using his cane to walk.

Over time his medications were gradually reduced from twelve to six. Our clinic staff have come to know him over the years as one of the nicest, kindest people. Mr. Robinson now ambulates normally, without the need for a cane. His wife has stopped going to counseling. They recently celebrated their wedding anniversary, kindly inviting his neurologist to attend (graciously declined).

8.2.2 Patient B

Seventy-six-year-old Mr. Decker has a great life. He feels no medical concerns except for a disabling writing tremor which has worsened over the last 5 years. He played football in high school and college and admits to multiple concussions, which have not prevented him from becoming a successful CEO of several companies before his retirement. In his retirement he is elected to chair community clubs and committees. He has plans for acupuncture to address this writing difficulty but wanted to keep this appointment first to "see what I had to say." His neurological and brief mental status exams reveal no immediate concerns. On the cognitive battery he recalls 3 out of 5 objects and otherwise does well. I ask him to write the letters A to Z, the numbers 0 to 9, and apply his signature. He agrees to a tailored brain training session when I tell him we might know immediately after the session whether he would derive benefit or not (see Figure 8.1).

Since starting and completing his course of brain training sessions, Mr. Decker is no longer embarrassed to pick up and fill out a tab in the restaurant, write a check in the store, or sign important papers in front of his committee board members.

8.2.3 Patient C

A mother returns with her 5-year-old son Jack, who has autism, a year after a prior visit because he remains unable to be contained, is not toilet-trained, is nonverbal, and she is having great difficulty in finding help to care for him. He has become more difficult to manage over the year. His school is threatening to dismiss him unless his mom agrees to medical intervention. The mother continues to refuse any form of pharmacotherapy. Other than the absent speech and extreme autism profile the physical and neurological exams are unremarkable; he is climbing all over the furniture and needs constant redirection. So, I offer her a non-pharmacological option.

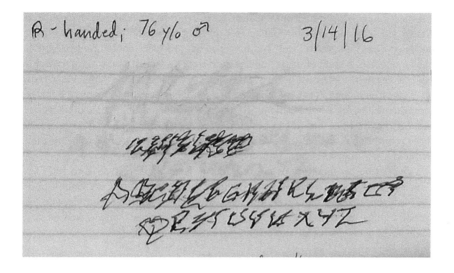

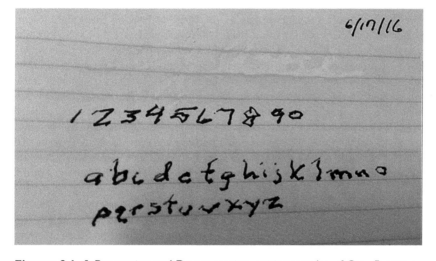

Figures 8.1 **A** Pre-session and **B** post-session writing samples of Case B over a three month period. (Signature concealed for patient privacy.)

It is challenging at first; the first session lasts just 10 minutes. The second 20 minutes. Thereafter, the child settles down. The mother states even after the first brief session she noticed a change in him; he seemed calmer that day and the next, which is why she came back. After a course of tailored brain training sessions this young man is toilet-trained, able to attend a special needs class, is reading and writing (below age level), and continuing to develop his verbal skills. The family is now able to go out for a meal at restaurants and to other public venues together without incident. Yes, challenges remain; Jack still has autism. The improved ability to communicate, easement of care for his daily needs, and the ability to keep him in school have impacted his and the family's quality of life for the better. He continues to come for neurofeedback sessions intermittently.

8.2.4 Patient D

A mother and father bring their 11-year-old daughter, Julia, to clinic, frustrated that her speech development has "never caught up," despite years of speech therapy from kindergarten to third grade. There are no other neurodevelopmental concerns; she is an excellent student. The EEG is normal. I offer a program of tailored brain training sessions; there is no pharmacological option. They (and their child) do not want her in speech therapy again. After 12 neurofeedback sessions their daughter makes an oral presentation in front of her whole classroom. Below is a drawing she made in the waiting room before one of her later sessions (see Figure 8.2).

8.2.5 Patients E1 and E2 (Representing Dissimilar Post-Concussion Cases)

E1: A father brings his 16-year-old daughter, Lisa, a high school soccer team player who used to be a straight A student until a sport concussion sustained a year ago. There is no pharmacological option. A tailored program of infra-low frequency

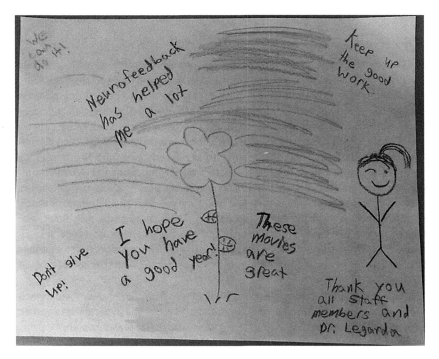

Figure 8.2 Case D's drawing (signature concealed for patient privacy).

brain training is adhered to. Gradually over time (six months) the patient restores her prior cognitive level of functioning; she is again the A grade student she was prior to the concussion. More on Lisa later.

E2: A mother brings her 19-year-old lacrosse-playing son, Philip, who has been arrested for juvenile delinquency and unlawful possession of regulated drugs while attending college. The mother is at her wit's end; her son used to be a very bright student but then got into the "wrong crowd." She is concerned about his future abilities for graduating college. He has a complex past medical history. At age 6 he had a significant head injury after swinging on the rope of a flagpole and falling onto concrete; he sustained a nondisplaced vertex fracture, a subdural hematoma, and a contusion of the left sylvian brain region. His symptoms were vomiting, headache, dizziness, and cognitive difficulties. He was observed for three days in hospital and recovered well. He was then diagnosed with Tourette syndrome at age 11; he is assessed with an atypical obsessive-compulsive disorder (OCD). He has unintended problems with authority. A neuropsychological profile discloses his superior intelligence and OCD. His physical and neurological exam are otherwise unremarkable. He has not responded to pharmacological interventions. We provide brain training. After 20 sessions Philip needs to move out of state to attend college on a scholarship playing lacrosse. When he comes home on break, he personally chooses to return for continuing neurofeedback sessions, driving himself to all his sessions instead of relying on his mother. He reports he is staying focused and out of trouble; he credits the ongoing positive changes in his life trajectory to the brain training.

8.2.6 Patient F

A 45-year-old female, Julie, with right spastic hemiparesis and wheelchair/walker activity after a stroke six months before, presents with her spouse, both frustrated that there is no further progress in healing despite completing physical, occupational, and speech therapies. She had a congenital cardiac defect, patent foramen ovale (PFO),[3] which was successfully closed in a procedure by a cardiologist colleague. He referred her to our clinic because of the remaining disabilities from her stroke. Further remediation is offered using infra-low frequency brain training and she is advised to restart all the modalities of rehabilitation therapy. Despite delays with third party payers in getting back into therapies, after 16 sessions she is ambulating fully using a cane with an ankle-foot orthosis of the right leg; her speech has normalized. She continues to gain functional improvements over time. A year after the stroke she experienced a focal seizure in the right arm that generalized, less than 2 minutes in duration. A 24-hr. ambulatory EEG was performed and the neurotherapy protocol further modified (see Figure 8.3).

Three weeks later the patient had a minor slip from her shower bench onto the shower floor without outside injuries. Later that day she experienced another brief seizure. Low dose topiramate (15 mg. twice daily) was prescribed; she remains seizure-free.

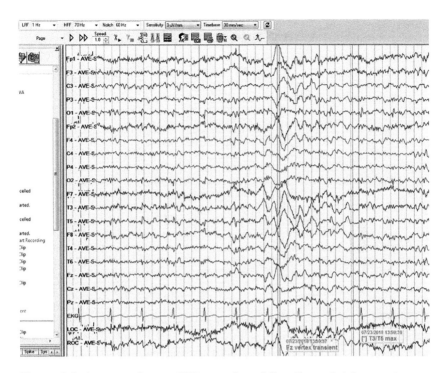

Figure 8.3 Average reference EEG recording of Case F reveals left posterior temporal slowing.

8.2.7 Patient G

A mother brings her 3½-year-old daughter Annabel, diagnosed with epilepsy, who has experienced adverse effects to all of the four medications we have trialed (lamotrigine, levetiracetam, oxcarbazepine, and topiramate) and continues to have frequent seizures. Her behavior has worsened over time and although she qualifies for pre-K she is not doing well with her peers and is doing poorly in class. Her EEG displayed left posterior quadrant dysrhythmias and spikes (see Figure 8.4). A personalized brain training protocol provides resolution of her seizures over time and she progresses neurodevelopmentally as expected for age. She completes 17 full neurofeedback sessions before moving to another distant city. We contacted her mother a year later; her child is doing very well academically and she has remained seizure-free.

8.2.8 Patient H

Parents bring back their 9-year-old son with epilepsy. His EEG study revealed biposterior slowing and spikes (see Figure 8.5). Isaac, who is seizure-free on lamotrigine and who still seems unable to learn anything new at school, has poor speech articulation, is beginning to isolate himself from his peers, and is becoming irritable and oppositional. A trial on stimulant therapy was not tolerated. There is no additional pharmacological option.

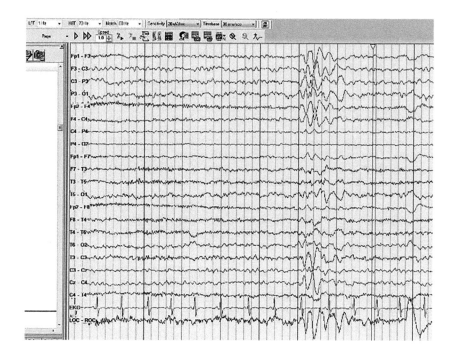

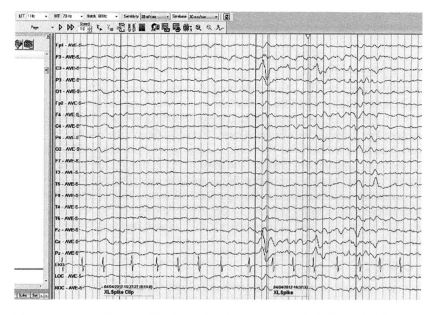

Figure 8.4 Case G's EEG (bipolar and average montage display) reveals left posterior quadrant dysrhythmias and spikes.

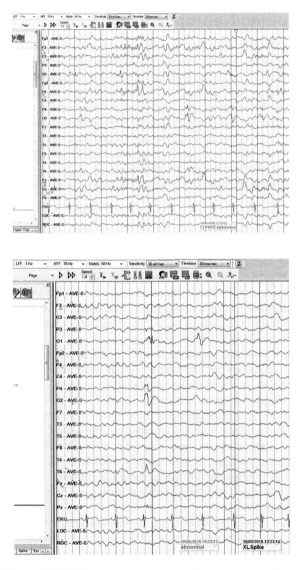

Figure 8.5 Case H's EEG (average montage) before lamotrigine therapy reveals biposterior slowing and spikes.

He adheres to a tailored program of ILF brain training. The positive results from neurofeedback are palpable both at home, where he remains stubborn but is more easily redirected, and at school, where his teachers are working with him to catch up with his peers. The child demonstrates growing self-esteem, a positive outlook, and has normal social interactions at this time.

8.3 Exploiting Neuroplasticity

In the recent past (pre-2010) such profile histories would too often raise regret, either because our therapeutic attempts failed or there was nothing but time and moral support to offer such patients in adapting (or mal-adapting) to their new reality. Today we have this evolving form of neurotherapy available, providing us with good reason for renewed optimism. All of the above cases serve to illustrate where targeted EEG-based neuromodulation and ILF brain training have proved to become a critical aspect of what we can do, as neurologists, in managing our patients with varied forms of acquired central nervous system dysregulated states or of maladapted neurodevelopmental disorders.

At the bioengineering level this is what takes place during every brain training session:

1. First, the prescribed scalp locations are located and named based on standard 10–20 electroencephalography (EEG) nomenclature for scalp placements.[4, 5] Recording electrodes are applied to the scalp using a mild abrasive lotion (e.g. Nu-Prep), to clean the skin surface first, then using electrode paste (e.g. Ten20 Conductive Electrode Paste) to keep the electrodes adhered to the scalp locations. Impedance checks (against biological tissue resistance) ensure the recording of brain signals satisfies technical standards and is equably met among the applied electrodes.
2. The patient's raw brain signal is recorded by the appropriately applied scalp electrodes, amplified, and digitized in the Cygnet® system software where it is processed according to the reinforcement frequency prescribed. Inhibit bands in the system serve to reduce unwanted brain signals and environmental artifact. The resultant signal is then relayed to partly drive the video monitor the patient is watching intently. Thus the patient engages with and reinforces their own brain signal, ostensibly their optimally regulating brain activity that is conveyed via the display monitor wherein the image projected fades or brightens and the audio diminishes or returns as the reinforcement feedback paradigm progresses either less or more proficiently, or merely progresses.
3. The patient's prevailing brain activity is monitored throughout the session by a Fast Fourier Transform-based trend graph of recorded delta, theta, alpha, beta and hi-beta frequencies in the EEG spectrum.

(Chapter 5 has a more detailed description of the clinical aspects of this.)

When the training protocol and optimal reinforcement frequency (ORF) are ideal, the EEG-based neuromodulation and infra-low frequency brain training methods promote a powerful re-regulation of the patient's brain networks, compelling them toward a recovery (or rediscovery or re-learning) of its inherent stability. This occurs after any productive session and may sustain only over the next day or two, thus requiring practice and repetition over time, as when learning a skill (like learning to play the guitar or to play golf), to eventuate toward a global brain homeostasis "reset" scenario wherein a new competence is incorporated in the system.

Synaptic adaptation (*Hebbian* learning) and homeostatic plasticity mechanisms are implicated.[6, 7, 8, 9] The responsive results in the above vignettes serve to demonstrate the capacity for neuroplasticity at any age. Children self-report (or their parents report) immediate benefits that sustain more readily; the "re-learning" in children appears precipitous. At any age, the more severely dysregulated the central nervous system (CNS) has become, the more immediately the desired anticipated response becomes observable, as the above cases for patients A and B illustrate in elderly adults.

The stable brain is a brain in healthy homeostasis and over time we witness that consistent exercise with neurofeedback empowers our patients to achieve this state of new or renewed competence. In our practice, we have learned over the years – and continue to learn from our patients – what works and what does not work for them. In our experience, a resolution of symptoms or a marked remediation of major complaints is achieved in most cases after 50 sessions (six months). This is most true of patients who consistently adhere to their scheduled sessions and other prescribed integrative therapies. With the evolution of the method into even lower reinforcement frequency ranges we find some patients, usually very young children and older patients who sustain an acute concussion, feel fully improved by their 20th to 25th session. We also have a few patients who continue to come for brain training long after they have completed 150 sessions.

This chapter describes the brain training protocols we frequently use for the more common neurological conditions. The reader should note that a few of these conditions are detailed further elsewhere in the book.

8.4 Patient Selection

A few words on the identification of patients for infra-low frequency brain training. First, elements of the patient's medical history and previous illnesses, past and present psychosocial history, and the review of systems are relevant in targeting the global brain needs. The patient may present with "headache" or "dizziness" for example, in which case the following questions need to be asked:

- Did you suffer from any previous injuries (i.e. in childhood, sports injuries, motor vehicular accidents, concussions)?
- Have you had any ER visits, hospitalizations, or surgeries, and what were the outcomes from these?
- Out of the below options, how would you rate your early growing up years?
  a) Great
  b) Normal, typical family dynamics
  c) Not so great
  d) Troublesome
- Do you have any difficulties at work; how do you think it could improve at work?
- Can you describe any earlier or current school difficulties?
- What is your medication history; what worked and what didn't work; what are your current medications?

The Review of Systems is critical; only here can disorders of arousal, gut regulation, sleep regulation, mood, cognitive functioning, and other symptoms offer clues to physiologic instabilities and specific cortical deficits. We find it useful to ask the patient to grade their adverse symptoms in order of greatest impact on their sense of well-being, which allows us to list the negative indicators on their quality of life in an order of difficulty for us to address. The history, when informed with these elements, in most cases will make it clear whether the patient would benefit from brain training.

The physical and neurological exam provide further clues on how to target the training. An elevated blood pressure and pressured speech indicate the need for parietal calming. Non-smooth pursuit in the eye exam, excessive involuntary motions, and seizures point to instabilities. Easy distractibility, left–right confusion, apraxias, and speech dysfluency, as well as overt focal deficits, all inform the neurofeedback clinician on how to prescribe the brain training protocol. Again, these findings are clearly listed in the initial assessment.

Not least, the patient's investment in self-healing must be taken into account. In our experience, when their insurance does not pay, the majority of adults will not pursue it, whereas most parents will do what it takes to better the lives of their children. To their credit, invested adults appeal repeatedly to their insurance carriers and many are successful in finding it covered.

In many cases it is more convenient to just pop a pill to feel better, than to commit the time, effort, and expense it takes for effective brain training to nurture results that sustain. Our current practice is to not put our patients through multiple medication trials. The reality is that those who seek neurofeedback have often tried all the pills and "nothing works," or they are the children of parents who refuse to medicate their children with psychoactive drugs; parental wisdom not wanting exogenous chemicals to interfere with actively peaking neurodevelopmental processes in the growing brain.

It is our practice to have follow-up medical visits after the first 5 sessions, after the next 5, and then after every 10 sessions. Brief within-session interactions are needed intermittently. It is important to provide anticipatory guidance before the first session. Brief patient feedback during the first two to three sessions allows for the identification of any immediate effects.

After the fifth and tenth sessions, the enduring problems become more readily identifiable and the protocol is further modified to address these. At the first follow-up visit the patient often needs to be reminded of all the complaints listed at the very first evaluation; they are not infrequently surprised to recall those symptoms that have now abated, and they feel encouraged to focus on the remaining difficulties they continue to experience.

Are we able to remediate everyone? No (see Tables 8.1 and 8.2). While this form of neurotherapy likely benefits us all, not all of us are suited to the therapy. It takes commitment, time, engagement with the process, patience in the chair (up to 50 minutes), and some patients need to rely on others to drive them to their brain training appointments. At some level a surrender is required to the mystery that remains in regard to the, as yet unidentified, full power of the brain to heal itself. There are also individuals who are fully identified with their disorder; to

Table 8.1 Patients with the following chief complaints not only benefit from ILF brain training but find the modality helped them "as nothing else has."

- Uncontrolled headaches head trauma sequelae stroke sequelae
- Academic learning difficulties memory changes
- Decline of executive skills
- Acquired and developmental speech disorders
- Uncontrolled tremors
- Uncontrolled seizures not candidates for surgery (and comorbidities)
- Sleep disorders
- Multiple sclerosis (and comorbidities) encephalitis and encephalomyelitis sequelae surgical
- Anesthesia sequelae
- Acute repetitive behavioral changes

Table 8.2 Neurological diagnoses we successfully remediate in our practice.

- Intractable posttraumatic headaches
- Post-concussion syndromes/chronic traumatic encephalopathy
- Post traumatic brain syndromes
- Post encephalitis syndromes and post encephalomyelitis syndromes
- Medically refractory seizures and epilepsy comorbidities
- Global academic learning disorders
- Cognitive impairments
- Speech dysfluency disorders
- Sequelae of cerebrovascular accidents
- Vascular Parkinsonism
- Poorly controlled Parkinson disease
- Intractable essential tremors
- Sleep disorders
- Chronic headache disorders
- Autism spectrum disorders
- Attention deficit disorder with or without hyperactivity
- Behavior disorders

heal would threaten their sense of identity. Last but not least, not all insurance carriers cover the service. When we started incorporating neurofeedback in our practice, no insurance carrier covered the service. Today more are providing coverage. The cost effectiveness of brain training cannot be denied; fewer emergency room visits, fewer physician visits, and reduced drug prescriptions are immediate benefits.

8.5 Prescribing Brain Training Protocols

In this section we make substantial use of standard 10–20 and derived inter-electrode 10–10 nomenclature to discuss some of the more common protocols we use in addressing brain instabilities (See Figure 8.6). We also make assumptions in referring the electrode scalp placements to underlying anatomic brain regions.[10, 11, 12, 13, 14, 15, 16]

Predictably, each brain is unique because every person's composite life experience, personality type, current neurodevelopmental stage (developmental and intellectual intelligence), and psychosocial stage[17, 18] (emotional intelligence) is differentiated from all others.[19] It will become clear, as each of the protocols mentioned below are described, that any one patient may have a profile, symptom(s), and diagnosis (or diagnoses) that fit more than one protocol. Therefore, each patient requires a tailored brain training protocol.

Each training session is limited to 50 minutes – too long for a few of our patients but most tolerate it well. We train a minimum of 10 minutes at each

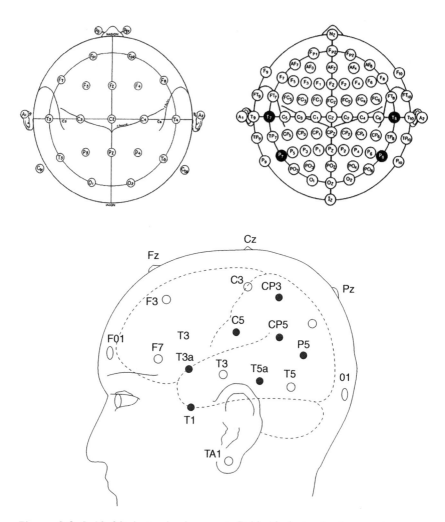

Figure 8.6 A 10–20 electrode placements **B** 10–10 electrode placements **C** Left hemisphere anatomic correlation of the central and parietal 10–10 electrode placements.[20]

prescribed scalp placement, which limits our sites to five, at most, per session. The following are the most common protocols we have found consistently applicable to the patient population we serve.

8.5.1 Post Concussion Syndrome/Post-Traumatic Brain Syndrome/Chronic Traumatic Encephalopathy

T4-O2.

T4-FP2.

T4-T3.

T3-O1.

T3-FP1.

Patients with a significant history of concussion(s) are trained in line with our "postconcussion protocol" (see Figure 8.7). We begin training at 0.01 millihertz (mHz), with 10 minutes at each bipolar site. We tend not to wait until the following sessions to move from one location in the scalp to the next; as long as the site is well tolerated, and the patient remains comfortable, we proceed to train at every

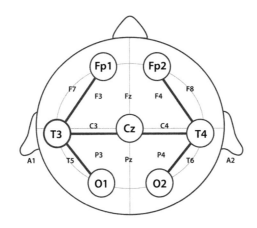

TIME	SITE A	-	SITE B	FREQUENCY
10	T4 - Cz	-	O2 - Cz	0.008 mHz
10	T4 - Cz	-	Fp2 - Cz	0.008 mHz
10	T4 - Cz	-	T3 - Cz	0.008 mHz
10	T4 - Cz	-	O1 - Cz	0.008 mHz
10	T4 - Cz	-	Fp1 - Cz	0.008 mHz

Figure 8.7 Head trauma/concussion protocol.

site in the first session. There is one caveat to this: in the case of a psychiatric diagnosis we train at one, or at most two, scalp placements in the first few sessions. Patients with psychiatric features are sometimes co-managed by a colleague neurofeedback practitioner who offers alpha-theta training,[21] a method available in most conventional neurofeedback systems that do not include ILF or synchrony training.

After 5–10 sessions or more, when improvements are noted (for example, fewer headaches, less anxiety, more engagement with life and social activities, less reactivity, diminished anger), we find that perhaps sleep is not fully restored or patients continue to complain of dizziness or fuzziness. We then add the following:

Infra-low frequency (0.05 Hertz or Hz) synchrony training at AFz + Pz. This overlies the anatomic regions of the Default Mode Network (DMN) – one of the major detectable active resting state networks, which exhibits oscillatory behavior in the range of 0.03–0.08 Hz.[22, 23]

We modify the protocol to T4-O2, T4-FP2, T4-T3, and T3-FP1 (the T3-O1 placement is removed).

Infra-low synchrony may not be well tolerated in children less than 13 years (pre-pubertal children). In reviewing the literature, it appears that uncertainty remains with regard to the developmental status of the DMN in the first years of life, whereas after puberty the typical adult posterior-anterior dimensions begin to consolidate in resting state functional MRI (rsfMRI) imaging.[24] This supports our current practice of restricting ILF synchrony training to older children and adults.

After a total of 15–20 sessions or more we then focus on maximizing frontal executive control in adult patients, adding fast or gamma (40 Hz) synchrony and, if we haven't yet done so, we drop the T4-FP2 scalp placement (many patients appear to tolerate only a few sessions at T4-Fp2 after its desired effects are achieved):

ILF synchrony (0.05 Hz) at AFz + Pz T4-O2, T4-T3, T3F-P1

Bi-frontal gamma synchrony (40 Hz) at Fp1+Fp2

Gamma synchrony is believed to optimize conscious connectivity (the "conscious pilot") and to promote the scavenging functions of microglia.[25, 26] In our experience, gamma synchrony is not well tolerated by children and we have abandoned the practice in this age group; it is known that the prefrontal networks do not mature organizationally until age 23–25 years.[27]

Hereafter, we address any specific cognitive complaints guided by the history and/or any neuropsychological report.

8.5.2 Acquired Specific Cognitive Impairments: Memory Deficits, Speech Dysfluency, Declining Executive Function

For patients with these diagnoses we first perform a cognitive battery; we use the mini-mental status exam (MMS)[28] and the Montreal Cognitive Assessment (MOCA).[29] For brain training in general we assume the starting protocol advised in the Othmer practice guidelines:[30]

T4-P4, T4-T3, T3-FP1.

We then add specific sites as follows:

T3-T5, T3-P3 – to promote memory, remediate dysnomia, and address forms of Wernicke network aphasias (language association areas).[31]

T4-F8, T3-F7 and T3-F3 – to remediate speech disarticulation disorders and Broca network aphasias (language production areas).[32]

T5-F7 and P3-F3 – to address conduction network aphasias (verbal initiative and maintenance of speech production).

After improvements are noted (trend graphs as well as patient reports), or after about 15–20 sessions, we begin to end each session in adults with Fp1+Fp2 gamma synchrony. Especially for patients with these disorders and lacking significant past medical histories for encephalitis or concussions, we are guided by the trend graph that monitors each session.

For complex cognitive impairments we do not infrequently obtain a full assessment from our clinical neuropsychologist, who furnishes us a comprehensive profile. This is especially useful in discerning the subtypes of aphasia and for delineating memory deficits, apraxias, visual spatial impairments, and higher executive dysfunctions, as well as determining the presence of mood dysregulation, emotional lability, inattention, arousal disorders, and general anxiety states. Some patients present with mixed neurological disorders, for example stroke and multiple sclerosis. The neuropsychological assessment guides us as to whether to train long tract pathways (true for multiple sclerosis) and/or regional cortical hubs (stroke-affected areas).

Psychiatric diagnoses are not a contraindication, however, their presence alerts us to the possibility of interference from psychoactive medications. We also proceed more slowly, often staying at just one or, at most, two sites in the first session. In our experience, most of the newer medications used in psychiatry (for example aripiprazole) do not hinder the brain training. Because this form of brain training promotes the inhibitory regulating networks in the brain, we do caution against the use of high doses of anti-dopaminergic agents for patients choosing this form of neurofeedback. As pointed out in other chapters, psychiatric patients are also likely to benefit from Alpha-Theta training, best practiced by our psychology and psychiatry professional colleagues. A last cautionary note in brain training individuals with strong psychiatric histories or early childhood trauma: they might report the training "made me worse" because they were unable to cope with memories, emotions, or an altered mood state that came up during the session. Likely this occurs because we are engaging with the earliest formed (and lowest frequency) networks in the brain. In this scenario we calm and stabilize them for 5–10 minutes at T4-P4 and at T3-T4 before they leave the clinic. Alas, there are times we don't see them come back. The presence of true psychosis is best served by our expert colleagues in psychiatry and psychology, but in general is not a contraindication to ILF brain training even in the neurologist's domain. Our neurofeedback colleagues in psychiatry report similar occurrences in their practice; they do have the more extensive training in this regard to address the issues that come up.

This is a good time to bring up the "rescue mode" we take when a patient reports not feeling well during a session (headache, dizziness, nausea, excessive sedation). When excessive sleepiness is experienced, we increase the reinforcement frequency in steps of 0.02 mHz to where they stay alert. The other discomfitures suggest that we are promoting some unexpected instability, so we train them at T4-T3 for 5 minutes or until their symptom(s) resolve – this is usually achieved readily – before continuing with the session We then modify their training protocol to exclude the scalp placement at which they experienced the unpleasant symptom. When patients report feeling anxious, we lower the reinforcement frequency. In general, these adverse occurrences are infrequent and most individuals tolerate their training well. There have been fewer adverse effects noted with the evolution of the software to allow for even lower ranges of infra-low frequency brain training. Additionally, it could also be the case that we practitioners have improved and are learning from experience. This truism needs to be stressed; those of us who practice infra-low frequency brain training are practicing at the frontier of non-invasive neuromodulation therapy.

8.5.3 Sequelae of Cerebrovascular Accidents

We start with the T4-P4, T4-T3 and T3-FP1 basic protocol.

We match the patient's reported and clinically detected deficits to scalp sites overlying the stroke-affected anatomic areas and extend the training to these identified correlated regions. For examples:

T4-C4 and T4-P4 for left-hand motor and sensory deficits. T4-C2 and T4-P2 for left leg motor and sensory deficits. T3-F7 and T3-F3 for expressive speech aphasias. T4-F8 and T4-Fp2 for abulia.[33]

We address other specific cognitive impairments as previously discussed.

Because we limit each session to 50 minutes, we modify the protocol over time to accommodate all the identified scalp placements needing to be incorporated in the training. We may also prescribe two protocols for profoundly affected patients and alternately train in them both (the second protocol every other session visit).

Many of these patients come because of persisting spasticity and gait disorders as well as because of speech disorders, inattention and disorganization, and abulia. While we have seen many successes, we also experience frustrations when patients do not achieve significant return of their functions. We see less benefit when a stroke has been established for longer than 10 years, although we do see some; in fact, the spouses and relatives of the patient often comment on how improved they see the patient, and it is the patient who does not see it or is frustrated by insufficient improvement. Always, we accept the patient's perspective above all. While most older patients improve in some faculties (spasticity is reduced, receptive speech is recoverable), the greater the age, the less complete the recovery of *motor function* tends to be. We persist when the stroke is recent in occurrence, however, even in these cases there is a sense that when the stroke involves a motor network hub extensively, then function is less likely to be restored. The neuroimaging studies guide us in this regard, but not as much as the patient's response to the training. We observe children and younger adults (less than 70) who had a recent stroke (less than 5 years past) to benefit greatly from ILF training. Young adults with cerebral palsy also appear to benefit greatly at any age, in terms of improving their quality of life in regard to speech articulation and spasticity, while full recovery is not expected.

8.5.4 Epilepsy and Its Comorbidities

Epilepsy by definition involves an intermittently overtly dysregulated network; it is likely that the interictal state is similarly, albeit more imperceptibly, dysregulated. Individuals with epilepsy do not infrequently report comorbidities like headache, depression, sleep disorders, and attention deficit states. Most of these comorbidities are addressed by the previously mentioned basic starting protocol sites T4-P4, T4-T3, and T3-Fp1.

Epilepsy connotes a significant brain instability, therefore we usually begin training patients with epilepsy at T4-T3 before going to other sites. Recent Cygnet software development, allowing for direct training of the Default Mode Network (DMN) by way of ILF synchrony at AFz + Pz, makes this an additional proposition in stabilization when managing older children and adults with epilepsies.

We use the patient's EEG findings to choose other discrete scalp placements with the aim to promote regional inhibitory control, keeping in mind that wherever we train on the scalp we are involving whole brain dynamics:

T4-T3 T4-P4.
    T3-C3 for left Rolandic spikes (T4-C4 for right).
    T3-F7 for left anterior temporal lobe spikes (T4-F8 for right).
    T3-Fp1, T3-F3, T3-F7 for left frontal and lateral frontal spikes.
    T4-Fp2, T4-F4, T4-F8 for right frontal and lateral frontal spikes.

In this section we enlarge on the difference between bipolar training and synchrony training. The bipolar scalp placement is better known to electroencephalographers (EEGers) and this is the same principle in neurofeedback use. Amplification of the signal *difference* between the two scalp sites is acquired during bipolar low frequency training. Synchrony training involves a new concept for EEGers; this is training by amplifying the *sum* of the two electrodes, connoted by the + sign. (See Chapter 5 for further details.)

We will also discuss in this section the developmental hierarchy that exists in the brain because of the way in which it continues to develop postnatally. At birth the brain is right-dominant; it is engaged with sleep regulation, gut regulation, sense of self in space and relating with self and with others, developing emotions, affect regulation, and first social nonverbal communications.[34, 35, 36] We also know the brain develops from caudal anatomic regions to anterior convexities, and thus from posterior occipital to frontal cortical regions. We follow this developmental hierarchy when we routinely start to train at T4-P4 (right parietal). With developmental speech disorders we train at T4-F8 before proceeding to train at the lateral sylvian networks of the muscles for speech and Broca's region (T3-F7 and T3-F3) on the left side. It may very well be that even during adulthood the right brain remains dominant in its regulatory role of the brain, even of the left brain.[37]

A personal note to end this section: In my practice as an epileptologist I do not readily refer children with epilepsy for infra-low frequency brain training unless they have significant comorbidities or additional neurodevelopmental challenges, as illustrated by Case H, or if they fail drug trials, as illustrated by Case G. The reason for this is that starting a medication, usually Lamotrigine (typically my first choice antiepileptic drug in managing any apparently idiopathic epilepsy in childhood), has a significant regulating effect and we can often observe the child to normalize in a global way – academically, socially, developmentally – as well as in terms of seizure control after reaching the target dose on the medication. Falling short of this desired outcome, I routinely recommend the brain training.

8.5.5 Intractable Headache (Not Related to Trauma or Concussion)

This is a surprising population of patients we enjoy offering brain training to and seeing their positive response. Typically, each patient is uniquely complex. Again, like epilepsy, intermittent formidable headaches that do not respond well to medication, or occur with such frequency that patients fear medication overuse, reflect a dysregulated state of affairs in the central nervous system. Thus, we start training at T4-T3 in these cases before moving to the other sites.

We cannot talk about the entity of "headache" in a chapter dedicated to the practice of clinical neurofeedback in a neurology specialty without expanding on this most common of complaints in medicine. The central pathophysiology of headache syndromes has a shared mechanism with arousal disorders[38] and with myofascial head and neck pain disorders,[39] accounting for frequent comorbidities. Headache invariably shows up in refractory extracranial disorders (e.g. autoimmune disease and chronic fatigue syndrome). Regardless of the association, chronic headache syndromes reflect an imminent or prevailing central dysregulation by whatever disease entity, effecting a consistent firing of afferents to the trigeminal complex (this largest of the cranial nerves serving a major sensory function to all anatomic structures above the shoulders, as well as providing motor efferents to the muscles of mastication). The spinal trigeminal nucleus, in particular, receives pain (and temperature) sensation from the head and facial structures and descends to the third cervical level, receiving nociceptive cervical afferents.[40]

Migraine mechanisms are elusive; peptides and neurotransmitter pathways remain targets of pharmacotherapy. Central sensitization is a factor in chronic headache syndromes; a frequent migraine attack from chronic nociceptive input in turn provides for persisting peripheral sensitization in a bidirectional feedback circuitry contributing to the chronicity of pain.[41]

Non-intuitively, very rarely are the causes for headache within the central nervous system itself. Many causes are sourced within the facial structures – teeth, gums, jaw bones and joints, neck muscles, and facial sinuses. Systemic instabilities may be the cause – hypertension (direct vascular mechanism), asthma (reduced blood return from intracranial contents), gastrointestinal distress (serotoninergic brainstem pathway), and direct effects from electrolyte, endocrine, and metabolic abnormalities may all provoke and even present as severe headache. The history must be obtained as outlined above and other treatable causes ruled out before proceeding with brain training.

Migraine and cluster headaches are the only true primary "head" ache disorders; the spinal trigeminal complex is dysregulated. Tension headaches remain the most common and have a musculoskeletal basis arising from chronically maladaptive neck dynamics (e.g. prolonged desk work, painting of ceilings) as well as from chronic stress. Posttraumatic headache syndromes are commonly associated with sequelae from facial injuries and/or neck shearing stress. While neurofeedback may help to alleviate symptoms, many headache disorders clearly require a multifactorial management approach. Neck stretching exercises, physical therapy, and preventive use of cervical collars are frequently recommended. Supportive counseling and life coaching form an important part of integrative therapy.

Stress and anxiety states are remediable by training further at T4-P4. The addition of ILF synchrony is likely beneficial. ILF synchrony is a fairly recent development that its mention here is made with mostly heuristic inference, however, in recent sessions we have found it of additional benefit when sleep regulation remains an issue. In sum, here is the initial headache protocol we follow:

T4-T3 T4-P4.
AFz+Pz ILF synchrony.

8.5.6 Pediatric Neurodevelopmental Disorders Affecting Academic Performance

Of all patient populations this group is perhaps the most gratifying to manage. It is a joy to watch a child's (and their parents') growing fears and anxiety about the future dissipate as she or he improves with neurofeedback. It cannot be emphasized enough that when children are not keeping up with their peers in school, they fail in far more ways than just academically – reduced self-esteem, lack of initiative, ambition and drive, and an inferiority complex all contribute to underachievement. These pre-adults can prove costly to society as they seek alternate realities through recreational drugs and excessive video-gaming, become vulnerable to hate group propaganda, or adopt criminal behavior for self-survival.[42] Troubled youth and adults should be referred to our psychology colleagues who are neurofeedback practitioners. Our over-burdened psychiatric colleagues benefit when such patients also train in neurofeedback. It is, as always, an integrative approach. School district counselors and workplace human resource support counselors should be invested with the ability to refer society's troubled youth and adults for these integrative services.

Focusing on the neuro-developmentally challenged young population we again ensure from their history there has been no head trauma and proceed with the starting protocol:

T4-P4.
T4-T3.
T3-P1.

As described above in Section 8.5.2 (see Figure 8.8), we use the trend graph as a guide to the patient's readiness for more discrete training.

For early expressive language developmental problems we remove T4-T3 and add the following sites:

T4-F8.
T3-F7, T3-F3.

For reading problems: T4-O2, T3-O1, T3-P3.
For memory: T3-T5, T3-P3.
For mathematics: T4-P4, T3-P3.
For attention deficit disorder: T3-Fp1.

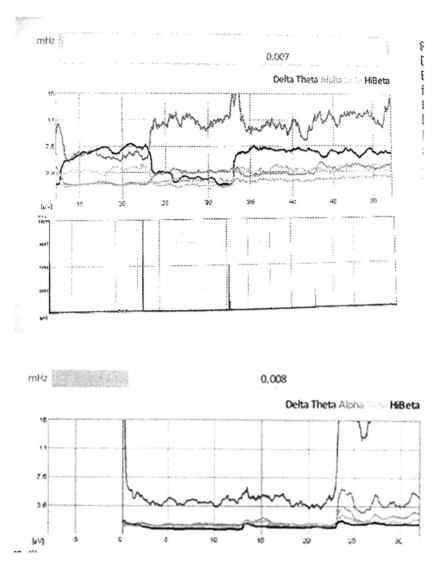

Figure 8.8 Session trend graphs. We monitor for a desired "flat-lining" of the hi-beta band (denoted by the heavy black line) before proceeding to bi-frontal gamma synchrony training.

For global learning difficulties we make use of psychoeducational evaluations from the child's school and when we note there is an average or above average global IQ score we feel confident she or he will benefit from neurofeedback. We find that parents and schools report back positively even with borderline to subnormal global IQ scores, so we do not have a cutoff; neither do we make anticipatory claims to parents that their child will improve (although we do find they invariably do). The key with this particular patient population is to not raise expectations but to maximize the child's potential.

8.5.7 Individualized Protocols

Now that the tools and the know-how have been covered, let us revisit the cases we met earlier and share their prescribed individualized protocols.

Patient A: T4-P4, T4-T3, T4-Fp2, T4-Fp1.

Initial protocol introduced was T4-P4 followed by T4-T3, with 10 minutes at each site on the first visit. Although this patient demonstrated marked instabilities, his severe anxiety appeared to override the physical instabilities noted, therefore parietal calming was elected first, followed by interhemispheric training. His wife's input was important; she had described him to be very anxious "all the time." In subsequent sessions we included T4-Fp2 to the protocol, and later T3- Fp1. He trained 15 minutes at each site and completed 55 sessions. By the 10th session he was walking without a cane. He was noted to still have a residual resting tremor, a mildly shuffling gait, and cogwheel rigidity, consistent with Parkinson disease. He was initiated on low dose carbidopa-levodopa, and today he is tremor-free. His wife tells us they tried to stop the carbidopa-levodopa; the tremors came back, so he has remained on the medication. Now 80 years old, his wife believes the neurofeedback stabilized his brain to the extent that there is no sign of his Parkinson disease progressing, "unlike our friends." We can neither support this statement nor refute it.

Patient B: T4-T3, T3-CP3, T4-P4, T3-T5, T3-P3, FP1+Fp2 synchrony.

The initial protocol introduced at the first encounter was T4-T3 followed by CP3-C3, with 10 minutes at each site. The choice was made based on the history of repeat concussions through the patient's high school and college years. It was suspected that he had sustained a mild degree of chronic traumatic encephalopathy, the marked writing tremor an overt sign of this instability. Subsequent sites included T4-P4, as his wife had described him to be worrying all the time about tomorrow and what might happen. She hated to drive with him because of his reactivity to poor drivers (T4-P4 training calms anxiety networks).

Currently 82 years of age, the patient has continued with memory changes; he was prescribed rivastigmine patch, which appears to help him. He returned for more sessions when I explained the evolution of the brain training technique to now include bifrontal synchrony training. We added T3-T5 and T3-P3 ILF training and Fp1+Fp2 synchrony to his protocol. His wife is astonished at his calm nature; his driving habits are markedly improved. He continues to come for sessions.

Patient C: T4-P4, T4-FP2, T4-T3, T3-FP1; T4-F8, T3-F7, T3-F3.

This 5-year-old boy had a severe form of autism and I had offered to address his behavior with pharmacotherapy. When his mother refused I was hesitant to offer the neurofeedback because of the challenges it would entail procedurally. We introduced Jack to the brain training room, chair, monitor, and allowed him to touch the electrodes. He watched me place the cupped ends on mom, on me, and then he allowed me to place them on his forehead. I explained the need to also put it in the hair area of his scalp and proceeded to place the cup there; I scratched his scalp gently with a Q-tip to let him know we would do this first and then add a glue to the cup, so it would stick to his head. He started well enough and it was a matter of sustaining his interest beyond 10 minutes thereafter. His mother helped greatly to secure his wandering hands. It only took about 5 sessions before Jack became fully engaged in the movies mom would bring and he ignored what we were doing. Truly, without the cooperation and assistance of devoted parents, the ability to train children with severe autism is a challenge. The initial protocol we used for Jack: T4-P4, T4-Fp2, T4-T3 and T3-Fp1. As we experienced his demeanor calm, heard his mother's report of his greater socialization (with family members at least, now playing with his sister instead of hitting her), and noting some irritability in him directly after training at the T4-Fp2 site in subsequent sessions, we removed this site at the 8th session and added T4-F8, T3-F7, and T3-F3 to address speech. He began to say intelligible words and mom reported he became toilet-trained. Jack remains very active to this day. When we train Jack lower than 0.008 mHz he loses bowel and urine control again, so we stay at 0.008 mHz. We tried to go lower after another 10 sessions and got the same result. This alerts us that any developmental regression in our patients who train with this technique may be a sign of training too low, as corroborated when the regressive trend reverses upon returning to the higher training frequency.

Now age 7, Jack is staying within the school system of special educational needs and they report progress with his participation in class and with learning. The biggest change we see is in the mother; she is beside herself with joy that there is now meaningful social interaction with her son – he now understands language, is better able to be redirected, and he is better able to state his needs (resulting in less behavioral outbursts stemming from frustration).

Children with autism benefit from ILF brain training long term. Offering an autistic child or adult this form of neurofeedback *first*, assists our ability to prescribe the most suitable pharmacotherapy to address residual symptoms. Jack's mom finally agreed to a ½ tablet of 0.1 mg clonidine as needed; she states she uses it only when he resists bedtime.

Patient D: T4-P4, T4-F8, T4-T3, T3-F7, T3-F3.

Julia was very cooperative with the brain training from the start. It was a real pleasure to work with her. We trained Julia in the following protocol: T4-P4, T4-F8, T4-T3, T3-F7 and T3-F3. She looked forward to coming to every session and her improvements with speech endure. She completed 50 sessions.

In this straightforward case we will take the opportunity to talk about initiating the training at 0.01 mHz, and how we are being guided to go lower. With few exceptions we find the trend graph of recorded brain frequencies during the session useful; we apply stronger, that is *lower*, frequency training sooner when we do not see good suppression of the upper beta-band frequencies, as long as the patient is comfortable and tolerating the training well. In this way, Julia was trained down to 0.007 mHz; at 0.006 mHz she had felt irritable and sleepy, so we stayed at 0.007 mHz.

Patient E1: T4-O2, T4-Fp2, T4-T3, T3-O1, T3-FP1, T3-T5, T3-P3.

Lisa was initially trained according to the developmental hierarchy because of her relative youth, however, she did not tolerate T4-P4. We started her at T4-T3. Then we found that she could tolerate T4-O2. Subsequently, we provided the full head protocol T4-O2, T4-FP2, T4-T3, T3-O1, and T3-FP1. As she improved with anxiety, sleep, and socialization issues we addressed her academic cognitive deficits. We added T3-T5 and T3-P3 for her short term memory and recall, removing the T4-Fp2 and T3-O1 derivations. Indeed, Lisa "taught" us what has become the post-concussion protocol we now use consistently.

A sense of fulfillment and deep appreciation is always felt when we see our patients able to return to their prior functioning through neurofeedback, even when the brain training is delayed a year after the concussion occurrence. Lisa came back to us recently because she sustained a repeat concussion through rough social interaction while playing with her peers, and she also hurt her right knee; it wasn't getting better and she wanted to know if the neurofeedback could help. This time she immediately came for treatment. We trained T4-O2, T4-T3, T3-C1, and T3-FP1. Right after the first session she reported her knee felt "good;" we dropped this site (T3-C1) by the third session, and continued training at T3-T5 and T3-P3. She required just 10 sessions before she felt back to her normal self again, performing consistently well in class. She has not returned, and we hope she stays well.

Patient E2: T4-O2, T4-FP2, T4-T3, T3-O1, T3-Fp1.
AFz + Pz ILF synchrony, Fp1 + Fp2 gamma synchrony.

Philip came to us after Lisa; he trained with the concussion protocol. Over time we stayed with the protocol, taking away T3-O1 and adding ILF synchrony to improve sleep. We later added bifrontal gamma synchrony to improve executive control, taking away T4-Fp2. He is succeeding in college, at lacrosse, and has stayed out of trouble with the law. His mother is thrilled; she refers other parents to bring their troubled children to us.

Patient F: T4-P4, T3-C1, T3-C3, T3-F7, T3-F3, T4-T3, T3-T5.

Julie was anxious and almost panicky about her physical well-being after the stroke which affected her dominant side. She had begun to teach herself to write and other dominant activities with her left hand and side. She was frustrated by her speech. We trained her with the following protocol: T4-P4, T3-C1, T3-C3, T3-F7, and T3-F3. Her speech recovered quickly and she no longer uses a walker, being adept with a cane. Although she has made great gains in independence, she is continuing the training, hoping to get back better right-hand function, which was most affected by the stroke. Although we have reduced the marked spasticity in the right hand through the neurofeedback training, the paresis remains. At this time, she continues with physical therapy and we recently referred her to occupational therapy. When she experienced the seizure (adult onset epilepsy frequently arises as sequela of a remote stroke), we modified the protocol to include T4-T3 and we added T3-T5, guided by the EEG findings of intermittent focal slowing recorded here, and removed T3-F7 because speech and swallowing functions had normalized. She remains on low dose topiramate daily and is prescribed lorazepam to be taken only as needed on an emergency basis (anticipatory management; the hope is she will not need it).

We do not give patients unrealistic expectations; we do allow them to train as long as they feel they are gaining benefit. We have one gentleman, 86-year-old Alan, who continues to come for neurofeedback sessions (220 and counting) after he sustained a concussion that significantly impacted his cognitive faculties two years ago. We are learning from our patients as we provide this neurotherapy to them and, therefore, do not attempt to project a finite number of sessions. Each session involves varied effort; those with the need and commitment to continue are supported.

Patient G: T4-P4, T4-FP2, T4-T3, T3-FP1, T3-O1.

Annabel is an important representative of young children with intractable epilepsy who do not respond to our typical medications. She had normal growth and development and was fully toilet-trained, a happy child, and then at age 3½ began to regress, becoming incontinent. Her mother thought she might have just had an accident here and there but then she noted her staring unresponsively during the episodes of incontinence and shaking her body softly. Over time her behavior began to change; she became aggressive and oppositional. She complained of frequent headaches. The episodes of incontinence progressed to occurring daily and she manifested mood swings. The first EEG was normal and as described in the vignette, we trialled her on several anticonvulsants without success. When she continued to have these episodes, we did a 24-hour ambulatory EEG a year later, after she was taken off all medications; this now revealed the left posterior regional slowing and rare spike paroxysms. This was her starting training protocol: T4-P4, T4-FP2, T4-T3, T3-FP1. When the EEG result became known we added T3-O1. We stayed at 0.01 mHz because she presented to us before the software upgrade allowing for lower frequencies, and then after only 17 sessions she had to move to Arizona. We called her mother for an update to include in her vignette. In grade school she is doing well academically. She is developing as expected without further seizure activity. Headaches still occur, but infrequently, responsive to acetaminophen. Were 17 sessions enough, we wonder?

Patient H: T4-O2, T4-FP2, T4-T3, T3-O1, T3-FP1, T3-T5, T3-P3, T3-F7, T3-F3

Isaac is a youngster with well-controlled epilepsy who had problems academically, behaviorally, and socially. We trained him in the following protocol, guided by his EEG findings: T4-O2, T4-FP2, T4-T3, T3-O1, and T3-Fp1. In subsequent sessions

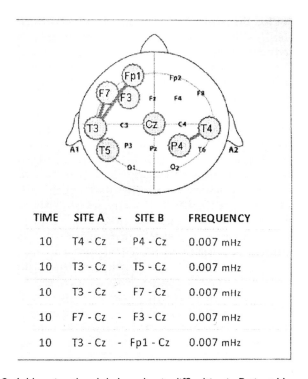

TIME	SITE A	-	SITE B	FREQUENCY
10	T4 - Cz	-	P4 - Cz	0.007 mHz
10	T3 - Cz	-	T5 - Cz	0.007 mHz
10	T3 - Cz	-	F7 - Cz	0.007 mHz
10	F7 - Cz	-	F3 - Cz	0.007 mHz
10	T3 - Cz	-	Fp1 - Cz	0.007 mHz

Figure 8.9 Addressing the global academic difficulties in Patient H.

we removed T4-Fp2 and T3- O1 and trained him at T3-T5 and T3-P3. The final protocol Isaac trained in is shown in Figure 8.9. As you can see, we addressed expressive speech last and replaced T4-O2 with T4-P4.

Isaac is managed with lamotrigine monotherapy long term. He remains seizure-free and his mother reports he continues to make great strides in the school setting. Isaac received a Most Improved Student award, not an unusual feat for this patient population who respond well to ILF brain training.

8.6 Viewpoints: Neurofeedback Practice in a Neurology Office

In the past five years, three neurologists have prescribed this form of neurotherapy for over 200 patients. A significant increase in "drop-out" rate is seen when insurance is restrictive, however, a significant number return when their coverage changes. Currently we anticipate at least 50% of new patients to become covered. Including the patient cases discussed here, we have about 45 "graduates." There remain a few who may choose to never graduate. At any given time, we have a total of between 90 to 110 active patients. We have two exam rooms devoted to this practice.

We do not feel the need to advertise our neurofeedback services. We have witnessed a steadily increasing demand for this form of neurotherapy over the last three years, and now see the need to expand the service.

It would be ideal to perform systematic outcome studies for these patients; case numbers are too small and variability in presentation is too great to allow conclusive judgments to be made at present. *Observation* and *trial and error* remain our methods of investigation, wherein the patient serves as their own control at baseline and throughout the training process.

It should be apparent that each patient's brain is unique and requires a tailored training protocol. The patient's progress (or lack thereof) should be noted between sessions and the protocol modified accordingly. We start everyone at 0.01 mHz and by session five we have everyone who tolerates it training at 0.008 mHz or lower. Children appear to tolerate the shifts to lower frequency training more readily. We find that most patients tolerate the same low frequency in both hemispheres, but we are prepared to double this frequency on the left side if needed, as per protocol guidelines. In general, the training is very well tolerated. In between their sessions patients are encouraged to work at their specific challenges, especially right after the session over the ensuing 2–3 days. For example, young children with reading and writing challenges are encouraged to work each of these skills, executing at least three 8.5 x 11 inch pages a day; adults with stroke symptoms to implement rehabilitative therapies of the affected part(s); and elderly adults with Parkinson's disease to do their prescribed balancing and other specific exercises repetitively. All patients are advised to take supplemental vitamin B complex and to maintain neurovascular health by performing non-strenuous aerobic exercise for at least 10–15 minutes three times a week, or 5 minutes a day.

It is emphasized this form of FDA-recognized neurofeedback continues to evolve, with more being learned with each software update. It will very likely be the case that any future writings on the experience with infra-low frequency and synchrony brain training will be modified from the last as software improvements and protocol evolution continue.

8.7 Summary Statement

Employing EEG-based neuromodulation and infra-low frequency brain training in a neurology practice empowers the inherent inclination for restorative healing present in each patient. Maladaptive developmental trajectories can be shifted towards healthier routes. Together with powerful drugs, prescribed to manage the varied severe neurological disorders (when these drugs are effective and well tolerated), the use of clinical neurofeedback is integrative. In the context of treating medically refractory central nervous system disorders of dysregulation, there exists no remediation that is less invasive. This "second-generation neurofeedback" is a compelling option to explore prior to surgical or other exogenous considerations (vagus nerve stimulation, deep brain stimulation, or transcranial magnetic stimulation).

We are proponents of the proposition that the dysregulated brain is remediable to its optimal homeostasis via endogenous neuromodulation, with ILF and EEG feedback exploiting latent neuroplasticity. At the time of this writing, advances in

ILF technology now allow for even more impactful low frequency training. The networks that are earliest to develop have the lowest frequencies; indeed, the routine EEG of a very premature infant (24–26 weeks age of gestation) is mostly flat, given the applied low filter cut-off at 0.5 Hz in standard AC recordings.[43, 44]

Incorporating the practice of neurofeedback in a neurology office requires additional training and learning, which currently entails a 5-day intensive course and extra readings. After the training course, annual summit meetings are held for active practitioners to stay informed with globally shared clinical experiences, updates in development, and advances in practice. Summit meetings can be attended by livestreaming and post-event viewing is also made available. There is online guidance 24/7 from the global professional community as well as technical support from the developers of the system. As an advocate for this tool in a neurology practice, I cannot emphasize sufficiently how taking this extra step has made a significant difference in what we can offer our patients with heretofore unmanageable and untreatable central nervous system disorders. It was a natural evolution for our practice to streamline our neurodiagnostic workflow with EEG-based neurotherapy.

The central nervous system's essential roles are correlation, adaptation, and homeostasis, allowing the whole organism to live in harmony with its environment. Homo sapiens' brains have additional prefrontal processing allowing for creativity, executive planning, and less reflexive responses to our environment as well as to psychosocial influences.[45, 43] The knowledge and practice of infra-low frequency neurofeedback requires a lifelong developmental perspective on the brain. Our aim is to recover a healthy homeostasis from prior untoward and current maladaptive influences acting on the brain. Not least, the practice empowers our patients towards that greatest of all therapeutic objectives, *self*-healing.

Notes

1 Othmer S, Othmer SF, Kaiser DA, Putman J. 2013. Endogenous neuromodulation at infralow frequencies. *Semin Pediatr Neurol* 20(246):257.

2 McMahon D. 2013. Notes from clinical practice: An MD's perspective on 9 years of neurofeedback practice. *Semin Pediatr Neurol* 20:258–260.

3 This congenital cardiac defect is well known to harbor blood clots. Blood clots break down into smaller clots called emboli that travel through blood vessels going to the brain. When brain vessels become occluded by emboli this results in lack of blood flow and subsequent death of dependent brain cells or "strokes" in the brain.

4 Jasper HH. 1958. The 10–20 electrode system of the international federation. *Electroencephalogr Clin Neurophysiol* 10:367–380.

5 Chatrian GE, Lettich E, Nelson PL. 1985. Ten percent electrode system for topographic studies of spontaneous and evoked EEG activity. *Am J EEG Technol* 25:83–92.

6 Zenke F, Gerstner W, Ganguli S. 2017. The Temporal paradox of hebbian learning and homeostatic plasticity. *Current Op in Neurobiol* 43:166–176.

7 Hellyer PJ, Jachs B, Clopath C, Leech R. 2016. Local inhibitory plasticity tunes macroscopic brain dynamics and allows the emergence of functional brain networks. *Neuroimage* 124:85–95.

8   De Pitta M, Brunel N, Volterra A. 2016. Astrocytes: Orchestrating synaptic plasticity? *Neuroscience* 323:43–61.

9   Thatcher RW, Palmero-Soler E, North DM, Biver CJ. 2016. Intelligence and EEG measures of information flow: Efficiency and homeostatic neuroplasticity. *Scientific Reports* 6(38890):1–10.

10 Acharya JN, Hani A, Cheek J, Thirumala P, et al. 2016. American clinical neurophysiology society guideline 2: Guidelines for standard electrode position nomenclature. *J Clin Neurophysiol* 33(4):308–311.

11 Towle VL, Bolanos J, Suarez D, Tan K, et al. 1993. The spatial location of EEG electrodes: Locating the best-fitting sphere relative to cortical anatomy. *Electroenceph Clin Neurophysiol* 86:1–6.

12 Blume WT, Buza RC, Okazaki H. 1974. Anatomic correlates of the ten-twenty electrode placement system in infants. *Electroenceph Clin Neurophysiol* 36:303–307.

13 Homan RW, Herman J, Purdy P. 1987. Cerebral Location of international 10–20 system electrode placement. *Electroenceph Clin Neurophysiol* 66:376–382.

14 Koessler L, Maillard L, Benhadid A, Vignal JP, et al. 2009. Automated cortical projection of EEG sensors: Anatomical correlation via the international 10–10 system. *Neuroimage* 46:64–72.

15 Kabdebon C, Leroy F, Simmonet H, Perrot M, et al. 2014. Anatomical correlations of the international 10–20 sensor placement system in infants. *Neuroimage* 99:342–356.

16 Legarda S, Jayakar P, Duchowny M, Alvarez L, et al. 1994. Benign rolandic epilepsy: High central and low central subgroups. *Epilepsia* 35(6):1125–1129.

17 Erikson EH. 1959. *Identity and the Life Cycle*. New York: International Universities Press.

18 Erikson EH, Joan M. 1997. *The Life Cycle Completed: Extended Version*. New York: W. W. Norton.

19 Goleman, Daniel. 1996. *Emotional Intelligence: Why it can Matter more than IQ*. London: Bloomsbury, 1996.

20 Legarda S, Jayakar P, Duchowny M, Alvarez L, et al. 1994. Benign rolandic epilepsy: High central and low central subgroups. *Epilepsia* 35(6):1125–1129.

21 Saxby E, Peniston EG. 1995. Alpha-theta brainwave EEG biofeedback training: An effective treatment for male and female alcoholics with depressive symptoms. *J Clin Psychol* 51:685–693.

22 Raichle ME, Macleod AM, Snyder AZ, Powers WJ, et al. 2001. A default mode of brain function. *PNAS* 98(2):676–682.

23 Seminowicz DA, Davis KD. 2007. Pain enhances functional connectivity of a brain network evoked by performance of a cognitive task. *J Neurophysiol* 97:3651–3659.

24 Power JD, Fair DA, Schlaggar BL, Petersen SE. 2010. The development of human functional brain networks. *Neuron* 67(5):735–748.

25 Sowell ER, Thompson PM, Holmes CJ, Jernigan TL, et al. 1999. In vivo evidence for post-adolescent brain maturation in frontal and striatal regions. *Nat Neurosci* 2(10):859–861.

26 Hammeroff S. 2010. The "conscious pilot" – Dendritic synchrony moves through the brain to mediate consciousness. *J Biol Phys.* 36:71–93.

27 Laccarino HF, Singer AC, Martorell AJ, Rudenko A, et al. 2016. Gamma frequency entrainment attenuates amyloid load and modifies microglia. *Nature* 540(7632):230.

28 Folstein MF, Folstein SE, McHugh PR. 1975. "Mini-Mental State". A practical method for grading the cognitive state of patients for the clinician. *J Psychiatr Res* 12(3):189–198.
29 Nasreddine ZS, Phillips NA, Bédirian V, Charbonneau S, et al. 2005. "The montreal cognitive assessment, MOCA: A brief screening tool for mild cognitive impairment". *J Am Geriatr Soc.* 53(4):695–699.
30 Othmer SF. 2019. *Protocol Guide for Neurofeedback Clinicians* (7th Ed). Woodland Hills, CA: EEG Institute.
31 Binder JR. 2015. The Wernicke Area. Modern evidence and a reinterpretation. *Neurology* 85:2170–2175.
32 Ardila A, Bernal B, Rosselli M. 2016. How localized are language brain areas? A review of Brodmann areas involvement in oral language. *Arch Clin Neuropsych* 31:112–122.
33 Siegel JS, Snyder AZ, Metcalf NV, Fucetola RP, et al. 2014. The circuitry of abulia: Insights from functional connectivity MRI. *NeuroImage: Clinical* 6:320–326.
34 Chiron C, Jambaque I, Nabbout R, Lounes R, et al. 1997. The right brain hemisphere is dominant in human infants. *Brain* 120:1057–1065.
35 Schore JR, Schore AN. 2008. Modern attachment theory: The central role of affect regulation in development and treatment. *Clin Soc Work J.* 36:9–20.
36 Schore AN. 2014. The right brain is dominant in psychotherapy. *Psychotherapy* 51(3):388–397.
37 Gogtay N, Jay N, Giedd JN, Lusk L. 2004. Dynamic mapping of human cortical development during childhood through adulthood. *PNAS* 101(21):8174–8179.
38 Holland P. R. 2014. Headache and sleep: Shared pathophysiological mechanisms. *Cephalgia* 34(10):725–744.
39 Conti PCR, Costa YM, Goncalves DA, Svensson PA. 2016. Headaches and myofascial temporomandibular disorders: Overlapping entities, separate managements? *J Oral Rehab* 43:702–715.
40 Piovesan EJ, Kowacs PA, Tatsui CE, Lange MC, et al. 2001. Referred pain after painful stimulation of the greater occipital nerve in humans: Evidence of convergence of cervical afferences on trigeminal nuclei. *Cephalalgia* 21(2):107–109.
41 Pizza V, Milano W, Padricelli U, Capasso A. 2017. Novel therapeutic Investigations in migraine pain. *PhOL Archives* 3:32–48.
42 Savage J, Ferguson CJ, Flores L. 2017. The effect of academic achievement on aggression and violent behavior: A meta-analysis. *Aggre Viol Behav* 37:91–101.
43 Hahn JS, Hannebre M, Tharp BR. 1989. Interburst interval measurements in the EEGs of premature infants with normal neurological outcome. *Clinical Neurophysiology* 73(5):410–418.
44 Tsuchida TN, Wusthoff CJ, Shellhaas RA, Abend NS, et al. 2013. ACNS standardized EEG terminology and categorization for the description of continuous EEG monitoring in neonates. *J Clin Neurophysiol* 30:161–173.
45 Teffer K, Semendeferi K. 2012. Human prefrontal cortex: Evolution, development and pathology. *Prog Brain Res* 195:191–218.

Part III

**Specific Applications
Areas of Neurofeedback**

Chapter 9

Early Development and Childhood Emotional and Behavioral Disorders

Roxana Sasu

9.1 Introduction

This chapter covers various aspects of neurodevelopmental disorders, as well as behavioral and emotional disorders of childhood and adolescence. It presents an overview of ten years of working with this population in our clinical practice of neurofeedback. It illustrates how our implementation of Infra-Low Frequency (ILF) Neurofeedback training, with emphasis on interpreting presenting symptoms in terms of basic failure modes, guides the clinical decisions made throughout the process. Several illustrative case studies are presented, some with similar formal diagnoses but strikingly different clinical presentations, highlighting the uniqueness of each case. The case studies also show how interesting and challenging this work with early childhood developmental and behavioral disorders can be for the clinician. At the same time, this work is satisfying and rewarding when the clinician can observe the positive impact of neurofeedback on all these disorders and see also how the neurofeedback complements and potentiates other interventions and modalities used to address such issues in children and adolescents.

9.2 Neurodevelopmental Disorders

Neurodevelopmental disorders are a group of neurologically based conditions with onset in the developmental period that can interfere with the acquisition, retention, or application of specific skills or sets of information. They may involve dysfunction in attention, memory, perception, language, problem-solving, or social interaction. Neurodevelopmental disorders include attention-deficit/hyperactivity disorder (ADD/ADHD), autism spectrum disorders, learning disabilities and intellectual disabilities. Neurodevelopmental disorders frequently co-occur, for example, individuals with autism spectrum disorder often have intellectual disability (intellectual developmental disorder), and many children with ADHD also have a specific learning disorder. Looking beyond the formal diagnoses, our clinical work focuses on the wide range of developmental, behavioral, and emotional symptoms for which the families of these younger clients seek neurofeedback.

In our neurofeedback clinic children and adolescents comprise about 50% of the clientele. Most of them seek help for a variety of issues, ranging from anxiety and depression to emotional reactivity and aggressiveness, from impulsiveness to obsessive compulsive symptoms, and so much more. Neurofeedback is being used for this population when traditional medicine is either not enough to alleviate their often chronic symptoms, or disturbing and dysfunctional behavior, or when the children's parents, fearful of adverse reactions and side effects, want to avoid the medication route all together. In broad generality, neurofeedback has proven to be an effective intervention to add to any other modality the clients are relying on to overcome their difficulties.

9.3 Risk Factors Associated with Mental, Behavioral, and Developmental Disorders (MBDDs) in Children

It has long been demonstrated that sociodemographic factors and environmental factors in early childhood have significant impact on development, mental health, and overall health throughout the lifespan. In a report published in March 2016, the Centers of Disease Control (CDC) offers some national data identifying significant associations of early childhood mental, behavioral and developmental disorders (MBDDs) with sociodemographic, health care, family and community factors.[1] The factors most strongly associated with early childhood MBDDs were fair or poor parental mental health, poverty and child care problems (for the 2–3 years age group). The analysis was based on data gathered through a parent-reported survey among parents of children between 2–8 years (National Survey of Children's Health 2011–2012).[2,3] While the report only included children with diagnosed disorders and was based on parents' reports that can be biased or contain errors, it revealed that 1 out of 7 U.S. children aged 2 to 8 years old had a diagnosed mental, behavioral or developmental disorder. The report highlighted the need to direct resources toward improving healthcare and supporting families and communities in order to prevent early childhood MBDDs and promote healthy developmental among all young children.

9.4 Prevalence of Behavioral, Emotional and Developmental Disorders in Children

The first comprehensive CDC mental health report from 2013 describes the number of U.S. children aged 3–17 years who have specific mental disorders, such as ADHD, disruptive behavioral disorder, oppositional defiant disorder, conduct disorder, autism spectrum disorder, mood and anxiety disorder, substance abuse and Tourette Syndrome.[4] The report used data collected from a variety of sources between the years 2005–2011, and the analysis of the data revealed the following:

Children aged 3–17 years identified as having a current diagnosis of:

- Attention-deficit/hyperactivity disorder (ADHD) (6.8%)
- Behavioral or conduct problems (3.5%)
- Anxiety (3.0%)
- Depression (2.1%)
- Autism spectrum disorder (1.1%)
- Tourette syndrome (0.2%) (among children aged 6–17 years)

Adolescents aged 12–17 years identified as having a current diagnosis of:

- Illicit drug use disorder in the past year (4.7%)
- Alcohol use disorder in the past year (4.2%)
- Cigarette dependence in the past month (2.8%)

Suicide, which can result from the interaction of mental disorders and other factors, was the second leading cause of death among adolescents aged 12–17 years in 2010. The number of children with a mental disorder increased with age, except for autism spectrum disorders which is highest among the 6–11 years age group.

The National Alliance on Mental Illness (NAMI)[5] citing statistics provided by the National Institute of Mental Health revealed a different, more severe situation:

- 20% of youth aged 13–18 years live with a mental health condition
- 11% of youth aged 13–18 years have a mood disorder
- 10% of youth aged 13–18 years have a behavior/conduct disorder
- 8% of youth aged 13–18 years have an anxiety disorder

Considering that the average delay between onset and intervention is 8–10 years, one can understand the importance of addressing emotional, behavioral or developmental concerns as early as possible.

In a state-by-state ranking for 2017, Mental Health America states that 11% of youth (age 12–17) report suffering from at least one major depressive episode (MDE) in the past year.[6] Major Depression is marked by significant and pervasive feelings of sadness that are associated with suicidal thoughts and impair a young person's ability to concentrate or engage in normal activities. The data indicate a significant increase in the number of depressed youths across the country over time.

- 7.4% of youth (or 1.8 million youths) experienced severe depression. These youths experienced very serious interference in school, home and in relationships.
- 5.13% of youth in America report having a substance abuse or alcohol problem.

The report continues with another sobering fact: 64% of youth with major depression do not receive any mental health treatment, which means that 6 out of 10 young people who suffer from depression, and who are most at risk of suicidal thoughts, difficulty in school and difficulty in relationships with others, do not get the treatment needed to support them. With such a high number of youths suffering from various severe and debilitating symptoms there is a great need for treatment modalities that can prevent and restore optimal function, and neurofeedback can play a central role here.

9.5 Diagnosis-based versus Symptom-based Treatment Approach

As discussed above, often MBDDs go undiagnosed until later in life. This explains why some of the youngest clients we see for neurofeedback training don't come with a formal diagnosis. They are brought to us because teachers or parents have concerns about them. Even among the ones who have been formally diagnosed, with our thorough assessment we reveal a variety of symptoms that oftentimes challenge the boundaries of the label. That allows us to build training protocols to include all the client's needs and this integrative approach leads to a better regulated nervous system, with positive consequences across the board.

In our long experience working with children on the spectrum, we have learned that an integrative approach will always yield the best results.[7] While neurofeedback can make a significant difference in symptoms, as it helps the brain self-regulate and function more optimally, other modalities can complement it and provide support while the brain rewires. Speech therapy, occupational therapy and music therapy, as well as ABA (Applied Behavioral Analysis) or Floor Time therapy, are just some of the more mainstream interventions used with this population, and it is well documented that the earlier the interventions, the better the outcomes. Less well-known, perhaps, but also very effective, are the various biomedical interventions, along with special diets to address underlying sensitivities, allergies or inflammatory processes. Music therapy as another way of training the brain into self-regulation has acquired a solid reputation for addressing the sensory processing and integration issues that often accompany spectrum disorders. Another aspect known to make a great difference is related to parenting. While support and love are important as they are for any child, setting appropriate limits is equally important, and failing to do so does more harm than good for this population, for which structure and predictability may well make the difference between chaos and a somewhat settled existence.

In our practice we get to work with a lot with clients who suffer with attachment disorders and symptoms related to it. Often children are brought to us due to escalating aggressiveness that is frequently directed towards adoptive parents. Attachment is the deep connection established between children and their primary caregivers—one that profoundly affects the child's development, their ability to express emotions and to build meaningful relationships later in life. If this core skill fails to develop early on, either due to neglect or abuse, the child will never learn to feel safe and secure in their environment and won't develop trust in others. This will have a significant impact on all aspects of later development, with the child presenting with poor self-confidence and self-esteem, an inability to build and maintain relationships, difficulty with emotional control and so much more. Neurofeedback training can restore that core sense of self and moderate the fear response to calm the brain and relieve the hair-trigger emergency response. That will have a profound impact on emotional regulation and control and will allow the child to develop a stronger sense of self and better relationships with others.

Anxiety is a normal physiological response to a threat in the environment. In anxiety disorders, however, the response to things that one should be able to cope with easily become out of proportion. Despite the 17% increase in anxiety disorder diagnosis in children and adolescents reported by the 2018 Child Mind Institute[8] report on children's mental health, anxiety remains untreated in 80% of this population. Described as the "invisible condition," anxiety is mistaken for other conditions and its symptoms minimized or ignored. Unfortunately, untreated anxiety leads to greater risk for depression, school failure, substance abuse and difficulty transitioning to adulthood. The average age of onset for separation anxiety is 11 years old, while the average age of onset for social anxiety is around 14 years old. Anxiety disorders are linked to a two-fold increase for substance abuse disorder. Anxiety and depression often coexist and in teenagers this is associated with more suicidal ideation, suicide attempts and more depressive symptoms.

Beyond the suffering of many children and adolescents we need to consider the socio-economic implications of unrecognized, undiagnosed and untreated mental health conditions in youth, knowing that 37% of students with a mental health condition age 14 and older drop out of school.[9] This is the highest dropout rate of any disability group. It is also noteworthy that according to the National Institute of Mental Health,[10] 70% of youth in state and local juvenile justice systems have a mental illness.

9.6 Case Studies

The case studies that follow are complex cases with a mixture of different symptoms in the realm of behavior, emotional and developmental disorders. They are, however, quite representative of what we encounter in our clinic.

When working with children who present symptoms of MBDDs, the neurofeedback process focuses on the right hemisphere to impact arousal levels. In some cases, it includes inter- hemispheric training to increase stability of function. That is not surprising given the fact that many symptoms in this realm stem from disruptions in early development that can interfere with learning how to self-regulate and self-soothe. The right brain is involved in early development of self-regulation; training this side of the brain allows for grounding and calming, which results in better emotional regulation and allows meaningful attachments.[11]

9.6.1 Case Study #1

This 6-year-old boy was brought to us for a variety of presenting symptoms. The official diagnosis was Asperger's Syndrome, or high functioning autism. His developmental history revealed a difficult pregnancy after in vitro fertilization (IVF), with the mother being placed on bed rest for most of the pregnancy. He was born prematurely at 31 weeks, weighing only 3.7 lbs, and then spent 21 days in NICU while isolated from his mother.

The first two years of life were described as difficult by his parents. Developmental delays in walking and talking, as well as poor eye contact and little meaningful communication, were concerns early on. When he arrived in our clinic, he presented with significant sensory processing and integration difficulties, which manifested as long periods of spinning and seeking pressure on his body—bumping into things or people. He had a very limited diet and avoided certain smells and textures. He wouldn't eat if different foods touched each other on the plate. Stimming behaviors were reported; he would move his toy cars back and forth and close his eyes for long periods of time. He was described as inflexible, having difficulties with transitions and changes in his routine. He was easily frustrated and any emotional dysregulation increased the intensity of motor tics, like blinking and twisting fingers or toes etc. When becoming anxious, he would tense up his body and would experience increased agitation, with his speech becoming more repetitive. With an increase in agitation and anxiety he could become aggressive. He had to be pulled out of three different schools due to violent behavior toward his peers.

Compulsions were another big concern; he always wanted his toy cars with him and would refuse to engage in other activities if he didn't have them. Repetitive hand washing was another presenting problem. Limited social interaction and poor expressive and receptive language skills were reported as well. He exhibited a variety of fears, which seemed to change over time. He was often constipated and parents suspected food allergies to be the reason for periodic skin rashes.

He came to us for intensive training and the training effects became obvious early on in the process. Following the developmental sequence, we focused on providing physical calming and emotional regulation and control, which called for two of the primary protocols. He calmed down significantly and after only three sessions he tried a new food and became more affectionate toward his mother. One of the first symptoms to respond to the training was constipation, which resolved quickly as a result of the calming effect of the training. He was in a significantly better mood and more easy-going with transitions. By session 6, speech patterns started changing from repetitive speech unrelated to ongoing discussions to more appropriate and diversified responses. At the end of the intensive training he was calmer overall and was less engaged in seeking sensory input. He was more adventurous in trying new foods and much less compulsive. He could still get upset with changes in his routine, but he was bouncing back faster; fears were less of a problem and he displayed increased interest in communicating with others. He was showing more affection to his parents and exhibited improved eye contact. He was more aware of others and tics were not as intense with heightened emotions. Sugar cravings and stimming behaviors had diminished as well. Parents suspected an underlying undiagnosed inflammatory disease and wanted to investigate complex biomedical testing and a diet based on the findings before continuing neurofeedback training, but it was clear after only 20 sessions that neurofeedback was a valuable tool in their toolbox.

9.6.2 Case Study #2

This 4-year-old girl, diagnosed with autism, was brought to us for training mainly to improve verbal communication. Born into a bilingual family, the child had very little language. There was poor eye contact, she would not answer when called, presented with short attention span and echolalia. She was highly sensitive to sugar intake, which made her very hyperactive. At the same time, she had limited her food choices and her appetite awareness was poor. Before starting the training she couldn't count, drawing was more like a scribble, and she threw frequent tantrums when things wouldn't go her way. Her developmental history revealed regression following a vaccine administered at 18 months. At the time of the vaccine she had about 10–20 words, but she stopped talking altogether after having it. She also exhibited some aggressive behaviors—hitting and screaming when not getting her way. She was not engaging with peers and didn't quite understand reciprocity when interacting with others.

After just a couple of sessions the girl started using more language and was recruiting new words. Her mother also reported that her appetite appeared to be better regulated and that she tried a food she had disliked in the past. By her sixth session the teacher reported that the child started counting and was now naming objects and organizing them by category. Soon thereafter she started writing her name and continued to experiment with new foods. In later sessions it was reported that her separation anxiety had moderated, and she was able to sit on her own in sessions instead of having to sit on her mother's lap. While it may seem minor, this was a significant step forward toward independence. All these changes were observed within the first set of 20 sessions, when the emphasis of the training was on calming her nervous system down.

9.6.3 Case Study #3

A 6-year-old boy, adopted at 18 months, presented with frequent tantrums, fear of anything new, hypervigilance and inflexibility. He was behind in reading and sometimes displayed immaturity in both behaviors and emotions. He had difficulties falling asleep and had frequent nightmares, all related to his feeling unsafe. He was manipulative and defiant, would lie a lot and was insensitive to others. He was obsessed with trying to control things in his environment, and he carried a lot of anger and was subject to mood swings. Teachers were concerned about his disruptive behavior in class, his distractibility and difficulty following directions and staying on task. 20 sessions into the training he had no nightmares or difficulties in falling asleep. Teachers and parents were seeing some significant improvement in his behaviors—he was less moody and much less worried, hypervigilance had lessened and he didn't feel the need to control everything around him as much anymore. Anger outbursts became less frequent and less intense and he experienced fewer mood swings. He was better with trying new things, not as fearful as he had been. There was some improvement in his ability to follow directions and stay on task, but it was clear that much more training was needed to consolidate these gains and further work was required on some of the behaviors that were about the same as before training. He was more connected and was displaying an increased ability to process things in a more mature manner.

9.6.4 Case Study #4

This 9-year-old boy had suffered hypoxia during birth. He was first in foster care and was then adopted, but his first two years of life had been rather traumatic. The parents' main concerns were his emotional reactivity and negative self-talk, the tantrums and oppositional behaviors as well as high anxiety that would make him shut down. Aggressiveness and sometimes rage were reported as well. He would get easily frustrated over homework and would start negative self-talk that would continue for a while. He had a difficult time recovering after being triggered. He suffered from constipation, which often is a consequence of living in fight-or-flight mode. He had a restless sleep and sometimes would complain of headaches and stomach aches. His sustained attention was poor and he needed constant redirection in order to complete his work. Impulsiveness was also a reported concern. He had had several physical injuries and concussions. The first QIKtest revealed difficulties with task maintenance when performing under both low-demand and high-demand conditions, and confirmed the difficulty he had in recovering after being pushed in high-demand situations for a longer period.

Already four sessions into the training he was much less reactive, and even said he was feeling happier. Constipation was improving. The teacher noticed that class-work was easier to complete and was impressed with his progress. He was calmer overall and was responding much better to being told "no," becoming less reactive and able to bounce back more easily. By session 13 he was better organized and able to plan his day, was completing schoolwork on his own in a timely manner, and continued to be in a better mood. He maintained good emotional control while the family went through a crisis, which would have been unimaginable before neurofeedback. While he will need more training to consolidate and maintain these training outcomes, it is exciting to see how quickly and dramatically he responded to training. No doubt the significant changes in symptoms will be reflected in the QIKtest when it is time to re-assess.

9.6.5 Case Study #5

The parents of this shy 7-year-old boy were seeking help for his debilitating anxiety, combined with physical agitation and obsessive worries that interfered with everyday life. During intake his parents described rituals and compulsions as well as emotional overwhelm when having to perform under pressure. He presented with low self-confidence and low self-esteem and had difficulties making friends. With increased anxiety sometimes he would shut down; at other times he would burst into tears or start compulsively cutting paper and chewing on it. Testing was a major anxiety trigger and any unstructured assignment would also result in increased anxiety. Stomach aches and sleep walking were also part of his clinical presentation. School days were mostly bad days in his perception, as he always feared failure and inability to complete tasks in given time. Over the course of the training, which spanned several years during which he came to sessions on and off, he went from being a withdrawn, fearful child to being happy and more confident and having mostly great days. His emotions were in better control, while thoughts and compulsions lessened. There were no more complaints of stomach aches and the anxiety, when emerging, was more manageable. With every big transition in his life—changing school and teachers, for instance, he still experienced some anxiety and would come in for maintenance sessions as needed. He has completed over 100 sessions to date and while the core of the training was directed towards calming all the aspects of his anxiety, we also worked on focus and frustration, self-confidence and ability to socialize. He became more flexible in new situations and less fearful of what the future would bring.

9.6.6 Case Study #6

This 5-year-old girl presented with difficulties following directions in school and at home, difficulties completing homework and disruptive behaviors in class. Some hyperactivity, emotional reactivity, tantrums and rage were reported by her parents. She would talk back to teachers and was bossy in interactions with her peers. Episodes of sleep talking and bruxism were also part of her clinical presentation. She was becoming self-conscious upon realizing she was often getting in trouble at school and her parents were concerned about her confidence being shattered. She presented as an energetic, happy and very talkative child that appeared hyperactive at times and seemed to lack self-control. She presented with obsessive worries about death and went through a period during which she displayed poor attachment toward her mother, being mean and distant. At times she would pick at her fingers. She responded quickly to sessions and the training allowed better self-regulation and optimal brain function. After less than 20 training sessions she was no longer grinding her teeth and was less hyperactive. She was now able to follow directions better at school, and her attention and hyperactivity greatly improved, to where she is now enjoying classwork and is performing quite well. Her previous attachment issues are gone and she no longer throws tantrums or rages. She is still coming in for tune-ups every now and then to maintain optimal function.

9.6.7 Case Study #7

This 15-year-old boy came in to seek help for his debilitating anxiety and OCD. He had a long history of difficulties controlling his emotions and taking responsibility for his actions. He described his anxiety manifesting as tension in his body, loss of appetite and feeling that everything is wrong. He would often worry about school and homework and this would interfere with his ability to complete the tasks. He reported feeling that he wouldn't remember things and having urges to constantly check everything. Ruminating on negative thoughts, vocal tics and pacing were also part of the presenting symptoms. His parents described him as an angry child with difficulties in school. He had been bullied for over a year and didn't tell anyone for all that time. The symptoms worsened towards the end of that year and he developed panic attacks and fears to the point that he had to be homeschooled for a while.

His baseline QIKtest revealed a very fast response time but poor accuracy, with many commission and omission errors and high variability of response times. His accuracy score was well below average. He had a hard time initiating a new task and had difficulties performing under pressure, especially when having to maintain being on task. Recovery was difficult as well, with more errors and high variability, as seen in Figure 9.1.

Two other tests were administered, after 10 and 20 sessions respectively, and there was a significant improvement in both, with the third one showing above average performance index and the accuracy index in the upper normal range. The overall improvements in brain performance as measured by the QIKtest are reflected in the results summary of test #2 and test #3, as shown in Figures 9.2 and 9.3.

Symptom-wise he had improved quite a bit after the first 20 sessions, feeling more relaxed and less anxious overall, reporting good sleep and better mood, with much reduced reactivity. His OCD had improved, but was still a big concern, and the reassessment revealed a need to continue training for symptoms related to that. After continuing training for another year, he was managing his stress levels very well and was doing much better overall. He went back into the school system without any problems.

Results Summary: .

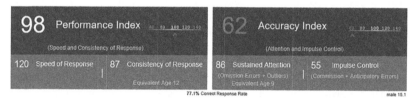

98 Performance Index			**62** Accuracy Index	
(Speed and Consistency of Response)			(Attention and Impulse Control)	
120 Speed of Response	87 Consistency of Response		86 Sustained Attention	55 Impulse Control
	Equivalent Age 12		(Omission Errors + Outliers) Equivalent Age 9	(Commission + Anticipatory Errors)

77.1% Correct Response Rate   male 15.1

Results	Data	Norm	Score	
M15.1 Total Test	Measured Value	Median of Distribution	Standard Score	Percentile
Omission Errors	10 errors	2₆ errors	82	12 %
Outlier Responses	5 errors	1₉ errors	89	24 %
Commission Errors	54 errors	8₅ errors	55	1₀ %
Response Time	319₆ ms	369 ms	120	90 %
Variability	106₆ ms	81 ms	87	19 %

RAW DATA	Period 1 Sect. 1 Low Demand	Period 2 Sect. 1 Low Demand	Period 3 Sect. 2 High Demand	Period 4 Sect. 2 High Demand	Period 5 Sect. 3 Low Demand	Sect. 1	Sect. 2	Sect 3	Total
Omissions(#)	6	0	0	3	1	6	3	1	10
Outliers	1	0	2	1	1	1	3	1	5
Commissions(#)	4	3	10	25	12	7	35	12	54
Response time(ms)	439	419	302	269	351	428	287	351	320
Variability(ms)	141	113	106	87	86	126	99	86	107

Figure 9.1 Initial QIKtest for case study #7.

Results Summary: .

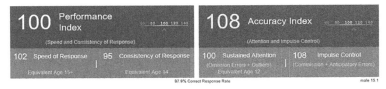

RAW DATA	Period 1 Sect. 1 Low Demand	Period 2 Sect. 1 Low Demand	Period 3 Sect. 2 High Demand	Period 4 Sect. 2 High Demand	Period 5 Sect. 3 Low Demand	Sect. 1	Sect. 2	Sect 3	Total
Omissions(#)	0	1	0	0	0	1	0	0	1
Outliers	0	1	1	1	1	1	2	1	4
Commissions(#)	1	0	2	2	0	1	4	0	5
Response time(ms)	388	436	352	347	450	411	350	450	372
Variability(ms)	100	77	97	100	98	93	99	98	95

Figure 9.2 Test #2: Case study #7 after 10 sessions

Results Summary: .

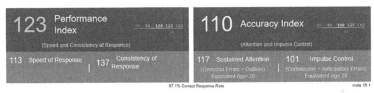

RAW DATA	Period 1 Sect. 1 Low Demand	Period 2 Sect. 1 Low Demand	Period 3 Sect. 2 High Demand	Period 4 Sect. 2 High Demand	Period 5 Sect. 3 Low Demand	Sect. 1	Sect. 2	Sect 3	Total
Omissions(#)	0	0	0	0	0	0	0	0	0
Outliers	0	0	1	0	0	0	1	0	1
Commissions(#)	0	0	1	4	3	0	5	3	8
Response time(ms)	359	384	329	306	357	372	318	357	332
Variability(ms)	29	30	59	59	58	32	60	58	47

Figure 9.3 Test #3: Case study #7 after 20 sessions.

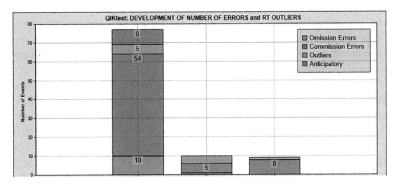

Figure 9.4 The development of number of errors and response time outliers.

9.6.8 Case Study #8

This teenage girl was seeking neurofeedback for severe anxiety and depression. She had a generalized anxiety disorder (GAD) and an ADHD diagnosis. Her birth had been problematic as she was oxygen-deprived during the process. She was diagnosed with severe separation anxiety at the very young age of two and had struggled with anxiety her entire life. Her anxiety manifested as physical tension and racing negative thoughts. She had poor emotional control and would experience rage and anger very frequently. The debilitating anxiety had led to depression, suicidal thoughts and one suicide attempt (by way of ingesting anti-anxiety medication). At times she would become aggressive when fear and anxiety escalated. Sleep was disrupted and she also had night-terrors and sleep walking episodes. Stomach pain, low appetite, headaches, bruxism, constipation and reflux were reported at the beginning of the training, and she also had irregular periods and severe PMS symptoms that would mostly impact her mood. Social anxiety, some compulsions and addictive behaviors completed the clinical presentation. She appeared fragile and thin, had dark circles under her eyes, and felt hopeless and fearful. She had been on several different medications, some of which resulted in the worsening of some of her symptoms. The training had a strong impact on her symptoms early on. Anxiety and sleep were the first symptoms to improve and gradually she started reporting a decrease in worries and depression. Her family also reported better emotional control. While coming in for sessions she started becoming more independent and more willing to take charge. She returned to school and started driving herself to appointments and to the gym. Soon her periods became regular again and she gained some weight, with her appearance changing to a healthier version of herself. She was smiling more and felt calmer and more confident. 20 sessions were just the beginning in her case, but the significant and profound changes she and her family had noticed were persuasive to them that significant improvement was possible. While undergoing neurofeedback training she was also in cognitive behavioral therapy, and the combination of the two, along with her parents' strong support, were probably the key to her success.

9.6.9 Case Study #9

This 10-year-old boy arrived with a dual diagnosis of ADHD and OCD. He was brought to training for impulsivity, rage and high anxiety, which was expressed as obsessive worries and negative thoughts about people getting hurt, especially those really close to him. He was described as a very bright and strong-willed child who was argumentative and very reactive, quick to anger and sometimes aggressive. Frustration would often spiral into negative self-talk, and once started it would take a long time to calm down. He sometimes took a long time to fall asleep when worries would escalate, and occasionally he would have nightmares. He was addicted to electronics and would become reactive and aggressive when screen time was restricted. Always very fast-paced, he was hyperactive and had little impulse control. Headaches and some sensory-seeking behaviors completed the clinical presentation. He was on a stimulant and an antidepressant when we started training. These were helping but not completely controlling his symptoms. He had suffered a traumatic birth and never learned to crawl. He had always been a poor sleeper and had sensory processing and integration issues of longstanding.

In this case the multitude of physiological issues, along with the varying effects of medication changes, made it almost impossible to fold neurofeedback in successfully. While some symptoms improved quickly others proved to be more difficult to get to, especially because this young brain proved to be highly sensitive and easily destabilized. A complex clinical presentation like this requires more patience and a very systematic approach that might take longer to implement than in other cases. And sometimes clients simply won't want to wait for neurofeedback to reveal their true potential, either because the symptoms are too disruptive or perhaps because the medication route is faster and easier. That was the case with this boy, as the family gave up after 15 neurofeedback sessions and before we were able to fully develop and implement the treatment plan. That, too, is a reality in fee-for-service clinical practice. However, we did get a glimpse of what can be achieved in this case, and often clients find their way back to us later when they are ready to undertake this longer and more demanding process.

9.6.10 Case Study #10

The following report represents an almost ideal case to review in that the child at issue benefited from having very competent, concerned and caring parents who spared no resources in getting the child the help that he needed. The parents faithfully pursued numerous therapeutic options for several years before encountering ILF training. One likely causal contributor to the problem in this case was high mercury levels in the entire family due to fish consumption in Asia, where the family resided at the time.

Difficulties were noted with the child from the time of birth in 2007. At fifteen months, there was a bad reaction to the MMR vaccine. Adrenaline and steroid injections followed. At two years of age the child was diagnosed with RSV (Respiratory Syncytial Virus), for which he was hospitalized. At age 2.5, the child was still unable to chew his food or to use a straw. He also exhibited stimming behavior.

Chelation was used for the removal of mercury. The child received Vitamin B12 injections and benefited from hyperbaric oxygen therapy. There was also an extended trial of conventional (EEG-band, frequency-based) neurofeedback that turned out to be unproductive, according to the parents. With the biomedical methods being employed the child began to use words, but this was clearly a matter of rote learning. There was no context and no novelty. The child did, however, develop some self-awareness. Speech therapy, which was pursued intensively, was largely unproductive. The speech therapist eventually capitulated, pronouncing in exasperation that the child was suffering from "rigidity of mind."

The child came to ILF training directly from speech therapy, at the threshold of entering school in 2013 at age six. Intensive training of 20 sessions was conducted over the course of two weeks. The child was judged incapable of taking the QIK test. He made observable progress with every training session. After the first session, his gait changed from unstable, quick walking to a more stable, calmer and slower paced gait. After the first day, the concept of "yesterday, today and tomorrow" was finally understood. The parents had been trying to teach that for a year.

The resting heart rate dropped from 125 to 85. At the end of the first day the child constructed his first novel sentence at dinnertime. The child became more aware of his surroundings, more attentive to events happening around him, and more connected with his parents. He did not have to be kept on a virtual leash all the time. By the end of the 20 sessions, the child was off all his medications and supplements (which had been more than 20), continuing only with conventional vitamins, enzymes and probiotics.

The family took the Cygnet® system home to Asia with them to continue training their child. He was accepted immediately into school with no concerns upon returning from Los Angeles.

Alternatively, there would have been no school option for him for another year. At this point, he was unable to say whether eight was larger or smaller than ten. He was still poor at social behavior and communication. Within weeks of returning to Asia, the diagnosis of autism spectrum disorder was replaced by "Social Communication Disorder," by the same developmental pediatrician who had originally diagnosed the autism.

By 2014, all biomedical treatments such as B-12 shots had been stopped, except for the occasional chelation. Parents concentrated on speech therapy and occupational therapy in addition to neurofeedback. The child passed his interview for acceptance into a new school. During the year, the parents returned to Los Angeles for more (brief) training of the child, and for additional speech therapy.

By 2015, chelation had been stopped as well. The parents returned to the U.S. for more neurofeedback (for the evaluation of additional protocols) and for speech therapy. The child was now able to do the QIKtest for the first time. He scored in the normal range across the board. He had conversations with staff during sessions, was engaged and happy, calm and focused. His mother described him as affectionate for the first time, as he had started hugging her without invitation, and he was making more eye contact. He was less obsessive and his language comprehension had improved, along with his fine motor skills (handwriting).

Near the end of the school year he earned a star student award (one of four meted out during the year in his class of 15) and was noted for "active listening" and being the "best reader in his class." In the fall he needed no more learning support and was at third Grade level in math. Prior concern with low muscle tone, poor coordination and poor spatial awareness had been replaced by commendations from physical education teachers. He was becoming a role model to classmates and was chosen to sing a brief solo in the Christmas musical. The year before he had been given a non-speaking role.

In the spring of 2016, he received another star student award in his second-grade class. His second QIKtest showed vast improvement over the first. In 2017, his QIKtest scores were superior all round. Percentile scores for all three tests are shown in Figure 9.5. The time series for reaction times are shown in Figure 9.6 for the first and last tests. It was in July of 2017 that the parents asked the child about the first airplane flight that he remembered as a coherent experience, and it was the trip home after his first ILF Neurofeedback sessions in 2013 at the age of six.

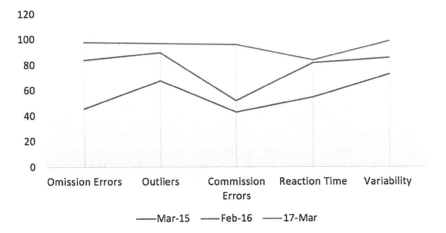

Figure 9.5 Percentile scores for three successive tests.

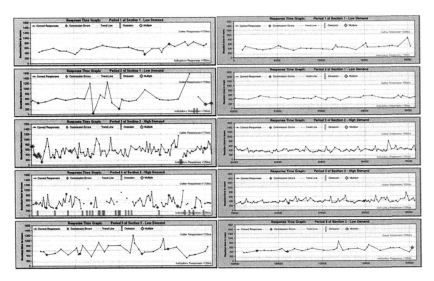

Figure 9.6 Time series of reaction times observed in the first test (2015) and the most recent test (2017).

In 2018, the parents introduced the latest protocol development—ILF Synchrony training—into the home training. The response was immediate. The attitude toward his mom became warmer. She was no longer seen primarily in her role of regimenting his life. A rash on his arm, which was being continually provoked, was observed to heal rapidly. Clearly, the youngster was experiencing a new level of calm.

The parents' reflection on their child's progress is instructive. They observed him questioning things that they thought he already knew—proof that the child's past verbal speech had been pure rote learning and did not reflect understanding. The same held true for concepts. He had fooled not only his parents but the speech therapist as well. The mother wrote: "We found that he had to relearn EVERYTHING again in a neuro-typical way. It was only after neurofeedback that our son was ready to absorb other therapies he was receiving (e.g. speech, occupational therapy). Neurofeedback really gave our son a whole new level of functionality that made it easier for his therapists to teach him. His natural gifts are coming to be expressed."

This case illustrates what can happen when all the necessary resources are being brought to bear on an autistic child. The linchpin of the therapy was clearly the ILF Neurofeedback, and it is noteworthy that all relevant functional domains—namely all that were previously deficited—were positively affected by the training. At this point, functionality is at age level or above in all relevant respects, and a new acquaintance would not be able to discern that the child had ever been autistic.

9.7 Conclusions

Working with the younger population often proves to be more challenging for several reasons. Most notably, very young children and non-verbal children won't be able to provide feedback to the neurofeedback clinician about training effects. This, in turn, makes it more difficult for the clinician to make appropriate changes to the training protocol to impact presenting symptoms, and lengthens the time needed to train to achieve desired results. In the younger population (below 6–7 years old) and in children with debilitating symptoms (like those related to the autism spectrum), the standardized computerized tests can't be administered. While those tests don't guide the actual clinical decisions on an ongoing basis, they can provide information on the strengths and weaknesses of one's brain performance, helping to track training outcomes.

There is also another important variable: medication. When medication is part of their baseline and is masking symptoms, it is more difficult to tell what impact the training has on those very symptoms. Sometimes medication changes, and the client's response to them, can blur the gauge of clinical outcomes and make it more difficult to implement a treatment plan. Beyond that, the individual's awareness, sensitivities and vulnerabilities will all play a role in the results we will see at the end of a certain number of training sessions. With therapies and other treatment modalities coinciding with the neurofeedback training, it is often more difficult to tease out the effects of each intervention. What has become clear, in all these years of working with children with behavioral, developmental and emotional disorders, is the fact that an integrative approach to their problems, along with support, will yield the best clinical outcomes.

Notes

1   Bitsko RH, Holbrook JR, Robinson LR, et al. (2016) Health Care, Family, and Community Factors Associated with Mental, Behavioral, and Developmental Disorders in Early Childhood—United States, 2011–2012. *MMWR Morb Mortal Wkly Rep* 65:221–226. DOI: 10.15585/mmwr.mm6509a1

2 2011/12 National Survey of Children's Health. Child and Adolescent Health Measurement Initiative (CAHMI), "2011–2012 NSCH: Child Health Indicator and Subgroups SAS Codebook, Version 1.0" 2013, Data Resource Center for Child and Adolescent Health, sponsored by the Maternal and Child Health Bureau. www. childhealthdata.org.

3 U.S. Department of Health and Human Services, Health Resources and Services Administration, Maternal and Child Health Bureau, The Health and Well-Being of Children: A Portrait of States and the Nation, 2011–2012. Rockville, Maryland: U.S. Department of Health and Human Services, 2014. www.mchb.hrsa.gov and www.cdc/nchs/slaits.htm.

4 Centers for Disease Control and Prevention (2013). Mental Health Surveillance among Children—United States, 2005–2011. *MMWR* 62(Suppl; May 16, 2013):1–35.

5 Any Disorder among Children (n.d.). Retrieved January 16, 2015, from www. nimh.nih.gov/health/statistics/prevalence/any-disorder-among-children.shtml.

6 2017 State of Mental Health in America—Youth Data. www.mentalhealthamerica. net/issues/2017-state-mental-health-america-youth-data.

7 Siri K, Lyons T. (2011). *Cutting-Edge Therapies for Autism 2011–2012* (2nd edition). New York, NY: Skyhorse Publishing, Inc.

8 Child Mind Institute (2018). *Children's Mental Health Report*. Understanding Anxiety in Children and Teens. https://childmind.org/our-impact/childrens-mental-health-report/2018report/ https://childmind.org/downloads/CMI_2018CMHR.pdf.

9 Any Disorder among Children (n.d.) Retrieved January 16, 2015, from www.nimh. nih.gov/health/statistics/prevalence/any-disorder-among-children.shtml.

10 Ibid.

11 Othmer S. (2019). *The Neurofeedback Clinician's Protocol Guide* (7th edition). Woodland Hills, CA: EEGInfo.

Chapter 10

Neurofeedback in Application to the ADHD Spectrum

Roxana Sasu and Siegfried Othmer

10.1 Introduction

The ADHD spectrum has been the primary clinical application of neurofeedback for over 30 years. In Chapter 2, review of the early research history established that the traditional SMR-beta protocols of EEG biofeedback were quite effective in managing the canonical symptoms of ADHD. Our own role in that development is covered in detail in two book chapters dating back to 1999.[1, 2] Six comparison studies have now been done that unanimously find an essential equivalence between EEG training in the classical manner and state-of-the-art pharmacological management. These comparisons typically relied strongly on the results of continuous performance tests of attention (CPTs), which primarily test for inattention and impulsivity. These tests don't give us a handle on the hyperactivity component or distractibility, for which one needs to rely on the observations of parents, teachers, or trained observers. These have their obvious shortcomings. Nevertheless, the essential findings are no longer in any doubt. Neurofeedback is competitive with standard medical treatment in the management of ADHD.

In recognition of this substantial body of evidence, the American Academy of Pediatrics rated neurofeedback as having Level 1 efficacy in application to ADHD.[3] (Under political pressure, the AAP subsequently softened this recognition without further investigation. Research support for the original assignment was never called into question.) In support, recent brain imaging research was cited in addition to the clinical studies.[4] This research documents the impact of neurofeedback training on the functional connectivity of neuronal networks. More recently, the adjudicating body in German psychiatry has likewise given recognition to neurofeedback in this application. The effect will be the gradual recruitment of neurofeedback into the arsenal of remedies for ADHD around the world.

The existing model of ADHD, however, remains in place essentially without alteration. The more ground-breaking implications of the effectiveness of neurofeedback in application to ADHD have yet to be recognized. The clinical reality as experienced by neurofeedback practitioners cannot be accommodated within the prevailing model of ADHD. By and large, the clientele that seeks out neurofeedback for ADHD is not looking merely to replace medication in the therapy. Neurofeedback is sought out because the medications are not resolving the issues that are actually compromising the child's life, or the side effects are not tolerated, or because the impetus is a related symptom such as bed-wetting, nocturnal bruxism, scary dreams, persistent head or stomach pain, or conduct problems. And yet, these are clearly ADHD children that have been medically diagnosed.

The case can be made that the very success of the medical remedies has resulted in a co-development of the conception of ADHD as being whatever is successfully treated with the medical arsenal, most typically stimulants. ADHD is what the medications treat. This has resulted in a kind of diagnostic tunnel vision that is unlikely to be called into question because it is working as intended. The synergy between the model and the remedy has led to ever more elaborate efforts to shore up the model rather than to move beyond it. There is a reluctance to recognize ADHD as the complex syndrome that it is. Developmental precursors are not given the attention they deserve. The complex etiology is not taken into account. The emotional context of attentional deficits has been completely ignored. There is no nexus between the behavioral model and emerging neurophysiological models of brain regulation.

This has not been an issue just for ADHD. With the development of the DSM-5, the initial objective was to seek more congruence with emerging neurophysiological models, as well as to increase reliance on biomarkers for diagnostic specificity. This nobly motivated effort failed, however, because the DSM model was hopelessly paradigm-bound. Plainly, the phenomenological basis of the DSM formalism 'does not carve nature at its joints.' The diagnostic partitioning does not line up with any biologically based organizational schema.

The clinical experience of the neurofeedback practitioner mandates a more inclusive conception. This is the *Dysregulation Model*. In this model, ADHD is seen as a disorder of cerebral dysregulation that crosses diagnostic boundaries and affects multiple systems. In this model, attentional dysfunction becomes a mere observable for the core dysregulation, one among many such observables. The issue can be illustrated with the following example. Within the classic DSM framework, Oppositional Defiant Disorder is comorbid with ADHD in some 60% of cases.[5] Since stimulants do not address this comorbidity, the dichotomous view is likely to be sustained. The more organic view would have it that emotional dysregulation clearly cohabits quite commonly with attentional dysregulation. One clearly impinges on the other. Emotionally based disorders often lie at the core of attentional disorders, and in such cases should have priority in therapeutic attention. A common mechanism may even underlie both. Alternatively, sensory processing disorders or specific learning disabilities may lie at the root of the apparent attentional deficit. Conversely, the attentional deficits seen in ADHD are ubiquitous in other clinical conditions.

The need clearly exists for us to move beyond a purely behavioral and phenomenological model. Since neurofeedback engages neural network organization directly, the canonical disorders need to be understood in the new framework. That project is aided by having a neurophysiological measure to go along with our neurophysiological remedy. The continuous performance test (CPT) that has been in use in our work since 1990 serves this purpose admirably. Whereas the results of CPTs have historically been interpreted in behavioral terms, they can equally well inform us with respect to behavior at the level of the neuronal networks. Refinements and new developments over the last 15 years have substantially increased the utility of the test.

At the same time, the clinical decision making by the neurofeedback practitioner remains based largely on behavioral and phenomenological observations, as these are available in real time. The distinction being drawn here is that a more physiologically grounded model allows the behavioral observations to be appraised differently. A more inclusive perspective is called for, one that accommodates not only the pharmacological model of ADHD but also the much broader implications of Infra-Low Frequency Neurofeedback (ILF NF). In essence, a few key failure modes are identified that line up with the basic protocols. These exist on a continuum, and at some level they afflict us all at one time or another, in sickness if not in health. Hence, they are no respecter of diagnostic boundaries. These basic failure modes are developmentally grounded. We all start out in life inattentive, distractible, and impulsive. Children only become capable of taking the CPT test during their fifth year, by and large. Full maturity is not reached until the twentieth year.

As described in Chapter 4, the clinical model is informed by considerations of functional neuroanatomy and is subject to selection through empirical findings. The results are consistent with current understanding of our intrinsic connectivity networks (ICNs) or resting state networks (RSNs). The quality of brain function is contingent on the steady-state functional connectivity of our ICNs, as well as on their dynamical interaction.[6] This is discussed further in Chapters 2 and 3.

The study of intra-individual variability of reaction time performance under various challenge conditions has revealed fluctuations in the range of 0.01 to 0.1 Hz.[7] Another such study found correlations between responses on the timescale of one second.[8] The study of event-related potentials (ERPs) under such challenges has shown differences on the timescale of 10 msec.[9] Each of these time domains can be targeted with a neuromodulation strategy. However, empirically it has been found that the broadest impact can be achieved by targeting the steady-state behavior of functional connectivity in the ILF range. This engages the foundations of our regulatory hierarchy.

Developments in the measurement of CPT data have enabled efficient collection of group data. These will be presented to consolidate the case for ILF NF in application to the classic symptoms of ADHD. The case histories that follow are intended to illustrate the breadth of impact of the method, and the particularity of its administration in each case. This supports the view that ADHD should be seen as a syndrome or spectrum. Heavy reliance is placed on CPT data in these case reports.

10.2 Refinements in the Analysis of CPT Data

All of the CPT data we published in the nineties was acquired with the Test of Variables of Attention (T.O.V.A.®). This pressured choice reaction time (Go/No-Go) test involves two periods of stimulus-sparse challenge, followed by two periods of stimulus-frequent challenge. The inter-stimulus interval is invariant at two seconds in order to maintain uniformly boring conditions. This presents a challenge to the maintenance of vigilance. Data analysis was based on Gaussian distributions and, therefore, dependent on norming populations that were, in turn, dependent on expert judgment.

In 2004 we acted upon the perceived need to make minor modifications in the test design that the T.O.V.A. team was not able to accommodate, and therefore new hardware and software were developed to emulate the T.O.V.A. design. The result was the QIKtest, developed by bee Medic in Switzerland. The basic features of the T.O.V.A. were preserved in the new design, even to the point that the norms carried over as well. The QIKtest provided for the return to a single period of stimulus-sparse challenge, in order to have an additional state shift to evaluate. Also, the threshold criterion for an anticipatory error was shortened from 200 msec to 150 msec for adults, and it has been age-adjusted for the young.

All subsequent data were stored on a central server, which then facilitated efficient evaluation of large data sets in systematic data mining. Analysis of reaction time data revealed reaction time outliers to be power-law distributed (i.e., $1/t^\alpha$). They would have to be considered separately so as to avoid contaminating the 'normal' reaction time data, known to be described by the ex-Gaussian distribution, the Gaussian with an exponential tail. These surveys also revealed that the discrete errors were not Gaussian-distributed and could in no way yield to parametric analysis (mean and standard deviation). Not only were the distributions long-tailed, but in the case of omission errors and reaction time outliers they were 'all tail.' That is to say, these were power-law distributed over the entire range. Commission error distributions could be fitted to a Gaussian component with a power-law tail.

The practical implications were multi-fold. Parametric analysis of the discrete error data was contra-indicated. Non-parametric analysis was mandated, with scores expressed in percentiles. To flesh out the entire distribution in order to make percentile scores meaningful, a large sample pool was required. Population-based norms were adopted for this purpose (as is customary in IQ-tests), with only the pathological extremes excluded from the analysis. The resulting norms are therefore relatively free of arbitrary human judgment. They were also fairly low in statistical uncertainty, being based in this case on a sample of 50,000 trials, with a sample size of 500 for each age and gender bin from age six to 70+.

There were theoretical implications as well. All three types of discrete errors were power-law distributed, which indicated that they were all subject to a chaotic failure mode. All three were also statistically highly correlated. They all scaled with dysregulation status. Thus, a common underlying failure mode could be reasonably postulated, enhancing the prospects that a small set of protocols could serve this disparate variable space adequately.

10.3 Results for the Evaluation of Group Data for ILF Neurofeedback

In 2017 a survey of training outcomes was performed in which 12,200 pre-post data sets were evaluated for a nominal 20 sessions of ILF NF. The survey included the contributions of more than a thousand clinicians to the database, and hence are representative of what is actually being accomplished in the clinical realm. The data were analyzed independently of any information about the clients beyond age and gender. Hence the results reflect attentional failure generally in the clinical population, not just among those labeled ADHD. However, that is in line with our present understanding, namely that a common failure mode is involved that cuts across clinical boundaries.

Results for the pre-post distribution of commission errors is shown in Table 10.1. Comparison of the two distributions yields the improvement in incidence as a function of the number of errors. The results indicate that improvements with training are achievable at any measurable level of deficit. If a child is capable of taking the test, improvements with training are the expectation. An average improvement by a factor of 2.4 characterizes the severely deficited region. A similar curve for omission errors reveals an improvement factor of 1.8. For reaction time outliers, an improvement factor of 1.4 is indicated.

The cumulative curve of commission errors is more revealing of what happens with the bulk of the population. The median number of commission errors declines in training by a factor of 1.9. The comparable factor for omission errors is 2.4, and for reaction time outliers it is 2.1. The results are summarized in Table 10.1.

The improvement factors are substantial, leaving no doubt about the robustness of the findings. The clinical significance of these improvements is not yet apparent, however. For that purpose, age-segregated data are drawn upon to fill out the picture. The tenth birthday was chosen to divide the early and late developmental periods. The twentieth birthday is the appropriate end point to the developmental phase. Conveniently, the normative data allow the median scores to be interpreted in terms of equivalent mental age. For the 6–10 age range, median mental age improves from 6 years to 10 for commissions, and from 6.2 to 8.5 for omissions. For the 10–20 age range, median mental age moves from 9 to 17 in commissions, and from 10.3 to 13.8 in omissions. The functional improvements are clinically significant for the discrete errors.

Table 10.1 Improvement factors

Improvement Factors	Commissions	Omissions	Outliers
Error Incidence	2.4	1.8	1.4
Median Score	1.9	2.4	2.1

Table 10.2 Ratios of improvement factors, comparing post-2013 with pre-2014 results

Ratios of Improvement Factors	6 through 9 yrs	10 through 19 yrs	20 years to 70+	Average
Commissions	1.12	1.18	1.09	1.13
Omissions	0.97	1.03	1.03	1.01
Outliers	0.96	1.11	1.22	1.10
Reaction Time	0.98	0.99	1.00	0.99
Variability	0.97	1.02	1.00	1.00

The problem being addressed with the discrete errors is much more the context out of which the action arises, as opposed to the execution of the action itself. The distinction between the two is particularly apparent in Parkinson's, and it's the heart of the story in Oliver Sacks' *Awakenings*. In the CPT we arrange for the most benign of circumstances. The challenge is a minimal one – the task can be readily anticipated, the choice is binary, and there are no external distractors. The failures thus identified, therefore, trace back to the brain's inability to maintain continuity of state or to random internal disruptors, or both. These two failure modes are the immediate targets of the ILF NF training process, and substantial success in that undertaking is in evidence.

Finally, it is of interest to inquire whether results have improved over the years with the ongoing refinement of protocols. For this purpose, the ten-year survey was segmented with the dividing line of the end of 2013. Comparisons are shown in Table 10.2 in the form of ratios of improvement factors for the two epochs. There have been improvements in outcomes with respect to commission errors and reaction time outliers, whereas results have been stable for all the other categories. These results testify to the existence of a robust training protocol with relatively predictable outcomes, at least in the statistical sense.

In the remainder of the chapter we shift toward a more clinical perspective on the performance of this work and the variety of symptom profiles that can be resolved with ILF NF.

10.4 Why Diagnosis Is Not Important from a Neurofeedback Perspective

Neurofeedback exercises the brain into self-regulation and improved function, irrespective of the modality. In ILF NF, the training is covert, and hence the exercise is self-generated by the brain in engagement with the signal. With proper protocols, improvements in performance should be achievable irrespective of baseline performance when initiating neurofeedback. There is usually a set of symptoms to work with that cues us with respect to self-regulatory status, and that set of symptoms might or might not fit into the diagnostic criteria for a particular condition. Even if nothing rises to the level of overt symptoms, there are relative strengths and weaknesses that may be discerned. Parents are often concerned that their children won't get the training because they don't have a formal diagnosis, and we quickly lay those concerns to rest. From a neurofeedback perspective, the more important aspect is 'who is this person that is presenting with these symptoms? How is that unique brain affected and constrained, given those specific symptoms? How is it dysfunctional and dysregulated?' The symptoms are the observable manifestations of the dysregulation status that we need to learn about and impact with the training.

A symptom is necessarily subjective, observed and appraised by the patient, and typically it cannot be measured directly or with much accuracy. Therefore, the same symptom is going to be perceived differently by any two affected individuals. This is not, however, a lamentable limitation. On the contrary, the specifics of how this symptom manifests in one brain or another is the information we need in order to decide how to train. The particularity and the context of symptom presentation are keys to the underlying pattern of dysregulation.

Having a diagnosis merely orients us towards one set of symptoms or another, but it doesn't give us any specifics on how those symptoms are related at a deeper level, or of the pattern of dysregulation that is affecting that brain and body. At the same time, not having a diagnosis simply means we get the information we need in the form of a list of symptoms the client describes during the intake. We then map those symptom patterns to principal failure modes of cerebral regulation, which in turn map to our training sites. We then lay out a training protocol that will target the identified failure modes, which implies that symptoms are being targeted only indirectly. The client will experience the training and will be able to notice and report on changes in symptoms as well as on shifts in functional status. These changes and shifts help us to understand in what way the training is affecting brain function, and we make continual adjustments to the training protocol to optimize results. Such adjustments may be made several times during one of the early sessions, before the training protocol settles down to a more predictable pattern.

10.5 The ADHD Spectrum in the Clinical Perspective

The clinical model distinguishes between two principal subtypes of ADHD for purposes of structuring a neurofeedback protocol: the *simple subtype* and the *complicated subtype*. The simple ADHD subtype is well described by the cardinal symptoms of ADHD: inattention and distractibility on the one hand; impulsivity and hyperactivity on the other. This pattern indicates the need to train two main areas in the brain – the left prefrontal cortex and right parietal. This bi-hemispheric strategy has served us well for many years, going back to the mid-nineties. It is traceable to the model of ADHD of Malone, Kershner, and Swanson,[10] which in turn is based on the model of Tucker and Williamson.[11] Representative clinical results obtained with the earlier SMR/beta training protocols at some 32 clinical practices are covered in Kaiser and Othmer.[12]

The left prefrontal cortex is a critical part of the executive control system that refers to directed attention, planning, reasoning, and judgment. It is involved in voluntary behaviors such as decision-making, planning and thinking, internally motivated attention, and inhibition of impulsive and compulsive behaviors. Good prefrontal function allows us to memorize information while planning and executing appropriate sequences of actions to achieve concrete goals. It is also crucial to good self-regulation by inhibiting primitive and immature reactions while time is allocated to consider possible outcomes and consequences of alternative courses of action. Whenever there is a lack of appropriate prefrontal control the person may have difficulty completing tasks, focusing for a longer period of time, and hewing to longer-term goals. They may also exhibit poor organization skills, be unaware of their own behavior, and unable to consider consequences of behavioral alternatives.

The right parietal cortex plays an important role in integrating information from our senses to build a coherent picture of the world around us. It is involved in visual-spatial processing, spatial and body awareness, orientation of the body in space, and motor coordination on the macro-scale. Impaired function of the right parietal cortex can lead to a lack of self-awareness and spatial awareness, and it can result in the inability of the subject to control body movement, leading to hyperactivity.

The complicated subtype of ADHD includes the above-mentioned symptoms as a result of poor function of the left prefrontal and right parietal cortex but adds physiological dysregulation and emotional symptoms to the picture. (Strictly speaking, ADHD is a disorder of exclusion, and thus the more complicated presentations should not be labeled ADHD. In the real world, however, this is what often happens, and that leads to the diagnostic tunnel vision already alluded to. The more complicated aspects may not be attended to because they don't fit the template.) The lack of emotional control resulting in oppositional or aggressive behavior requires training the right prefrontal cortex, while the symptoms of instability including headaches, mood swings, asthma etc. require left–right (i.e., inter-hemispheric) temporal stabilization. It is tempting to surmise that it is easier to work with the uncomplicated subtype. The problem is that the lack of self-awareness in ADHD makes it difficult for clients to report on changes occurring with the training. For the neurofeedback clinician this presents a challenge in making clinical decisions regarding training protocols. The complicated subtype, on the other hand, involves sensitive, touchy nervous systems with an abundance of symptoms that are easy to report on and easy to track. These people are well aware of what is bothering them. Our clinical adjustments to the training protocols are perceived promptly by the client and this helps the process of finding what is optimal. Fortunately, these clients are plentiful in our clinic.

In a clinical setting like ours, people who seek help have typically already tried numerous other modalities to resolve their issues, which explains why we tend to see the complex cases, where ADHD-related symptoms are part of a bigger picture. For those with uncomplicated ADHD, modern medicine addresses the problem well enough that further help with neurofeedback is unlikely to be sought. It's mostly when clients really want to avoid medication altogether that we get to see people in this category.

There are a few major differences between traditional treatment options and neurofeedback for ADHD. The most important one is the fact that neurofeedback is non-invasive and doesn't put anything into the system, while medication is invasive and has potentially significant, troublesome, and even lasting side-effects. The other difference is that while medication administration is limited by age, neurofeedback can be done at any age. Last but not least, allopathic medicine will consider the severity of the presenting symptoms when deciding on a treatment plan and a certain dose of medication to be administered. With neurofeedback, the severity of a symptom is not important in establishing how to train that brain. We also have the ability to be very specific in terms of which areas in the brain we target with the training and exactly how to fine-tune the frequency in order to obtain best results. Medication effects wear off in hours, while the changes promoted by neurofeedback can last a lifetime if sufficient training has been done.

In our assessment process we include the QIKtest in all cases in which the client is capable of taking it. The CPT is a gruelling challenge for the young ADHD child. It is administered at age six and up, provided that the client can understand and follow instructions and is able to stay with the task. The baseline test is a consistency check on what we learn about that brain's way of functioning during the intake. The client should also 'recognize himself' in the test results as they are explained to him. Results are presented in the more familiar form of standard scores rather than percentiles. A parent who feels reassured that her child is scoring at norms would be distressed to find out that this refers to the fiftieth percentile. We live in a Lake Wobegon world. Percentile scores are therefore converted to standard scores via the Gaussian distribution. The conditions under which the baseline test is taken (e.g., with or without any medication), will typically be replicated during the comparison test that is done 20 sessions later. It is expected that the second test will show improvement in most areas, with significant improvement expected in areas of initial deficit. Adverse outcomes in one aspect or another compel the training strategy to be redirected.

Often times, attention and impulse control issues are part of a more complex scenario that can present under a different name: PTSD, attachment issues, developmental disorder, addiction, depression, or anxiety. Our understanding of brain function allows us to interpret symptoms of inattention, impulsivity, or hyperactivity in the context of a certain layered and more complicated picture. The CPT test has historically been associated with the characterization of the ADHD brain, but we have put it to use much more universally. It is a test of nervous system status that is very revealing of the capacity for self-regulation. Whereas it is not prescriptive of training protocols, it is a truth test of sorts to index our approach to the goal of improved self-regulatory capacity.

10.6 Clinical Case Studies

10.6.1 Case #1

Christine, a 20-year-old woman, sought help for symptoms related to her ADHD diagnosis. During the intake interview, however, a much more complicated picture was disclosed – a picture that included trauma and a history of addiction. Adopted as an infant, she had a normal early life. Her adoptive parents divorced when she was 12 years old and she was raised by her mother, with whom she never really got along. The relationship with her sister, adopted as well, wasn't close until later in life. As her family life became increasingly more stressful, her academic performance suffered. She had been in several car accidents and had pain in her upper back and muscle tension in her neck and shoulders as a result. She had a history of multiple drug addictions, which she was able to overcome – she had been sober for two years when she came to us. She described how anything she put into her system had the power to get her hooked – she had abused cocaine, marijuana, and would even use Adderall to get high. Currently she was struggling with new addictions: food and cigarettes. She had suffered one seizure-like episode with a drug overdose. She complained of poor balance and motor coordination and her sense of direction was not good either. She described having difficulties falling asleep and found it impossible to wake up in the morning despite setting several alarms. She also had a history of sleepwalking.

Between the addictive behaviors and immense anxiety, her terrible sleep hygiene and thus disrupted sleep patterns, the obsessive fears of failure or becoming overweight, and the migraines, headaches and severe PMS, the fact that she came in with the diagnosis of ADHD seemed beside the point. She did have difficulties concentrating and had a hard time staying on task, would often zone out and was both hyperactive and impulsive. But, given the fact that her brain had been through so much, can we understand the latter symptoms as consequences of all the different traumas her brain had suffered or just another set of separate issues that happened to be experienced by the same brain?

Our improved understanding of brain organization and function has helped us refine our method of training the brain. It is a well-known fact that trauma to the brain means disruption in early development and interference with self-regulatory processes, particularly affect regulation and autonomic function. When core self-regulation is deficient, a person will be unable to feel safe or comfortable within themselves and in the world. An unmodulated fear response radiates throughout the regulatory regime, affecting regulatory status quite broadly. The right hemisphere is responsible for acquiring this skill and when things don't go as planned, for whatever reason, that puts the brain in emergency mode and makes it work overtime to try and keep the person safe and connected. The more urgent issue is the lack of core self-regulation and its consequences, which can emerge immediately or later in life in the form of anxiety or hyper-vigilance, attachment deficits or reactivity, aggressive or paranoid behaviors – all serving the same purpose of preserving life and assuring personal safety.

With the client described above, not only had she experienced trauma as an infant when she was adopted at four months of age, but then her sense of safety and bonding was shattered yet again when her adoptive family broke up. The self-destructive, addictive behaviors can be easily explained by her lacking a sense of core self, needing external stimuli to cope with life.

During her first QIKtest she found it quite challenging to stay awake, missed one target and almost missed 19 others (reaction time outliers), while also pushing the button for the non-target four times. She was slow and variable in her response times and accuracy suffered as well, as shown in Figures 10.1 and 10.2.

Results Summary:

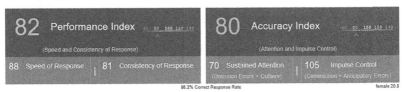

Figure 10.1 QIKtest Results Summary. (See a color version in the plate section.)

RAW DATA	Period 1 Sect. 1 Low Demand	Period 2 Sect. 1 Low Demand	Period 3 Sect. 2 High Demand	Period 4 Sect. 2 High Demand	Period 5 Sect. 3 Low Demand	Sect. 1	Sect. 2	Sect 3	Total
Omissions(#)	0	0	1	0	0	0	1	0	1
Outliers	1	0	1	14	3	1	15	3	19
Commissions(#)	0	0	2	1	1	0	3	1	4
Response time(ms)	393	440	394	444	482	417	417	482	423
Variability(ms)	61	91	90	125	83	81	110	83	90

Figure 10.2 Key scores, incremental and cumulative. (See a color version in the plate section.)

On more detailed analysis, as shown in Figure 10.2, we can see which parts of the test were more challenging. She started the period 1 low demand task and did pretty well, with only one outlier and no other errors, and she was fairly fast and consistent. As we kept boring her in the second period, she remained accurate but slowed down and became significantly more variable in her responses. Entering the third period of the test with the faster pace, she started making more mistakes, missed the target once and also had two commission errors. Maintaining the high demand task was an even bigger challenge for her, as she slowed down and became very inconsistent, and also had a significant number of outliers. Just as she described during the intake, she had a hard time staying on-task, which is obvious when we look how her performance degraded as she needed to maintain a task, boring or challenging. With increased performance pressure her anxiety level increased, and thus when making mistakes in the test she sped up instead of taking her time to consider before acting. Recovery in period 5 was difficult, with three outliers and one commission error, and she was both slow and variable.

The response time graphs in Figure 10.3 allow us to see the time course of events, where she made the mistakes, and in which part of the test her performance was better or worse. Clearly this client was able to perform fairly well when under pressure, as long as the stress was of a short duration. When the pressure continued her performance declined, and with increased stress her nervous system tended to shut down. She almost fell asleep during the test.

Compared to a normal distribution of response times for age group and gender, the distribution of her response times is much more spread out, with a mean of her test at 423 ms, compared to 362 ms for the norm (see Figure 10.4). When looking at the different parts of the test, it is evident that the performance decrement increases during the second high demand task, which was the most difficult for her to perform.

She had been medicated in the past but her sensitive nervous system didn't tolerate the different medications well, or she ended up abusing them, so eventually she just stopped taking them. The only medication still being used when we started our sessions was melatonin to help her sleep.

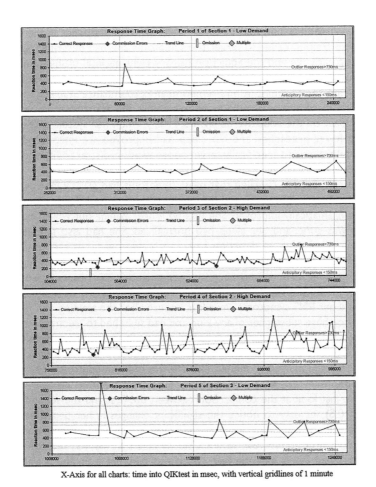

X-Axis for all charts: time into QIKtest in msec, with vertical gridlines of 1 minute

Figure 10.3 Response time graphs, QIK baseline test, case #1. (See a color version in the plate section.)

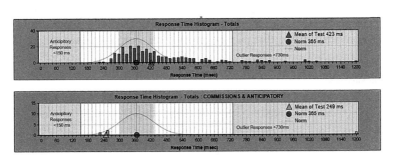

Figure 10.4 Response time histograms – totals, QIK baseline test, case #1. (See a color version in the plate section.)

We started training and one by one we added all the areas in the brain we needed to train in order to target the symptoms she had described. Given the traumatic early life and the addiction history, right parietal training for calming was crucial. At the same time, several instability symptoms indicated a great need for bilateral training at mid-temporal sites to enhance stability. Later, right prefrontal placement was introduced to address the attachment issues, as well as to impact on the addictive behaviors. Finally, when her system settled down, she had fewer headaches, and her sleep had improved, we introduced the left prefrontal training to specifically target concentration, distractibility, and impulse control.

The reevaluation revealed that most symptoms had greatly improved. Concentration was much better and her ability to stay on task for prolonged periods had dramatically improved. She was no longer zoning out while reading. The anxiety was gone, and her sleep had normalized. She had also stopped taking melatonin. Her sense of direction had greatly improved, but she continued to have difficulties getting to appointments on time. She rarely had any nightmares now and waking up in the morning had become easier. Her obsessive worries had moderated and she was less hyperactive. The headaches and migraines had vanished, and her PMS symptoms were less intense after the training. She felt less of an urge to abuse substances of any kind and had switched to electronic cigarettes to help her quit, after having already had success in reducing her smoking even before the start of training. The remaining concerns related to weight gain and being successful in life, but she felt like she was more in control of her thoughts and emotions.

If we just look at the comparison between the first and the second QIKtest (Figure 10.5), it's easy to notice the significant changes in her performance. This time there are no omissions or outliers, but interestingly she had seven commission errors, compared to just four earlier. One variable that day was her coffee intake; she hadn't had any before the test, which was different from the previous time. Coffee acted like a stimulant for her, waking her mind up and helping her focus, so the fact that she hadn't consumed any probably influenced her performance. Speed and consistency were significantly improved from the first test.

The greatest difficulty was still to perform under the pressure of the high demand task, she found, especially when maintaining that task (see Figure 10.6). She had similar difficulties during the first test, but this time she was faster and more consistent during that part of the test and that might have caused her to

Results Summary: .

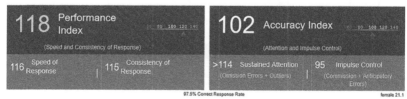

Figure 10.5 Results summary QIKtest 2, case #1.

RAW DATA	Period 1 Sect. 1 Low Demand	Period 2 Sect. 1 Low Demand	Period 3 Sect. 2 High Demand	Period 4 Sect. 2 High Demand	Period 5 Sect. 3 Low Demand	Sect. 1	Sect. 2	Sect 3	Total
Omissions(#)	0	0	0	0	0	0	0	0	0
Outliers	0	0	0	0	0	0	0	0	0
Commissions(#)	0	0	1	5	1	0	6	1	7
Response time(ms)	379	373	303	280	370	376	291	370	316
Variability(ms)	68	51	64	51	55	60	59	55	58

Figure 10.6 Raw data, QIKtest 2, case #1.

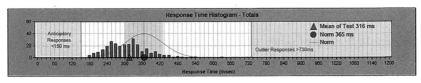

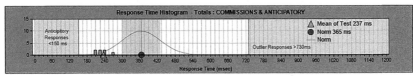

Norms: the blue line represents a normal distribution of reaction times for this age and group; compare by form and position to your data in red. The light blue area represents 68.2% (or ±1σ) of a normal distribution.

Figure 10.7 Response time histograms, QIKtest 2, case #1.

make more commission errors. With a mean reaction time more than one standard deviation above norms, she was performing at greater risk of commission errors (Figure 10.7). It's only at the very end during the recovery period that she speeds up instead of becoming more careful after the one commission error she made, but overall her performance had significantly improved (Figures 10.8 and 10.9). This is consistent with the perceived changes in her symptoms, which were all reduced in severity to allow for better performance in everyday life.

With such a complex case, 20 sessions is typically enough to see significant favorable change but not enough to be able to say, 'we're done training.' In fact, because of her complicated early life and the addictive behaviors, further training was recommended and other training modalities were needed to work on resolution of learned habits.

10.6.2 Case #2

George, a 33-year-old man, sought help for his ADD symptoms when the medication he was taking created new issues for him such as rebound headaches and palpitations. In other respects, the medications had been helpful.

Pre-Post Graphs

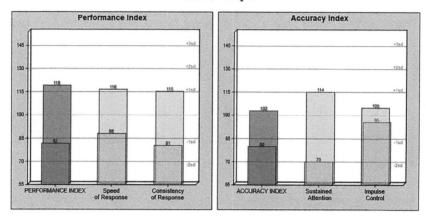

Figure 10.8 Pre-post graphs, case #1.

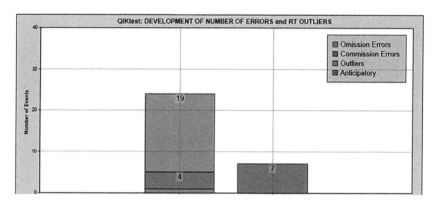

Figure 10.9 Development of number of errors and outliers, case #1.

In his developmental history there was nothing exceptional except for his parents' divorce when he was still an infant. He was raised by his mother and stepfather. In his family history he mentioned ADHD, along with autoimmune disorders, insomnia, depression, anxiety, obesity, alcohol addiction, and conduct problems. He was taking Adderall 10 mg/day, and occasionally up to 20 mg when he had to undergo some testing in school.

His main concerns before we started training were difficulties concentrating, getting on task, completing tasks, and impulsivity. About once a week he would have a hard time falling back to sleep once he woke up around 2am. He would experience anxiety as tension in his body and obsessive worries. He sometimes had neck tension and ground his teeth. He would overeat with stress and was sensitive to sugar – he would have a sugar-fueled high and then crash later. He had frequent headaches when not drinking coffee or not taking Adderall.

Results Summary:

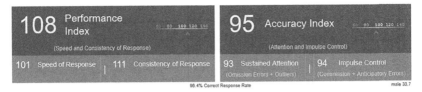

Figure 10.10 Results summary QIK baseline test, case #2.

RAW DATA	Period 1 Sect. 1 Low Demand	Period 2 Sect. 1 Low Demand	Period 3 Sect. 2 High Demand	Period 4 Sect. 2 High Demand	Period 5 Sect. 3 Low Demand	Sect. 1	Sect. 2	Sect 3	Total
Omissions(#)	0	0	1	0	2	0	1	2	3
Outliers	0	0	0	0	0	0	0	0	0
Commissions(#)	0	0	4	3	0	0	7	0	7
Response time(ms)	398	389	322	349	393	393	335	393	353
Variability(ms)	37	49	82	65	63	44	75	63	59

Figure 10.11 Raw data, QIK baseline test, case #2.

His only QIKtest was taken before we started training him (Figure 10.10), and he complained that it had been difficult to perform because he was getting distracted by the ticking of the clock on the wall. He missed the target three times during the test, twice in the recovery part of the test, period 5, and once during the high demand task, which is consistent with what we already knew about his difficulties performing under pressure and staying on task for long periods of time (Figure 10.11). His overall performance and accuracy were average. He hadn't taken Adderall the day of the test and didn't take it for the most part while doing the sessions in the clinic.

He started noticing positive changes in his distractibility early on with the training and was able to track results as he was studying for exams. It took a while to find the optimal protocol for him; he had a very sensitive nervous system and because of the Adderall and caffeine variables it was, at times, challenging to figure out what each was contributing to the reported shifts. He clearly benefited from the sessions and would report improvement in concentration and the ability to deal with stress and deadlines he had to meet, but usually the results faded a day or two after sessions. He didn't finish his 20 treatments and we didn't get to take a second QIKtest, so there is no measurable data to gauge brain performance. Given the inability to hold the gains, it was clear that a lot more training would have been needed before his brain would successfully stay on track and perform optimally on its own. One hypothesis for the failure to hold gains is that the infant had in fact been traumatized by the parents' divorce, and that the resulting impact on nervous system functioning had not fully resolved. This case also illustrates what can frequently happen as the client comes to terms with this novel method. An initial healthy skepticism may well transition to its opposite, heightened expectations, as the first good effects are felt. When the training procedure then fails to live up to those new expectations, the effort is abandoned.

10.6.3 Case #3

Aidan, a 16-year-old young man with a dual diagnosis of ADHD and dyslexia, received intensive neurofeedback training at our clinic. Over a two-week span he received 20 neurofeedback sessions, at a rate of two sessions a day, and he continued with home training.

The main concerns described during the intake with us were hyperactivity and distractibility, anxiety as worries, some frustration and compulsive organization, as well as difficulty with academic classes. Words would move on the page when trying to read. This problem was helped considerably with Irlen lenses. He had headaches with reading or when dehydrated and had some difficulties falling asleep. In the past he had been sleep-walking and had night terrors as well. Sugar sensitivity was described also.

He was born through emergency C-section with his umbilical cord around his neck and was described as a stressed baby. He walked early and talked late and wasn't much of a talker even later on in life. He was accident-prone and had a few falls and stitches growing up, and even had a finger reattached at 11 months. Around the time he was 4 years old his parents separated for a year. In his genetic history insomnia, postpartum depression, anxiety, OCD, dyslexia, and Asperger's were present.

Prior to the neurofeedback he had been on 54 mg of Concerta®/day, which he stopped taking while undergoing neurofeedback. His pre-training QIKtest (Figures 10.12 and 10.13) revealed an average performance index and an accuracy index well below average, with impulsivity scores in the 1st percentile, a high number of commission errors, and a significant number of omissions. The part that he found to be the most difficult was the high demand section, where his performance dropped significantly. After the first two sessions he reported falling asleep faster, and one session later noticed improvement in reading comprehension, although at the time the protocol wasn't yet focusing on reading issues. His mother also noticed him becoming less hyperactive even though he was off his medication for the duration of the neurofeedback training. By session 10 behavioral issues had subsided to where

Results Summary: .

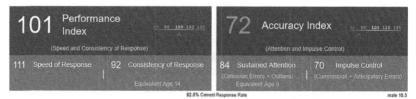

Figure 10.12 Pre-post graphs, case #1.

RAW DATA	Period 1 Sect. 1 Low Demand	Period 2 Sect. 1 Low Demand	Period 3 Sect. 2 High Demand	Period 4 Sect. 2 High Demand	Period 5 Sect. 3 Low Demand	Sect. 1	Sect. 2	Sect 3	Total
Omissions(#)	0	1	4	5	3	1	9	3	13
Outliers	0	0	0	1	1	0	1	1	2
Commissions(#)	2	0	18	14	2	2	32	2	36
Response time(ms)	398	398	280	326	429	398	303	429	335
Variability(ms)	81	48	91	111	124	67	104	124	91

Figure 10.13 Raw data, QIK baseline test, case #3.

Results Summary:

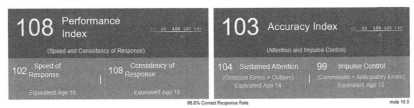

Figure 10.14 Results summary QIKtest 2, case #3.

RAW DATA	Period 1 Sect. 1 Low Demand	Period 2 Sect. 1 Low Demand	Period 3 Sect. 2 High Demand	Period 4 Sect. 2 High Demand	Period 5 Sect. 3 Low Demand	Sect. 1	Sect. 2	Sect 3	Total
Omissions(#)	0	0	0	0	0	0	0	0	0
Outliers	0	0	3	0	0	0	3	0	3
Commissions(#)	0	0	5	4	0	0	9	0	9
Response time(ms)	402	380	337	366	431	391	352	431	368
Variability(ms)	82	55	84	97	54	71	92	54	74

Figure 10.15 Raw data, QIKtest 2, case #3.

they would have been when he was on medication. Reading continued to improve, and he actually started reading more with – or even without – his Irlen lenses.

During reassessment progress was reported, which included a better understanding while reading and an improved ability to visualize what he read. He described more immediate and detailed imagery and was less fidgety and distracted. His sleep had gotten better with fewer nightmares and less anxiety or obsessive worries. He also noticed being more comfortable when having to deal with traffic.

The second QIKtest (Figures 10.14 and 10.15) showed some improvement in the performance index with a significant shift in speed and consistency. His speed of response decreased somewhat, which allowed for higher consistency of response and improved accuracy. In fact, accuracy went from a score of 72 to a score of 99. This kind of spectacular improvement becomes even more relevant in the prevailing context, since he had stopped taking his medication before undergoing treatments in the clinic.

It was decided that it would be appropriate for him to continue training at home, and he received 4–5 sessions a week while continuing to stay off the medication. A month into home training his mother reported further improvement in concentration and in his ability to make good choices, and he was better able to manage usual day-to-day events.

10.6.4 Case #4

Michael, an 11-year-old boy, was having a hard time in school. He didn't have a formal diagnosis but exhibited some of the classic symptoms of ADHD. He had a short attention span, was easily distracted, impulsive and disorganized, and couldn't sit still in school. Among the presenting symptoms there were some learning difficulties, like understanding math concepts and calculation and writing problems. He was described as being clumsy. He was inflexible and defiant mostly in a school setting; frustration and anger were issues as well. Occasional headaches and stomach aches, as well as teeth-grinding and sugar cravings, completed the picture. After being adopted at birth, his early life was unremarkable, except for some chronic ear infections that required tubes at age one until age two. As a result, he was sensitive to sound, especially to loud noise.

Taking the QIKtest (Figures 10.16 and 10.17) the first time proved to be quite a challenge for Michael. He scored below average for speed, consistency, and

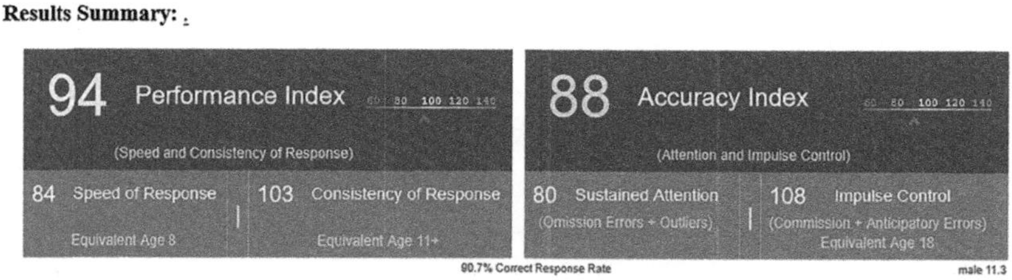

Results Summary:

Figure 10.16 Results summary QIK baseline test, case #4.

Results	Data	Norm	Score	
M11.3 Total Test	Measured Value	Median of Distribution	Standard Score	Percentile
Omission Errors	18 errors	5.0 errors	85	17%
Outlier Responses	24 errors	4.4 errors	77	6%
Commission Errors	8 errors	12.9 errors	108	70.5%
Response Time	543.3 ms	436 ms	84	14%
Variability	113.1 ms	112 ms	103	56%

Figure 10.17 Results summary data, QIK baseline test, case #4.

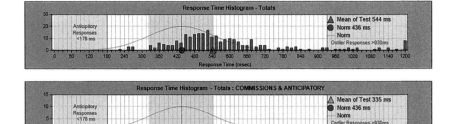

Norms: the blue line represents a normal distribution of reaction times for this age and group; compare by form and position to your data in red. The light blue area represents 68.2% (or ±1σ) of a normal distribution.

Figure 10.18 Response time histograms, QIK baseline test, case #4.

inattention with only one score, impulsivity, within the normal range. This indicates that he was slow and somewhat variable, and unable to stay on task. The response time histogram (Figure 10.18) reveals a broad distribution of response times with lots of outliers.

His training protocol targeted areas in the brain to promote physical, emotional, and mental calming as well as stabilization. T3-P3 was added for the learning difficulties. Over a five month span he completed 20 sessions of neurofeedback. His statement at the end: 'I'm not stupid anymore,' conveys his own sense of the progress he had made in just 20 sessions. The child was thrilled about his new way of relating to his peers. This sheds some light on how difficult it can be for people with these symptoms to fit in, how much harder they feel they need to work to keep the pace in school or at work, and how much their dysregulated nervous system can hinder function. During his re-evaluation his mother reported improvement in most initial symptoms, and his second QIKtest supported that with measurable data.

He was enjoying school and was more optimistic now that his attention and impulse control had significantly improved. In place of his earlier defiance, he was less frustrated and angry, and much more flexible and cooperative. He was much more organized and improved his writing and math skills. He didn't have any headaches or stomach aches and wasn't grinding his teeth anymore. He was less clumsy and was now able to sit still in school, so he wasn't distracting others as he had been before.

His first test reflected the above described difficulties mostly in attention and, to a certain degree, in impulse control. Twenty sessions later, a second test showed significantly improved overall scores, with a superb leap towards the upper limit of normal accuracy index scores (Figures 10.19 and 10.20). Both sustained attention and impulse control were much better, and the performance index greatly improved as well.

In light of these impressive gains, we suggested retesting Michael after three months to see if the results were holding. This is not always assured after training only for 20 sessions. Although the impulse control continued to improve, the performance index dropped back to the level measured prior to the neurofeedback. The need for additional sessions is indicated by these results (Figures 10.21

Results Summary: .

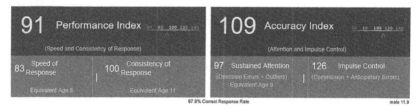

Figure 10.19 Results summary QIKtest 2, case #4.

Results	Data	Norm	Score	
M11.7 Total Test	Measured Value	Median of Distribution	Standard Score	Percentile
Omission Errors	0 errors	5.0 errors	>122	max
Outlier Responses	1 error	4.4 errors	115	84 %
Commission Errors	4 errors	12.9 errors	116	86.9 %
Response Time	457.9 ms	436 ms	96	40 %
Variability	108.4 ms	112 ms	106	66 %

Figure 10.20 Results summary data, QIKtest 2, case #4.

Results Summary: .

Figure 10.21 Results summary QIKtest 3, case #4.

Results	Data	Norm	Score	
M11.9 Total Test	Measured Value	Median of Distribution	Standard Score	Percentile
Omission Errors	4 errors	5.0 errors	102	57 %
Outlier Responses	9 errors	4.4 errors	90	26 %
Commission Errors	2 errors	12.9 errors	125	95.5 %
Response Time	549.6 ms	436 ms	83	13 %
Variability	113.3 ms	112 ms	100	51 %

Figure 10.22 Results summary data, QIKtest 3, case #4.

and 10.22). Since the brain showed itself capable of operating at the higher performance level, it should be able to do so again. Other factors that could explain the failure to hold gains should also be looked for. Figures 10.23 and 10.24 show the development of errors and outlier response times for the three different data sets.

Pre-Post Graphs

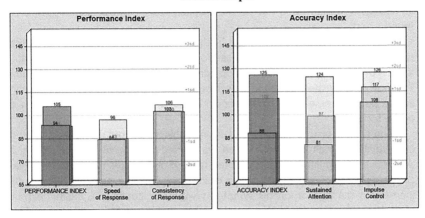

Figure 10.23 Pre-post graphs, case #4.

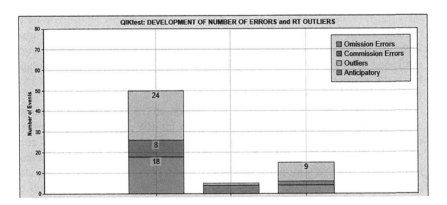

Figure 10.24 Development of number of errors and outliers, case #4.

10.6.5 Case #5

Nicky, an 8-year-old boy, had been diagnosed three years prior to coming to see us for ADHD symptoms. His mother described him as a very smart child who was highly impulsive and hyperactive, had poor self-control, and a short attention span. He had difficulties organizing, was distractible and forgetful, and was impatient and easily frustrated. He was always rushing through tasks which led to him making mistakes and had some difficulties with math and spelling. He always wanted to do as little as possible to get by and had poor self-confidence. He was playing the class clown in order to feel accepted and would manipulate anyone to get his way by lying and cheating, about which he never exhibited remorse. He was fearless, selfish and careless, and never personally at fault. Most recently he had gotten in trouble in school for aggressive behaviors. He was also biting his nails, mostly when under pressure. He had stomach aches with constipation, and sugar cravings were an issue as well. Bedwetting had been a problem in the past but had stopped a few months back.

Noteworthy is the fact that the birth process had been a breach presentation that required an emergency C-section, and Nicky was born with the umbilical cord around his neck. All developmental milestones were reached on time. His mother described herself as a perfectionist and would push him just as hard as she pushed herself. In consequence, Michael blamed her for wanting him to be perfect.

The genetic history revealed addiction problems, thyroid disorders, and bipolar disorder, as well as ADHD. When we started training, he was on 10 mg of Adderall a day, which had been doubled three months prior to the start of neurofeedback treatments due to a lack of improvement in symptoms. Despite the increase in the medication his symptoms were not controlled, and his parents were concerned he would have to take more and more of it until, eventually, it wouldn't work for him at all.

During the first QIKtest (Figure 10.25) Nicky had a difficult time staying on task and had to be prompted several times to continue, as he was becoming increasingly restless and bored. At the end he was able to report on the number of mistakes he had made. The test report revealed all scores within the normal range, with high scores in sustained attention and consistency of response times, while the speed of response was normal. Whereas his impulse control score was high, he clearly struggled with stopping himself from impulsively pressing the button for the non-target.

In designing his training protocol, we considered basic placements to target most of the described symptoms: stabilization for the sugar cravings; physical calming for anxiety, hyperactivity, self-awareness, and constipation; emotional control for self-confidence, frustration, anger, and aggressive and manipulative behaviors, as well as social-emotional awareness; mental calming to address impulse control, organization, attention and forgetfulness, and also attention to details to help with math and spelling. We did a total of 21 neurofeedback sessions in the clinic and after the reevaluation they continued with home training for another two months.

He responded quickly to the training and subtle changes in symptoms were noticed early on. By session 4 he was mellower, less easily frustrated, and not

Results Summary: .

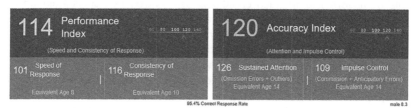

Figure 10.25 Results summary QIK baseline test, case #5.

getting in trouble as much in school, something that the teacher had commented on. He was less impatient and less forgetful, not rushing through tasks all the time. He also didn't need to be told to stop misbehaving that often. He was even able to report feeling calmer and felt good about not getting in trouble in school much anymore.

Nicky was still taking his medication on school days, but his parents decided to try to stop it on the weekends to observe his behavior without it. Prior to doing neurofeedback, going off the medication on the weekends was impossible due to his being really 'out of control,' however, after just six sessions, he did pretty well with the drug holiday. Soon his math improved, and he became more thoughtful and calmer, while remaining well-behaved without medication during the weekends. During his treatments we adjusted the protocol as needed, according to his response to the training, and took on more areas to work on as we continued to calm and stabilize his nervous system.

The reevaluation revealed significantly improved performance with the QIK-test (Figure 10.26) and, according to his parents, the following changes in symptoms: he was less hyperactive, less impulsive, and less easily frustrated. He hadn't displayed any aggressive behaviors in weeks, was biting his nails less, and his mathematics performance had improved considerably. He had been off the medication during the weekends and was observed to maintain good behavior without it. He was doing much better in school both with performance and behavior – a change that his parents and his teachers had noticed. Several symptoms had not changed significantly: he was still rushing through tasks and was still using manipulative behaviors to get his way. Spelling was still problematic, and he needed repetitions and prompts to follow instructions. These concerns, along with the goal to help lower his medications while supporting brain function with neurofeedback, were the reasons we recommended home training.

All the scores in the second test were significantly better than the scores in his first test, and interestingly he didn't have any anticipatory responses or outliers in the retest. This reflects a readiness of his nervous system to attend to the task at hand and respond appropriately. Also noteworthy is the fact that although his performance during the first test scored within the normal range, he improved it during the second test in all evaluated areas. Summary data are shown in Figure 10.26). Corresponding data for the principal measures are shown in Figures 10.27 and 10.28.

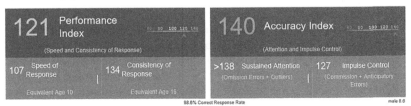

Figure 10.26 Results summary QIKtest 2, case #5.

Pre-Post Graphs

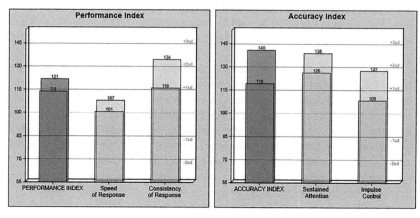

Figure 10.27 Summary data, Standard Scores, Case #5.

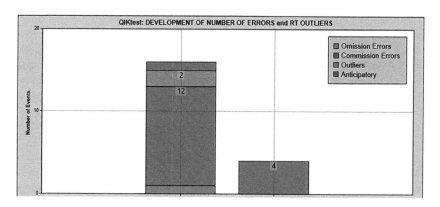

Figure 10.28 Improvement in incidence of discrete errors, case #5.

The home training allows for longer, more frequent sessions, utilizing the protocols that were established in the clinic. By reinforcing the training further, on an almost daily basis, the expectations are to see further significant gains and help the brain to hold those gains. They did about four sessions a week in the two months following the treatments in the clinic before returning the system, to a total of 32 sessions in addition to the 21 we had completed here. While doing the home training Nicky was only taking half of his 10 mg of Adderall and he continued to improve. His teacher was impressed with his good behavior, and he even got an award for his creative writing. The teacher pointed out that his spelling had improved, and that he really had taken a lot of time and put a lot of effort into this project, something he would have absolutely not been able to do before neurofeedback. He continued to benefit from the sessions at home and, when they returned the system two months later, he was a different child, according to his mother. During the summertime, while on vacation, he went off the medication and continued to do well without it.

With all the clinical cases described above, as well as with all the other clients we continue to help with neurofeedback, the individuality and specificity of our method, as well as the individual response for each person we train, become ever more obvious. It is within the brain's scope to enhance its own functional capacity if it is merely given information on its own behavior, to which it is normally blind. By facilitating this process, we allow enhanced self-regulation to emerge and to consolidate. Beyond the diagnostic label, what needs to be fully understood is the uniqueness of each case and the many variables that come with it.

10.7 Summary and Conclusion

This chapter reflects the evolution in the understanding of the ADHD spectrum that needs to occur. First of all, the behavioral features of ADHD are here embedded in a more comprehensive dysregulation model that draws attention to commonalities rather than distinctions. The responsiveness of the entire repertoire of behavioral sequelae of ADHD to a simple training technique points to a modest set of underlying mechanisms. The fact that this technique relies entirely on information derived from the extreme infra-low frequency domain implies further that we are engaged with the tonic regulation of our intrinsic connectivity networks. The fact that this training occurs while the brain is being minimally challenged argues further that our primary concern is with the internal organization, the functional connectivity, of the task-negative network, the Default Mode. A secondary concern is with the interaction of the task-negative with the task-positive control networks.

The review of the case reports illustrates the individuality with which matters need to be approached clinically, even within the overall homogeneity and commonality of approach. We may be seeing here one of the early exemplars of the coming age of personalized medicine. In the application of infra-low frequency training, the adaptation of the protocols to each case is obligatory. Nevertheless, the statistical data document the breadth of impact of this method on attentional deficits across the clinical spectrum

Notes

1 Othmer, S., Othmer, S.F., & Kaiser, D. (1999). EEG biofeedback: An emerging model for its global efficacy. In *Introduction to Quantitative EEG and Neurofeedback*, Evans, J. R. & Abarbanel, A., eds., Academic Press, San Diego, CA, 243–310.
2 Othmer, S., Othmer, S. F., & Kaiser, D. (1999). EEG biofeedback: Training for AD/HD and related disruptive behavior disorders. In *Understanding, Diagnosing, and Treating AD/HD in Children and Adolescents, An Integrative Approach*, Incorvaia, J. A., Mark-Goldstein, B. S., & Tessmer, D., eds., Aronson Press, Northvale, NJ, 235–296.
3 American Academy of Pediatrics. http://pediatrics.aappublications.org/content/125/Supplement_3/S128.full.pdf+html
4 Levesque, J., Beauregard, M., & Mensour, B. (2006). Effect of neurofeedback training on the neural substrates of selective attention in children with

attention-deficit/hyperactivity disorder: A functional magnetic resonance imaging study. *Neuroscience Letters*, 394, 216–221.

5   Biederman, J., Newcorn, J.,& Sprich, S. (1991). Comorbidity of attention deficit hyperactivity disorder with conduct, depressive, anxiety, and other disorders. *The American Journal of Psychiatry*, 148(5), 564–577.

6   Broyd, S. J., Demanuele, C., et al. (2009). Default-mode brain dysfunction in mental disorders: A systematic review. *Neurosci Biobehav Rev*, 33, 279–296.

7   Castellanos, F. X., Sonuga-Barke, E. J., et al. (2005). Varieties of attention-deficit/ hyperactivity disorder-related intra-individual variability. *Biol Psychiatry*, 57(11), 1416–1423.

8   Esterman, M., Noonan, S. K., et al. (2013). In the zone or zoning out?: Tracking behavioral and neural fluctuations during sustained attention. *Cerebral Cortex*, 23(11), 2712–2723. doi:10.1093/cercor/bhs261.

9   Mueller, A., Candrian, G., et al. (2010). Classification of ADHD patients on the basis of independent ERP components using a machine learning system. *Nonlinear Biomedical Physics*, 4(1), 1–12. www.nonlinearbiomedphys.com/content/4/S1/S1

10 Malone, M. A., Kershner, J. R., & Swanson, J. M. (1994). Hemispheric processing and methylphenidate effects in attention-deficit hyperactivity disorder. *Journal of Child Neurology*, 9, 181–189.

11 Tucker, D. M., & Williamson, P. A. (1984). Asymmetric neural control system in human self-regulation. *Psychol Rev*, 91, 185–215.

12 Kaiser, D. A., & Othmer, S. (2000). Effect of neurofeedback on variables of attention in a large multi-center trial. *Journal of Neurotherapy*, 4(1), 5–15.

Chapter 11

ILF Neurofeedback and Alpha-Theta Training in a Multidisciplinary Chronic Pain Program

Evvy J. Shapero and Joshua P. Prager

11.1 Introduction

Chronic pain has been a persistent challenge to the field of medicine. By virtue of its unique aspects and complex presentation, it has yielded best to treatment in a multi-disciplinary approach. This chapter describes such a program, with emphasis on the role of Infra-Low Frequency (ILF) Neurofeedback and Alpha-Theta Neurofeedback. Application is largely focused on cases of Complex Regional Pain Syndrome (CRPS) and Post Laminectomy (Failed Back Surgery Syndrome). The pain program has evolved over a period of more than 20 years, benefiting in particular from the introduction and maturation of the infra-low frequency training. Alpha-Theta training has been utilized throughout.

11.2 Acute Pain vs Chronic Pain

The International Association for the Study of Pain (IASP) defines pain as "an unpleasant sensory and emotional experience .... [A]ssociated with actual or potential tissue damage.... Pain is ... always a psychological state even though ... pain ... has a proximate physical cause."[1]

> While acute pain is a normal sensation triggered in the nervous system to alert you to possible injury and the need to take care of yourself, chronic pain is different. Chronic pain persists. Pain signals keep firing in the nervous system for weeks, months, even years. There may have been an initial mishap—sprained back, serious infection, or there may be an ongoing cause of pain—arthritis, cancer, ear infection, but some people suffer chronic pain in the absence of any past injury or evidence of body damage.[2, 3]

Chronic pain is a devastating phenomenon that affects not only the body part that is involved but also substantial portions of the nervous system, especially the brain.

The consequences go beyond the patient, to include family and loved ones.[4] The total cost of chronic pain in the United States annually is estimated to be over

600 billion dollars, including the costs of medical care, medications, and lost productivity in the workplace. Chronic pain likely affects at least 100 million American adults.[5] Many rely on opioids just to be able to move. As the trend toward the use of opioids for pain has increased, so has the risk of chemical dependence and abuse. The recent recognition of the epidemic of opioid abuse in the USA has led to the development of guidelines for monitoring the drugs. Therefore, alternative therapies have become even more important.[6]

11.3 Gate Control Theory

Chronic pain has come to be recognized as a disease process in its own right. On the one hand, there are known physiological processes that over time allow "normal" somatosensory signals to be recruited into nociceptive pathways, which radically expands the range of sensation perceived as painful. On the other hand, there are central mechanisms that effectively apply a weighting factor to the pain signals, assigning salience to the perceived signals. This modulatory role was first proposed as the "gate control theory of pain" by Ronald Melzack and Patrick Wall in 1965, and has since been further elaborated.[7] There are many stories of how people are injured on the battlefield or in sports games and do not feel any pain until sometime later. This has to do with the brain being engaged with higher priorities and shutting the gate until it can pay attention to the messages. A major study by Beecher in the 1940's demonstrated that a significant number of soldiers at Anzio Beach in World War II who lost a limb and made it to safety did not require analgesic while in the battlefield.[8] The gate control theory helps explain how the brain influences the experience of pain.

11.4 Pain as an Alarm Signal

In consequence, pain signals may be corrupted at the source as well as "wrongly" interpreted at the central nervous system. Moreover, as pain is by its nature an alarm signal, our biological system arranges for the alarm to become even more compelling and intrusive over time if it is not attended to. Since chronic pain cannot be "turned off" by endogenous mechanisms in the general case, it can take patients to the limits of their tolerance.

11.5 Components of Pain

There are three components of pain. There is the sensation—how much it hurts; the emotional—that is the suffering, how unpleasant the experience is; and the cognitive dimension—how we interpret the pain, based on our previous experience.[9,10] There is a vicious cycle in which pain causes disability and emotional distress, which in turn worsen the perception of pain. How patients think about their pain, their beliefs, experiences, environment, mood, involvement in the "sick role," and coping skills can all influence the severity of pain and play a role in the patients recovery.[11,12]

Pain can be viewed as a signal of danger in the body until it reaches the emotional level. It is important to distinguish the sensation of pain from the experience of suffering as a result of the chronic nature of pain. The limbic system, where emotions are processed, modulates the level of pain experienced. The pain alone is often not responsible for the suffering. Anxiety, fear, a sense of loss, and anger contribute to the suffering. Suffering also occurs when relationships with family members are strained, with loss of financial status, and with loss of identity. So suffering can be a manifestation not of pain itself but of the losses that occur when pain persists.[13] High levels of emotional stress caused by the constant pain can lead to somatization and hypochondria. "Fear-related experiences such as catastrophic thinking and avoidance are especially significant in exacerbating pain perceptions."[14, 15] According to Main et al (2010), "Pain catastrophising is a better predictor of pain-related disability and activity intolerance than pain itself."[16] Eliminating pain behaviors such as guarding, rubbing, or grimacing leads to improved pain perception.[17] Failing to address psychological issues in chronic pain patients may result in prolonged disability.

11.6 Multidimensional Nature of Pain

Ranking equal in importance with all of the above considerations is the question of who the person is that is coming for help with a chronic pain condition. "Chronic pain is associated with a high prevalence of psychiatric disorders."[18] It has become abundantly clear that patients with a history of early trauma or adult trauma are at a high risk of developing chronic pain.[19, 20] Patients with a history of sexual abuse are also at a high risk of having pain related disorders.[21] Predisposing factors include temperament, anxiety and depression, elevated fear response, negative thinking, uncertainty, sense of helplessness, and substance abuse—all vulnerability factors for chronic pain. Illness perception predicts depression/anxiety, consequences of being ill and effects on identity and emotional functioning.[22] Suicidal ideation is a significant risk factor for patients with CRPS and related to depressed mood, decreased functioning, and pain severity.[23] Neurobiological variables have also been identified, including the finding that immune function and inflammation are activated by pain states.[24] Cognitive impairment is also common in people with chronic pain—pain causes an alteration of the brain structure affecting attention and memory,[25] decision making,[26] processing speed,[27] and loss of gray matter.[28]

Seen in the new paradigm, chronic pain preferentially afflicts those whose nervous systems were already dysregulated, for whom this event is not the first, or even the primary, insult to their cerebral organization. The recovery capacity or resilience is compromised in these individuals and, when subjected to the challenge of persistent pain, the cerebral regulatory system is overtaxed and a descent into chronic pain ensues.

The consequences of chronic pain are brain-wide, and thus compromise cerebral functionality across various domains of function. With the affective domain and autonomic regulation compromised in first instance, the consequences then extend to cognitive and executive function, exacerbated by the consequences of poor sleep architecture that follows directly from the relentless experience of pain.

The fallout extends beyond the patient to include the family, other loved ones, and activities within the workplace. As relationships suffer and productivity declines, there are further feedback loops that lubricate the slide into dysfunction and perhaps even into personal isolation and disengagement from life. An unhealthy lifestyle, lack of support, withdrawal from social connection, and substance abuse represent additional compounding factors.[29]

11.7 Influence of Culture in Understanding Pain

Culture plays a significant role in the perception of pain and its treatment. The Institute of Medicine of the National Academy of Sciences "Report on Health Care Disparities"[30] concluded that there are significant racial and ethnic disparities in pain perception, assessment, and treatment, which are found across settings and pain diagnosis. Pain treatments rely on scientific evidence, which often has not included individuals from diverse backgrounds.[31]

11.8 Functional Rehabilitation Program

Comprehensive interdisciplinary functional rehabilitation (FRP) is the gold standard for the treatment of many pain syndromes.[32, 33, 34] This involves the participation of multiple disciplines that address both the sensation and suffering components of the pain, the psychological context, the lifestyle issues, and the need for concomitant physical rehabilitation. The majority of the patients seen at the California Pain Medicine Center have either Failed Back Surgery Syndrome or suffer from Complex Regional Pain Syndrome (CRPS). Hence, they are among the most challenging of chronic pain patients. The core of the program consists of medical management, physical therapy, neurofeedback, and psychotherapy.

Each discipline involved in rehabilitating the patient, both in terms of reduction of pain sensation and reduction of suffering, plays a different role. As part of the intake process, psychological assessment of the patient's emotional state is performed to accurately determine suitability for invasive pain treatments, such as spinal cord stimulation and drug delivery pump implantation.[35, 36] Specialized psychological tests have been developed to help identify risk factors. Cognitive dysfunction is also very common with pain patients; therefore, neuropsychological evaluations may be utilized if the patient demonstrates cognitive impairment, which may interfere with the treatment. "Psychological events are both risk factors in and consequences of chronic pain."[37]

One key to treatment success is the communication among the various professionals jointly working to motivate the patient, and to modify treatment if necessary. At each team meeting, patients progress is reviewed to determine other risk management strategies. Each component is essential, and collaboration with participating providers is absolutely required to provide optimal quality patient care. This integration of multiple modalities in an intensive program has led to substantial and significant improvement for patients suffering from chronic pain. The multidisciplinary approach allows for more accurate diagnosis and characterization, combined with a wider array of treatment options.[38]

11.9 Pain Psychology

Knowledge of the psychology of pain can greatly improve the treatment of chronic pain. Many pain patients are involved in litigation as a result of accidents, work-related injuries, or medical malpractice. Negative experiences further interact and impact treatment, therefore, treatment should include management of psychological problems. Various types of psychotherapy methods are incorporated depending on the needs of the patient. No single psychotherapeutic approach is effective and appropriate for all patients, problems, and contexts of pain.[39, 40] Therefore, it is best to utilize a combination of psychotherapeutic orientations.

11.10 Physical Therapy

Physical therapy focuses on mobility, strengthening, and functional exercises to help re-establish muscular control for pain-free lateral movement and regular physical activities. Physical therapy may include mirror box therapy, graded motor imagery, and virtual reality to desensitize the patient from lateralized pain. Inactivity is a serious impediment to improvement in chronic pain, and can produce concurrent myofascial pain. Obesity is also a problem in chronic pain. Additional methods of care are provided when appropriate. These include restorative yoga, mindfulness meditation, nutritional counseling, massage, aqua therapy, chiropractic, substance abuse treatment, psychopharmacology, and other subspecialty consultations.

11.11 Neurofeedback

Infra-Low Frequency Neurofeedback training addresses itself to core regulation of arousal, affect, and of the autonomic nervous system.

Once a more stable physiology is established with ILF Neurofeedback, Alpha-Theta training is introduced for the resolution of psychological traumas, and to help eliminate learned fears and adverse behaviors. As a prerequisite to Alpha-Theta training, patients are also taught diaphragmatic breathing, relaxation techniques, heart rate variability training, grounding techniques, and self-regulation strategies.

The focus of the remainder of the chapter is the contribution to functional recovery made by the neurofeedback component. Neurofeedback contributes to recovery via two primary modalities. First, through infra-low frequency training it provides a pathway for recovery from acquired neural dysregulation. Infra-Low frequency Neurofeedback training addresses itself to core regulation of arousal, of affect, and of the autonomic nervous system. Once a more stable physiology is established with ILF Neurofeedback, Alpha-Theta training is introduced for the resolution of psychological traumas, and to help eliminate learned fears and adverse behaviors.

Because of the existence of this program over a period of 20 years, an unusual opportunity exists to survey the contribution made by neurofeedback over the course of its evolution to include the infra-low frequency region, and to discern trends. At the outset, the primary emphasis was on the Alpha-Theta component of the neurofeedback experience in order to resolve trauma formations and help with the psychological fallout of the pain experience. EEG-band training was always employed prior to the Alpha-Theta experience, however, in order to calm and stabilize the physiology.

The status in the 2006 time frame was captured in a book chapter in *Weiner's Pain Management*.[41] What could be accomplished with neurofeedback in application to CRPS at the time was presented in a survey of outcomes published in 2007.[42] Since the patients under study were undergoing multiple therapies concurrently, and also were no longer naive to neurofeedback, the chosen outcome measure was the change in pain level before and after a single neurofeedback session. Fortuitously, this made possible direct comparison with a prior study using neurofeedback on resting state functional magnetic resonance signals. The results were comparable, with a slight advantage in favor of the EEG neurofeedback.[43]

Single-session effects, however, do not tell the story. Typically, a degree of symptom regression would be experienced over some time frame in CRPS, necessitating occasional booster sessions. Entry into the infra-low frequency region (0.1 Hz and below) took place in 2006. Protocol placements remained the same, and the training procedure remained identical. The thrust into the ILF domain had been driven all along by the most challenging clients, pain patients among them. Whereas clinical results were quite generally improved with respect to EEG-band training, there was particular benefit for trauma syndromes. ILF Neurofeedback, therefore, offered greater symptom relief across the board, while also preparing the ground better for the Alpha-Theta training to follow.

Overall, the program patients experienced reduced pain, severity, improved coping strategies, positive stress management, increased endurance and stamina, improved emotional health, and restored positive outlook. We next focus on the Alpha-Theta experience of patients, both because it is so central to the overall treatment program and because this complement to the ILF neurofeedback is most appropriately treated in the context of chronic pain management.

11.12 Alpha-Theta Training

After sufficient gains have been made with ILF training in stabilizing and calming the brain, Alpha-Theta training is introduced to most clients. Those who are suspicious, fearful, skeptical, or still hyper-vigilant are not encouraged to undertake it. Clients who are open to the exploration, on the other hand, are encouraged to try it. Alpha-theta training is yet another tool for promoting calming of the nervous system. By giving feedback on the alpha and theta bands of the EEG, Alpha-Theta training moves patients toward engagement with their inner experience. With the aid of technology that illuminates the journey, the client enters a slightly altered state in which the conscious mind encounters the subconscious reality that has been forming throughout the life of the person. The encounter is typically non-verbal, but unsurprisingly it either speaks to the moment or resurfaces events from prior history in a compelling way. The authenticity of the experience is typically apprehended immediately by the patient.

The work can only flourish when the client feels safe, and progress is contingent on a non-judgmental, caring rapport between the client and the therapist. Nevertheless, if some degree of resolution begins to take place, the client can rightfully and proudly "own" his own progress toward mastery of his condition. There is, of course, precedent for all of this in ancient practices such as chanting, drumming, or other rituals. These may involve isolation of the individual, sensory deprivation, carefully modulated hyper-ventilation, and possibly even the aid of hallucinogenic agents. More recently, methods of low-level auditory and visual brain stimulation—all frequency-based—have also proliferated. What all of these methods have in common is the preferential promotion of low-frequency EEG activity that promotes access to deeper states of the individual.

Alpha-Theta is also referred to as deep state training. As this experience becomes increasingly familiar, the encounter with the core self becomes a resource for the patient to support recovery. Alpha-Theta training has been utilized as a therapeutic tool for trauma conditions, PTSD, and addictions, since the late eighties, although early research goes back to the seventies.[44] However, it is also known to be a useful tool in peak-performance training; in the promotion of creativity, self-discovery, and insight; and in the enlargement of the scope of awareness. It is a question of whether one adopts a deficit-focus or an optimum functioning orientation. In application to chronic pain conditions, the patient is likely to migrate from an initial deficit focus to a positive orientation to the experience.

In their ground-breaking book, *Beyond Biofeedback*, Alyce and Elmer Green showed that theta training made material from the unconscious accessible. Falling into a theta-dominant state can produce detached thoughts or a stream of vague images that are not necessarily connected. They may not make immediate sense in the prevailing narrative of the conscious life. Nevertheless, there is typically a sense of connection to these experiences. The closest one comes to having experiences such as this in ordinary life is during the transition from wakefulness to sleep, where it is referred to as hypnagogia. Typically, this state in transition is very brief, but with the reinforcements involved in Alpha-Theta training the hypnagogic state can be sustained. The client typically migrates between alpha-dominated and theta-dominated states throughout the session, with the respective states of consciousness each contributing to the experience.[45]

Persistent alpha dominance typically represents a state of both physical and emotional relaxation—a distancing from engagement, most particularly of visual engagement. Theta-band dominance, by contrast, is a state that facilitates the recall of early childhood experiences, of learned behaviors, traumatic events, and other "stuff" that we hold on to. Theta dominance is thought to be the bridge between the conscious and the subconscious. With vigilance subdued, the edge of sleep onset represents a state of heightened suggestibility and of hypnotizability. (Advantage was taken of this connection quite early in the history of the field. In what was perhaps the first clinical use Alpha-Theta training, Tom Budzynski used the method to resolve thanatophobiathe—fear of death.[46] This may have occurred as early as 1966–7). While Alpha-Theta training is not really about self-regulation per se, clients nevertheless report that they feel more whole, more content, and more confident, with an enhanced sense of well-being. One client described Alpha-Theta as "the frosting on the cake."

Alpha-Theta opens the brain to learning new behaviors and allows the old scripts to be rewritten. Most clients report deep insights, heightened self-awareness, and meaningful self-discovery that becomes integrated in their life. This tool can be beneficial for the client who is defensive, resistant, and controlling, yet remains open to change. It is the client doing the work without the therapist being directly in charge.

As an agitated physiology quiets down, resistance declines and the client becomes more open. When clients encounter past traumas, they are not reliving the experiences but rather witnessing the events benignly. There is typically no sense of existential threat. Moreover, the experience typically surfaces no more than the client can readily handle. Many clients experience a shift in energy and a transformation in appearance and behavior. One is even tempted to refer to this as the mini (non-surgical) face lift! Core beliefs are shifted; a decrease in pain is felt; a reduction in psychological stress and a trend toward feeling more confident is experienced.

Scenes from the past may appear by surprise. Imagery that seems odd to ridiculous is not uncommon. Having conversations with relatives who have passed is not unusual. Exploring these scenes and images with the client typically leads to some meaningful insight and element of self-discovery. Many times over, the recall of some very small moment of insight translates into a huge impact on healing and growth. One must not underestimate this experience and should, perhaps, establish it as a base to open the door to deeper resources within.

Commonly the Alpha-Theta experience is punctuated by experiences that are transformational in character. This may involve insight into connectedness with others; a surge of unconditional love and forgiveness; an illumination of gratitude and appreciation; the expanding and dissolving of boundaries; a deeply certain feeling of knowing; and connecting with spiritual beings or deceased family members. Also not uncommonly observed, small nuggets of insight in Alpha-Theta training can lead to large transformational shifts. This testifies to the unique—and in fact indispensable—contribution of the Alpha-Theta experience to the therapeutic journey. We have witnessed transformations in personality and character traits even after a single Alpha-Theta session.

11.13 Alpha-Theta Imagery

One client reported baffling imagery of ants and crabs. While he was totally embarrassed about these images and shrugged them off as absurd, he was encouraged to take a look more closely and was asked some questions: What do ants do? Where are the crabs? What do they look like? How do you see them? Is there any connection to them in your life? His replies: Ants are workers that are always busy. "Oh my gosh, that's me in my life." Crabs on the beach were walking sideways: Silence and then a smile. "That's me always being side-tracked and not moving forward." This was a moment of pure revelation and transformation for him. The language of the unconscious is a symbolic one. What is so poignant here is that words are unnecessary to communicate a message. The symbol, the representational picture or image, conveys the complete thought, concept, or idea without the use of words to describe it; we have here the proverbial "picture that is worth a thousand words."

Another client saw herself, in almost all of her Alpha-Theta sessions, on a zip line going to this tree house with a fireplace and hot tea waiting for her. After drinking the tea and relaxing for a bit she would take the zip line back to a place of chaos. In talking about the imagery, tears appeared, and she disclosed the affair that she was having and the guilt she felt. She had been in therapy for almost six months and had not disclosed this bit of information. Relief and resolution were on their way! And her CRPS chronic pain started to be less intense.

Another client saw a mask in her imagery. Upon discovery, it was her unborn child that had died in utero and had now come back to assure her she was OK. A gentleman in his late 60's, highly anxious, with panic attacks, a sleep disorder, and OCD about certain things in his home, very much wanted a loving and committed relationship but was very shut off. During one of his Alpha-Theta sessions, he left his heart on a rock and in return he received love. The following week he met a lovely woman while walking his dog on the beach. You could call it a coincidence; more reasonably, it is only too likely that the Alpha-Theta training had prepared the ground.

Another severe chronic pain patient saw herself in a beautiful white, flowing cotton dress dancing on the beach, enjoying the sun and the feeling of joy. She said it was the only time she had not experienced pain in the last five years.

Steve Fahrion, collaborator with Elmer and Alyce Green in the original research into Alpha-Theta, describes the journey as one of "exploration and discovery," in contrast to "active coping."[47,48] It is apparent that the sheer unpredictability of these journeys sets them apart from what typically transpires in psychotherapy. And yet, very clearly, subsequent psychotherapy becomes more productive: coping skills are enhanced; defense mechanisms dissipate; and insight is more apparent. The Alpha-Theta experience helps to break down defenses and resistance to therapy, thus allowing talk therapy to reach another dimension of value and insight.

Of course, profound Alpha-Theta experiences do not happen with everyone. Commonly reported is a state of deep relaxation without any notable remembered experiences. Yet others simply slide off into sleep. This can happen with the many who show up in a sleep-deprived state, or with those still dealing with unresolved ADHD. There can be negative experiences as well, such as pain-inducing imagery and troubling or mysterious body sensations. When that happens, it is usually a sign that not enough calming of the brain with infra-low frequency had been achieved prior to the Alpha-Theta training.

11.14 Case Presentations

Alpha-Theta training can be performed with either a single channel or a dual-channel montage. When the work was begun years ago the single-channel configuration was standard, and it has been retained throughout for reasons of simplicity and consistency. The active electrode is placed at PZ, the reference is placed on the mastoid behind the ear, and the common connection (called ground) is placed on the forehead for convenience, although it can go anywhere on the head.

All patients were taught Heart Rate Variability training and diaphragmatic breathing prior to initiating alpha-theta training. Some autogenic phrases were incorporated in the 5–8 minute guided imagery segment at the very beginning of the session. Sensory deprivation was used to facilitate entry into deep states and headphones were utilized for the auditory feedback. Peniston worked with his alcoholic patients to create an image of their desired outcome, which typically was a scene in which they would reject the alcohol.[49] This helped to clarify their intension. However, with chronic pain patients, the guided imagery presented was designed to allow the body to relax, and the mind to enter into a journey of exploration, while healing the emotional and physical aspects of the self. This is geared to result in an experience of insight. The unconscious mind gives us subtle information that we may or may not be aware of or that we tend to avoid. The following case studies clearly demonstrate the power of healing and transformation with Alpha-Theta.

11.14.1 Patient 1

A personal reflection by a client best illuminates the issue of sudden insight and redirection:

"This was a profoundly healing experience for me. Sharing the experience was as important in the healing as the internal cognitive journey that took place during the Alpha-Theta session.

The session started with my picking a shell from a collection in a basket. I picked a fairly small snail shell. During the guided imagery we were to examine the shell in our minds. I noted its roughness on the outside but also the cool, sheltered interior. As I did this, I realized that much of my life I had tried to live in such a shell. I attempted to be tough on the outside while often seeking the safety of retreat. And suddenly the shell no longer felt right. It was too small, too confining, too cumbersome. Then the shell spoke to me, saying 'You don't need me anymore.' With these words I felt lighter, freer but also curious, social, and confidently vulnerable.

I then found myself walking along a beach. It was beautiful, warm, and peaceful. I felt the roughness of the sand and the touch of a light breeze. My mother, who had recently died, was walking with me. We held hands. She was her old self, healthy and cheerful. We talked indistinctly for a while, and then about missing each other. Finally, she said she had to go. Before she left, she looked me in the eyes and said, 'Don't forget to laugh!,' and then she did a little dance she used to do. She had often thought I was too serious.

Subsequently, probably with this encouragement, I was flying, happy, excited, and adventurous. I stopped at various places to play, dancing with folks in a small village in Spain, laughing and talking with people in a bar in Amsterdam, kayaking on an unrecognized river.

Finally, I landed on a beach. I came into the session struggling with the question of what would anchor me in the world now. My wife, my long-time friend and I had just spent the last several years caring for our aging mothers, who lived in the same elder care development. In the fall, my mother died. The funeral of my friend's mother had taken place the day before this session. My wife's mother had just been admitted to hospice the week before. Suddenly the people who had organized our lives would be gone. The three of us were standing at the water's edge, enjoying the sunset. On the horizon, standing above the waves, our mothers appeared as their earlier vibrant and healthy selves, smiling and waving at us. We waved back, excited to see them and then they faded away. What came to me at that moment was that I was looking for something that I already had. The three of us had been each other's anchor and were continuing to be so. We had supported each other through the many tough decisions of long illnesses, battles with the health care system, and disheartening days. But we were also lucky enough to have these capable and strong women who had faced life with courage, humor, and kindness as our role models. It was our turn to take our place as the older generation, giving to each other and our children what our mother's had given to us."

11.14.2 Patient 2

A 32-year-old married female, with three young children, suffered from failed back surgery and severe chronic pain. A year after the surgery she was no longer able to work as a teacher, take care of her children, or have any quality of life. She became severely depressed and anxious, addicted to the pain medications that had all proved ineffective in controlling her pain. She was in bed 24/7 and could not function in any capacity. In addition, she discovered her husband had been having an affair. During the pain program she went through detox, in addition to the daily modalities of physical therapy, psychotherapy, neurofeedback, and medical management. After completing 12 sessions of ILF Neurofeedback, she was ready for Alpha-Theta. She was guilt-ridden that she had been unable to take care of her kids. Two very close relatives passed away in quick succession and she was unable to attend the funerals. She had so much anger toward her husband, and she felt God had betrayed her. After all, she had been a Sunday school teacher.

"Feelings of hopelessness and the ever-present debilitating pain overwhelmed me the night before I was due to start neurofeedback. 'What even is Neurofeedback? If it can help me, how come I haven't heard of it before?' I wondered to myself. After six years of struggling with back pain and nerve damage, I was willing to try anything for some relief. After exhausting all the methods doctors offered me, this seemed to be my last hope before looking at a lifetime not only in pain, but on pain medications which lent themselves to undesirable side-effects. I was staring at a lifetime of the vicious cycle of pain, restless sleep, depression, and anxiety. Already having to resign from teaching and my marriage falling apart, I was left with no hope and no choice but to give this neurofeedback thing a fighting chance.

My first training session was very interesting. As I sat in a comfortable chair, sensors were pressed onto my scalp with a kind of sticky paste. Watching a computer monitor, I was to relax and 'move' the rolling ball across the screen as it collected dots and revealed a picture from nature scenes. After clearing a board, another screen filled with dots appeared and I was to do the process again, without a remote control but with my mind, or my brain. I began to feel sleepy after about 20 minutes, which is when the sensors were removed and the 'gel' was cleaned up from my scalp with rubbing alcohol. 'That's it? That's the training?' I thought. For 20 days I was to come in, get 'hooked up,' and basically play video games with my mind for 30 minutes. This was the plan to calm down my central nervous system and get my chronic pain under control. Bring it!

After the first several sessions of neurofeedback my central nervous system began calming down. My opiate pain medications were being titrated down, eventually to zero, sleep was improving (I slept through the night and dreamt for the first time in over three years), my appetite was improving, and hope was returning—hope for this 'neurofeedback thing,' hope for healing, hope for a future.

It wasn't until I had completed about 15 awake-state neurofeedback training sessions that I was introduced to another form of neurofeedback: deep-state alpha-theta training. This was to be a completely different experience from what I had done up until that point. Lying back in the chair, sensors were placed on my scalp in different positions, an eye mask placed over my eyes, and headphones over my ears; the session began. I was encouraged to breathe deeply and easily, let go of tension and discomfort, and to focus inside and allow any fleeting thoughts to come and go. Using guided imagery, my neurofeedback clinician led me on a visual journey to the ocean. To this day I remember it vividly, like it was yesterday. In this visualization I made my way down steps on a cliff, walked down the beach where children were playing, the ocean waves crashing gently into a cave, where I found an empty, crystal box. I was instructed to place all my worries and fears in that box and place it back in the cave, where I could visit it anytime to add more emotions to the box. After leaving the cave, I was left to enjoy the rest of my time in deep-state Alpha-Theta by the ocean.

Through the headphones I heard alternating sounds of crashing waves and a babbling brook, and rhythmic tones of 'gongs' and 'dings.' However, what was happening in my mind, or brain, was such a powerful experience I believe vital to not just my physical healing, but my emotional healing. During this and subsequent Alpha-Theta sessions I was able to visit people from my past, learn about myself and my journey with God, and discover things about myself, enhancing my emotional well-being.

During one session I visited with my grandmother who had been my best friend and had passed away a couple years before. We talked and laughed together, looked through her family picture albums that were black and white pictures taken in the early to mid 1900s—pictures I don't recall ever seeing while she was living. The pictures were so detailed and accurate in my mind during the session. My grandmother told me the names of the people pictured and I can still remember the clothes they were wearing and the expressions on their faces.

It was such a meaningful experience for me—not only did we get one more moment together where we laughed and talked with ease, but I came away with the message that my absence during her passing was okay with her. She knows how much I loved her and how much I miss her; how much I regretted not telling her those things when she was dying. She reassured me that I had told her many times while she was living and the times we spent together were some of the best in her life. Wow. I came away from that session with the knowledge that my grandmother does know how much I love her and I feel completely at peace with the circumstances of her passing. No regrets!

During another powerful Alpha-Theta session I had an opportunity to visit with a friend who was a second mom to me and had died suddenly at a young age of a brain aneurysm. Through guided imagery I was encouraged to visualize a forest where a white glowing light floated above me and led me near a waterfall, where my friend was waiting to offer me advice. At the time I was going through a divorce, re-entering into the workforce, and raising three children. The advice my friend gave me led me to be at peace with the entire situation. She urged me to let go of some of the daily things in life that 'had' to be done, to break the rules every now and again and allow the kids to eat ice cream before bed on a school night, to not take everything so seriously. This session was the turning point for my happiness because now in life, with my kids and my job, I truly enjoy every moment and break the rules more often than not.

Unfortunately, during my lifetime dozens of people close to me have passed away, either suddenly or in very tragic circumstances. Beginning at the age of eight, when my Godfather committed suicide, to the dozens of people who have passed since, I suffered some emotional trauma regarding death and life. Alpha-Theta training has been the key to the resolution of such traumas and now, almost three years after my first session, the effects are lasting.

Using guided imagery that led me to a high cliff, I had an encounter with a beautiful bald eagle during another memorable Alpha-Theta session. At first the eagle was far in the distance and I watched it fly, almost float towards me. The eagle was carrying something in its beak and as he approached, I realized it was a piece of paper I was to take from its beak. On the paper was a message for me. The neurofeedback and Alpha-Theta training happened at a critical time in my life. There was so much physical and emotional healing to take place and so many components of my life were at forks in the road. It was decision time for me and whatever decision I made, it would not only affect myself, but my children, my husband at the time, my health, and my future. Somehow I did know what I had to do but leading up to voicing the decision was daunting. It was during this Alpha-Theta session that I realized everything was going to be okay because the message in the eagle's beak read, 'You can do it!' It was at that moment when I knew, truly believed I could … and I did.

I have also experienced Alpha-Theta sessions where no guided imagery was used. These sessions were powerful all the same and left me feeling deeply relaxed and at ease with my current circumstances. My mind was able to drift in and out of various thoughts, go to various places such as revisiting the forest from a previous session. These sessions also left me feeling completely rested and revitalized my outlook for the future.

Neurofeedback training gave me my life back. It calmed my central nervous system, which allows me to manage my pain without opiate medications, thus enabling me to return to the workforce and participate in my children's lives. It facilitated restful, uninterrupted sleep at night and eliminated my depression and anxiety. Although it couldn't save my marriage, the Alpha-Theta training gave me the ability to be courageous and confident in my future. There is a greater sense of peace about my life and an underlying joy in every situation I face. Since doing Alpha-Theta I have not stopped smiling. Life is to be lived and now, thanks to neurofeedback and Alpha-Theta training, I can live it to the fullest."

11.14.3 Patient 3

"My Alpha-Theta session began with some sounds consisting of music in the background, binaural beats, a gong sound, an occasional ping, white noise, ocean waves, and a brook.

As I heard the music, I started to take deep, cleansing, and calming breaths to help my mind and body relax. As I was doing this, my inner voice was coaching me to pay attention to the feeling of the air going in and out of my nose. While I did this I was also reminding myself that I was not here to meditate but to relax and allow my mind to open up and go where it wanted. This was difficult at first.

As I concentrated on the sounds flowing from the headphones, I noticed my mind drifting and then returning to paying attention to what was going on in the room. I coached myself to take a few more deep, relaxing breaths and focus my attention inward and relax. Soon I was able to let go of the room and start to let my mind wander.

At first it wandered to work-related tasks. When I noticed this, I coached myself again to take a few more deep, cleansing breaths. Soon thereafter my thoughts went to a place I had created a short time previously, something called a 'safe place.' It was a place had I made up that had all of my favorite things. It was beautiful, calm, and relaxing. My safe place is a crescent shaped cove with a house nestled up at one end of this cove between a high cliff wall that sheltered the cove and the beach. The entrance point was a natural staircase that begins at the opposite end of the cove from the top of the cliff to the beach floor.

Then the image began to fade. My attention was back in my body and I could see the darkness behind my eyes. I took another deep breath. In my heart, I was hoping that my mind would wander back to my cove. I coached myself to just relax my mind and try not to hold onto my own wants and expectations.

After another deep breath, I found that I was thinking about my cove again, but this time there was a girl on the beach. She was dressed in a full length, white Mexican style dress that covered her legs and feet as she sat on the dry, warm sand with her legs tucked up to her chest. She was looking out at the ocean. I knew the sand was warm and comfortable. I also knew that what the girl was looking at was unsettling. I knew this before I was able to see what she was looking at. I seemed to have this awareness that the girl was me. The next image that came to me was of a violently stormy ocean, with dark foreboding clouds thick with lightning. The ocean itself was dark, tumultuous, and swelling. The image started to fade out again.

This time I noticed a tightening at the top of my throat and a slight pain. The kind of pain one gets when they are so full of emotion it stops their ability to speak. I wanted to swallow and make it go away, but a feeling sense told me to pause, to notice this sensation in my throat. I had this feeling sense that I was supposed to feel and recognize this pain and pay special attention to where it was, not to simply alleviate the uncomfortable feeling and move on. So instead I took another deep, slow breath to try and relax again and go back to letting my mind wander.

I quickly came back to the beach, and this time the girl was standing. She was standing and I felt her fear and worry. I could see it in her stance. She was staring out at the ocean. Her hair now caught up in the wind that was blowing firmly in all directions. Then I saw this huge tsunami wave standing like a wall of water. It wasn't moving but it threatened to consume the girl and the cove. The ominous and threatening clouds were above and behind this huge tsunami wave. I/the girl felt some water droplets on my face from the thrashing wind. Then I saw the girl hold up her hands like she was wielding magical power to hold the tsunami at bay. It looked and felt like she was using all her strength and then some. As she was doing this I could see and feel her yelling and grunting from the exertion. Then the image faded out again.

I was back in the chair and I could feel tears coming from my eyes. I could feel the lump in my throat. I was surprised that the image was so moving. I was also a little confused as to why I was so moved by this short scene that played out. I took a few more deep breaths. This time I felt a deeper sense of relaxation from my breaths.

My mind quickly and easily returned to the cove again. The same scene was still playing. This time when I looked at the tsunami I didn't see it as a tsunami. I recognized it as my fear. The girl put her hands down, threw her head back, and just screamed with all her might at the huge wave. She then threw her hands straight back and to her sides as her *head fell back. Her chest lifted and I felt this heavy sort of feeling leave her chest and go into the big wave. The scene then calmed. The image faded again, and I was seeing the darkness behind my eyes. I noticed that my cheeks felt wet and my throat ached slightly. The pain and lump in my throat softened. I now felt that it was okay to swallow to help make my throat more comfortable. I took a few more deep breaths and I was back at the cove.*

The storm and the wave had gone. The girl was now dancing like a little girl on the beach, running back and forth with the water. It was then that I (the girl) had this sudden impulse to lie down on the beach and let the waves wash up over my feet and spill on to the rest of my body. And that is what the girl did. She did so, and I felt her joy and absolute freedom. Then I caught myself thinking, 'I would never have done that in real life.' I would be too afraid to. I don't do things like this because my mind would always irrationally focus on how unsanitary that may be. How annoying it would be for the sand to wash up your legs and get stuck in the bathing suit or get lodged in body parts most uncomfortably. It was then that I had another realization. My whole life, I allowed my fear to hold me back from so many things. My fear was immense like the tsunami and I wasn't able to even enjoy the most simple and innocent of pleasures. I cried again, a good cry. The session ended."

11.14.4 Patient 4

This next case vignette remains the best example of how healing and integration can occur within the Alpha-Theta experience.

A 54-year-old male with a history of depression—decreased energy, negative thoughts, overwhelmed, irritable, and socially isolated. His diet was poor; he did not exercise; he used marijuana every night to calm down; he suffered occasional panic attacks, and carried Xanax just in case. He had been very anxious as a child. He was resistant to medications, having tried many for his depression. He had been in analysis for two years at a rate of five sessions per week. He understands why he may be depressed, but he still cannot get past it. After twenty sessions of stabilization with ILF Neurofeedback the panic attacks diminished, cognitive functioning improved, mood improved, there was no longer a need for marijuana, and he started exercising. Still, some issues with negative script remained from childhood. His father had been negative and his mother distant.

After several, very positive, Alpha-Theta experiences, one was most profound: Imagery of going to his childhood home where he had grown up. He met his inner child who comforted him and reassured him that "It's going to be OK." A lot of forgiveness was extended, and love expressed. After the session he remarked: "Now I know what it really feels like to be psychologically integrated." Soon after, his relationship with his kids became more intimate and playful. His comments below are from after his completion of neurofeedback.

"I went from wanting to die to wanting to live ... having treatment-resistant chronic depression, and dysthymia with the occasional panic attack is no picnic ... In September I left psychoanalysis because it was simply not making me as happy as I needed to be and as quickly as I needed to be (of course my analyst would say I was 'resisting' or some other thing Vienna made up to keep patients on the couch) and began neurofeedback. Within three sessions, my wife noticed improvements in my mood and irritability (I didn't

notice anything yet, but 'the fish can't see the water'). Within twelve sessions even I noticed a 'break in the clouds' that had been my lifelong companions. In under 40 sessions I was able to discontinue neurofeedback ... I now no longer smoke pot nightly just to escape my head and get a whiff of happiness (I don't smoke it at all) ... and I'm walking 30 minutes a day—just so I can live longer—and that is a very different head to be in ... How do I know it was neurofeedback that catalyzed the change? Simple ... I've tried everything else and nothing else worked for very long ... The dirty little secret I had which I told my NF therapist was that I did not want to get better ... at least I didn't want it enough to put any effort in ... NF required no active effort, no affirmations, no heavy emotional lifting—it just required that I show up, sit in a chair, and watch the video ...

Because of my experience my wife began going (and it had a great impact on her in fewer sessions, but then women are superior beings) and then my 9-year-old with anger and impulse issues began going—and his issues have also been almost completely resolved ... my youngest son is blessed by having no issues (and believe me, we looked) ... It's not that NF will make you suddenly like butterscotch, but being given butterscotch will no longer make you want to shoot somebody (or yourself) ... Even my relationship with my MOTHER is good now (and that, my friend, is the longest shot of all!) ... Without NF I do believe my marriage, my children's family, and in all likelihood, my life would have come to abrupt ends ... I'm not being dramatic, just calling it like it is ... Every mental health professional should—if they truly want to help their patients—be able to offer or refer to NF, as either a replacement or adjunct to other therapies ... there is no longer any excuse for them to continue to refuse to become experts in its application ..."

11.14.5 Patient 5

"My first A/T experience: A couple months ago I had awakened from a nightmare about an event that never took place but the feelings felt real. I felt guilty for not protecting my younger brother from our abusive dad. The guilt continued to linger no matter how I tried to convince myself how wrong my thinking was. My A/T session cleared all that up! I started sitting comfortably with no idea what was going to happen and no expectations. There was a guided imagery that I started with and I was told to leave a gift and receive a gift. I left behind Acceptance and I received Love. The next thing that I can recall was having a dialogue with my brother. I was telling him how much I hated our father and how sorry I was for not protecting him. He told me that it was ok, that he is ok. He told me that this was in the past and that I need to accept it and move on. There was back and forth dialogue about this and as soon as I told him he was right and that I accept it, a huge blue light came shooting out of my chest. I immediately felt relaxed and calm. Then I was freezing, shivering, while also pouring sweat. I was not sure how much longer I was going to be in this process and needed to find a way to warm up. I ended up imagining a campfire and everyone that loved and supported me through some of the roughest years of my life was around that campfire with me. They took turns hugging me and telling me how much I am loved. When the time ended I was tearful and happy. I felt a peace that I had not felt in a while. I forgot about the gifts until I was asked what they were. The idea of acceptance has followed me since, and I am more accepting of people that are different. Less opinionated.

I had another session that, in the moment, didn't make any sense. The entire session food just kept popping up, a muffin, chow mein, etc. About a week later I realized that I had not been thinking about food much during the day. I realized that previously I had been obsessed with food and had thought about it all the time. I didn't realize that this was not normal or that I even did that until it was gone. I am now food-obsession free. I talked to my mom about it, she said that I was hungry a lot as a kid and she felt guilty for not feeding me more when she thought that I had had enough.

In another session with Evvy I was obsessing over what to do about work, I felt conflicted, sad, angry, torn, etc. I currently live in a not-so-great neighborhood and try to run every morning, I have developed hyper-vigilance and am frequently looking over my shoulder. I recently noticed that my hands are always cold.

Beginning A/T, I started with a guided imagery, walking down a busy loud street and I felt my anxiety shoot up. I was then told to turn down an alley, I felt immediate fear—something bad could happen and no one would see. I remembered that I was with Evvy and this was all in my head and I was safe. I then walked down some steps. As I walked down each step it seemed magical. The step would light up with flowers and greenery like in a Disney movie. I then approached a room with a book where I was asked to write everything that I wanted to change about myself. I immediately wrote fear and job and then tried to force myself to come up with more things. Soon after I felt like I was floating in water, only not getting wet. Jesus was holding me while telling me 'I've got you,' 'You don't need to worry about anything,' 'I've got you, I will protect you.' I immediately felt calm, peaceful, lighter, and safe. I felt like this massive energy poured out of me.

I don't remember what happened next, but soon after I saw images of two administrators whom I neither like nor respect because of past experiences with them. They flashed repeatedly about 10x and then vanished, and I was flying on a large animal over a town in a valley. I tried to analyze this and lost it. Time was then up. 30 minutes later while driving home I decided to quit my job and felt at peace about it. It has been seven days since I made that decision and it still feels good. I have not thought much about it; the obsessive thoughts are gone. I am less hyper-vigilant in places and I feel safe. I have also noticed that my hands are not as cold all day anymore. AT is transforming my life. Thank you so much!!'"

11.14.6 Patient 6

Clinical history: 49-year-old female, literary agent, with severe burning in left foot—rated 7– 8/10. Symptoms began approximately eight months after the death of her mother and death of her beloved cat. She was treated with steroid injections, orthotics, insoles, walking boot, and toe separator. The pain worsened when treated by a body worker and the pain spread up her leg to her buttock. Hypersensitivity, walking, stress, and wearing snug clothes all aggravated the condition. She participated in physical therapy for three months with little relief. She felt no relief from Neurontin, Prozac, Cymbalta, Lexapro, and Vicodin. She was seen by a psychologist for several months, however reported it worsened her condition.

Medical treatments were numerous, including by a neurologist, orthopedic surgeon, hematologist, and rheumatologist. Several MRI's were all unremarkable. Trauma history at age 10, as she witnessed the Iranian revolution; at age 17 she lived alone in Paris; she had a history of eating disorder and of body dysmorphia. After her father suddenly passed away her mother came to America to live with her. For seven years she was the sole caregiver for her mother, who was battling cancer. She felt extreme abandonment from her sisters during this caregiving period and loneliness was a tremendous issue for this patient.

She was extremely anxious about any pain sensations, catastrophic thinking, and any physical sensation felt life threatening, despite evidence to the contrary. Living with a lot of guilt for putting her mother in a hospice and blaming herself for her mother's death was a daily theme. All medical interventions exacerbated her symptoms. ILF Neurofeedback calmed her physiology and she began to feel more hopeful, however, Alpha-Theta imagery was most profound for her. An eagle appeared and told her "she was on her way to robust health." The eagle appeared again and sent her a "message of love." She was still experiencing pain but without the emotional attachment. Next came imagery of a rock being taken out of her backpack on a hiking trail. She concluded the "rock represented her heavy heart," and she suddenly understood the connection of the physical pain with the emotional pain.

In her last Alpha-Theta session the guided imagery took her through a house room by room. This imagery suggests seeing a house which symbolically tends to represent the self. Each room represents a different aspect of the self. Living room—how we receive and connect with others, dining room—how we nurture others, kitchen—how we nurture ourselves, bedroom—our sensuality, bathroom—our pride and physical appearance.[50]

The patient was invited to go into the attic (which typically represents the past and what may suggest needs resolution). She was asked to find something in the attic and bring it to whatever room she wanted. In the attic she found a red stone heart—she took it to the bedroom and placed it in the middle of the bed. With wide eyes and a smile her response was: "I get it."

Our job is to search for hidden messages and honor the symbols without judgement—they often contain valuable information. This client came away with the insight and understanding of how her highly charged emotions created a major role in her experience of pain.

11.15 Final Thoughts

Recently, a very stoic student in the Alpha-Theta practicum for professionals stated that he had done a lot of therapy over the years and had even experienced many Alpha-Theta sessions; he was certain there were no issues left to be resolved. Nonetheless, he was encouraged to do the sessions in order to receive his Continuing Education Unit. The theme of the imagery was forgiveness. At the end of the session, surprisingly, tears were flowing and in a very humble tone he remarked: "I guess I'm not finished!"

After 20 years of doing this amazing work, we continue to marvel at physical, emotional, and meaningful responses from the clients as they enter into that "ah ha" moment.

As team members of the Multidisciplinary Chronic Pain Program, it is our responsibility to offer tools to the patient that will help them find their way out of the vicious cycle of pain and anxiety that feeds and exacerbates their suffering.

Guided imagery incorporated with Alpha-Theta is one such tool that has been most effective. It often starts by grazing the surface of our life and suddenly progresses to lurching deeper into the subconscious, where we hold our stuff and perhaps find some resolution. We must remember: "Pain may be inevitable, but the suffering and debilitation are optional."[51]

> The witch doctor succeeds for the same reason all the rest of us succeed. Each patient carries his own doctor inside him. ... We are at our best when we give the doctor who resides within each patient a chance to go to work.
>
> Albert Schweitzer[52]

Notes

1 Mersky H, & Bogdul N. (eds). (1994). *Classification of Chronic Pain: Descriptions of Chronic Pain Syndromes and Definition of Pain Terms.* 2nd ed. Seattle, WA: IASP Press, p. 210

2 The American Academy of Pain Medicine. https://www.medicinenet.com/chronic_pain/article.htm#chronic_pain_facts.

3 Zacharoff K L, Pujol M L, & Corsini E. (2010) PainEDU.org *Manual: A Pocket Guide to Pain Management.* 4th edition, Newton, MA: Inflexxion Inc, pp. 51–60.

4 Silver J. K. (2004). *Chronic Pain and the Family.* Cambridge, MA: Harvard University Press, pp. 4–14.

5 American Pain Society. (2012). Chronic Pain costs U.S. up to $635 billion, study shows. www.sciencedaily.com/released/2012/09/12091191100.htm.

6 Miotto K, Kaufman A, Kong A, Jun G, Schwartz J. (2012). Managing co-occurring substance use and pain disorders. *Psychiatr Clin North Am.* 35(2):393–409.

7 Melzack R, & Wall P. D. (1965, November 19). Pain mechanisms: A new theory. *Science* 150(3699):971–979.

8 Pain in Men wounded in battle LT.t CoL. Henry K. Beecher, M.C., A.U.S. *Annals of Surgery* (1946) Volume 123 Number 1.

9 Louw A. (2013). *Why Do I Hurt? A Patient Book about the Neuroscience of Pain. International Spine & Pain Institute.* Minneapolis, MN: OPTP, pp. 1–48.

10 Engel G. (1977). The need for a new medical model: A challenge for biomedicine. *Science* 196: 129–136.

11 Engel G. (1977). The need for a new medical model: A challenge for biomedicine. *Science* 196: 129–136.

12 Gatchel R J, Noe C E, et al. (2002). A preliminary study of multidimensional pain inventory profile differences in predicting treatment outcome in a heterogeneous cohort patients with chronic pain. *Clin J Pain.* 18(3):139–143.

13 Cassell E. J. (2003). The psychology of suffering. In Haas L J, (ed) *The Handbook of Primary Care Psychology.* New York: Oxford University Press.

14 Hasenbring M, Hallner D, Klasen B. (2001). Psychological mechanisms in the transition from acute to chronic pain: Over or underrated? *Schmerz (Pain)* 15(6):442–447.

15 Vlaeyen JWS, Crombez G. (2007, August). International association for the study of pain: Pain clinical updates: Fear and pain: Volume XV(6), pp.1–4.

16   Main C J, Foster N, Buchbinder R. (2010, April) How important are back pain beliefs and expectations for satisfactory recovery from back pain? *Best Pract Res Clin Rheumatol.* 24(2):205–217. doi: 10.1016/j.berh.2009.12.012

17   Jensen M, Turner J, Romano J, Karoly P. (1991). Coping with chronic pain: A critical review of the literature. *Pain* 47: 249–283.

18   Knaster P, et. al. (2012). Psychiatric disorders as assessed with SCID in chronic pain patients: The anxiety disorders precede the onset of pain. *General Hospital Psychiatry* 34(1):46–52.

19   Burke N, Finn D, McGuire B, Roche M. (2017). Psychological stress in early life as a predisposing factor for development of chronic pain: Clinical and preclinical evidence and neurobiological mechanisms. *Journal of Neuroscience Research* 95: 1257–1270.

20   Fishbain D A et al. (2016). Chronic pain types differ in their reported prevalence of post-traumatic stress disorder (PTSD) and there is consistent evidence that chronic pain is associated with PTSD: An evidence-based structured systematic review. *Pain Medicine* 18(4):711–735.

21   Sachs-Ericsson, N. (2007). Childhood abuse, chronic pain, and depression in the National Comorbidity Survey. *Child Abuse Neglect* 31(50):531–547.

22   Costa ECV, et al. (2016). Illness perceptions are the main predictors of depression and anxiety symptoms in patients with chronic pain. *Psychology, Health & Medicine* 21(4):483–495.

23   Do-Hyeong L. et al. (2014). Risk factors for suicidal ideation among patients with complex regional pain syndrome. *Psychiatry Investigation.* Psychiatry Investig., 11(1):32–38.

24   Zhou W, Dantzer R, Kelly K W, Kavelaars A. (2012). Comorbid chronic pain and depression: A search for common neuroimmune mechanisms. *Brain Behav Immun.* 26(1):S45.

25   Dick BD, Rashiq S. (2007). Disruption of attention and working memory traces in individuals with chronic pain. *Anesth Analg.*, 104:1223–1229.

26   Aparian AV, et al. (2004). Chronic pain patients are impaired on an emotional decision-making task. *Pain* 108(1–2):129–136.

27   Hart R P, et al. (2007). Cognitive impairment in patients with chronic pain: The significance of stress. *Curr Pain Headache Rep. Anesth Analog.* 7(2):116–126.

28   Valet M, et al. (2008). Patients with pain disorder show gray-matter loss in pain-processing structures: A voxel-based study. *Psychosomatic Medicine* 71: 49–56.

29   Living with Chronic Pain. *Cleveland Clinic*, (2014). http://my.clevelandclinic.org/disorders/chronic_pain/hic_living_with_chronic_pain.aspx.

30   Institute of Medicine. (2003). *Unequal Treatment: Confronting Racial and Ethnic Disparities in Health Care.* Washington, DC: The National Academies Press.

31   Tait R C, & Chinbnall J. T. (2005). Racial and ethnic disparities in the evaluation and treatment of pain: Psychological perspectives. *Prof Psychol Res Practice* 36(6):595–601.

32   Singh G, Willen S N, Boswell M V, Chelimsky T. C. (2004). The value of interdisciplinary pain management in complex regional pain syndrome type 1: A prospective outcome study. *Pain Physician* (April)7(2):203–209.

33   Bosy D, Eltin D, Corey D, Lee J. W. (2010). An interdisciplinary pain rehabilitation program: Description and evaluation of outcomes. *Physiother Can.* 62: 316–326.

34 Arnold B, Brinkschmidt T, Casser H R, et al. (2009). Multimodal pain therapy: Principles and indications. *Schmerz* 23:112–120 (PubMed).

35 Prager J P, & Jacobs M. S. (2001). Evaluation of patients for implantable pain modalities: Medical and behavioral assessment. *Clinical Journal of Pain* 17: 206–214.

36 Manchikanti L, et. al.(2002). Understanding psychological aspects of chronic pain in interventional pain management. *Pain Physician* 5(1):57–82.

37 Gamsa A, & Vikis-Freibergs V. (1991). Psychological events are both risk factors in, and consequences of, chronic pain. *Pain* 44(3):271–277.

38 Bosy D et al. (2010). op cit.

39 Stricker G. (2010). Psychotherapy Integration. www.apa.org/pubs/books/4317208. aspx.

40 Zarbo C. (2015). Integrative Psychotherapy Works. www.ncbi.nlm.nih.gov/pmc/articles/PMC4707273/.

41 Othmer S. (2006). Efficacy of neurofeedback in pain management. In *Weiner's Pain Management: A Practical Guide for Clinicians*. 7th edition, Boswell M V, & Cole B. E., editors. Boca Raton, FL: CRC Press, pp. 719–740.

42 Jensen M P, Grierson C, Tracy-Smith V, Bacigalupi Stacy C, Othmer S. (2007). Neurofeedback treatment for pain associated with complex regional pain syndrome type 1. *Journal of Neurotherapy* 11(1): 45–53.

43 deCharms R C, Maeda F, Glover G H, Ludlow D, Pauly J M, Soneji D, Gabrieli J D, Mackey S. C. (2005). Control over brain activation and pain learned by using real-time functional MRI. *Proc Natl Acad Sci U S A*. 102: 18626–18631.

44 Martins-Mourao A, & Kerson C. (2017). *Alpha-Theta Neurofeedback in the 21st Century: A Handbook for Researches*. Foundation for Neurofeedback and Neuromodulation Research, pp. 317–343.

45 Green E, & Green A. (1977). *Beyond Biofeedback*. New York: Delacorte Press, pp. 124–134.

46 Budzynski T. H. (1994). The New Frontier, Megabrain. *The Journal of Mind Technology* 2(4): 58–64.

47 Fahrion S L, Walters E D, Coyne L, Allen T. (1992). Alterations in EEG amplitude, personality factors and brain electrical mapping after alpha theta brainwave training: A controlled case study of an alcoholic in recovery. *Alcoholism: Clinical & Experimental Research* 16: 547–552.

48 Fahrion S. L. (1965). Human potential and personal transformation. *Subtle Energies* 6: 55–88.

49 Peniston E G, & Kulkosky P. J. (1990). Alcoholic personality and alpha-theta brainwave training. *Medical Psychotherapy* 3: 37–55.

50 Leviton C D, & Leviton P. (2011). *The Journey into Self*. USA: Trafford Publishing, pp. 195–200.

51 Unknown. www.quotationspage.com/quote/2089.html

52 Cousins N (1979) *Anatomy of an Illness as Perceived by the Patient*. New York: WW Norton & Company. p 78

Chapter 12

Effect of Infra-Low Frequency (ILF) Neurofeedback on the Functional State of the Brain in Healthy and Depressed Individuals

Vera A. Grin-Yatsenko and Juri Kropotov

12.1 Overview

Over the last decade, Infra-Low Frequency Neurofeedback (ILF NF) has established itself as an alternative or complement to classical neurofeedback within the EEG spectrum. The modulation target of ILF NF is rhythmic fluctuations of the slow cortical potential that lie below 0.1 Hz.

Despite growing clinical utilization and research interest, the organization and functional role of this low-frequency rhythmic activity remains undetermined. The question of mechanisms underlying low-frequency, quasi-periodic activity is now regaining research interest after a significant hiatus, under the impetus of fMRI research. This domain was extensively studied in animals in the fifties and sixties.[1, 2, 3] In the subsequent focus on the EEG domain, the higher- amplitude ILF range needed to be suppressed in analog recordings. Effectively, the field blinded itself to the phenomenology of the Slow Cortical Potential (SCP) for many years. When interest was revived, the SCP was mainly exploited as a baseline for time-domain events – the evoked potential and contingent negative variation, etc. This even led to the utilization of the SCP as a baseline for transient neurofeedback challenges, starting in the eighties.[4, 5, 6, 7] The steady-state behavior of the SCP remained suspect as a fruitful area of research until findings in fMRI forced attention back to that topic.

Previous studies have reported a good effect of ILF training on the subjective perception of enduring positive psychological change, as well as improved functionality in the cognitive and executive function domains.[8, 9, 10, 11, 12] This chapter will discuss the results of two pilot studies, both of which demonstrate a significant change in functional state after 20 sessions of ILF NF, with a view toward elucidating mechanisms.

12.2 Background

There have been anecdotal reports on the benefits of EEG neurofeedback for depression going back to the earliest days of work with human subjects. Depression was not the focus at the time, so the reported improvements were not formally tracked, quantified, and reported. The same held true when the method transitioned to clinical work.[13] In the days when SMR-beta training was being done rather exclusively, depression was parsed along the arousal dimension, with low-arousal depression at one end and agitated depression at the other. Low-arousal depression was redressed with low-beta training on the left hemisphere with a frontal bias (e.g., T3-F3), and agitated depression with SMR-band training on the right with a parietal bias (e.g., T4-Pz).

With the migration into the ILF regime, recovery from depression became more predictable. However, the parsing into high- and low-arousal conditions ceased to be determinative. A single training frequency, the optimal response frequency (OR), turned out to be sufficient, and it was person-specific rather than diagnosis-specific. Further individualization could be achieved by means of adding different placements.

It was fMRI research that drew attention back to the regime of the Slow Cortical Potential, which revealed dynamics that dominated in the 0.01 to 0.2 Hz regime. The fMRI signal is a direct measure of cortical activation (as indexed by oxygen uptake), and the surface potential has been shown to be a correlate of cortical activation as well (see Chapter 2). The two variables are correlated – but one of them requires a $3 million scanner for data acquisition. For feedback purposes the SCP not only suffices, but is preferable to the fMRI signal, because of the exquisite resolution that is available with this measure. It is also more directly reflective of neural activity. The fMRI signal also reflects vascular contributions in the above spectral band that for present purposes represent a confound to be avoided.[14] Yet another advantage of relying on the SCP is the larger parameter space available for ILF training in the frequency and spatial domains. That allows for a specificity and particularity in targeting that is simply not available in fMRI feedback.

The fMRI signal has an advantage in being an absolute measure, whereas potentials are always with respect to a reference. This presents no problem in ILF training because a bipolar montage is preferred in any event, as it focuses attention on relative activity between two sites, giving us access to the dynamics of network interactions. The subtlety with which fluctuations in activation are revealed in this measure allow it to be used effectively in continuous, closed-loop, covert feedback.[15] That can lead to subjectively perceived state shifts in as little as a few minutes, and observable shifts in functionality and symptom status in as little as 30 minutes. Such rapid responding enriches the clinical experience and allows for fine-tuning of the parameters of the training, the target frequency, and placement.

12.3 The Pilot Studies

In the first of the pilot studies, changes in the SCP within the salient 0.01 to 0.5 Hz range were systematically characterized before and after a sequence of 20 ILF NF training sessions. Curiously, even with more than a decade of clinical experience with ILF NF, the impact on the spectral distribution within the SCP range has never previously been formally evaluated. This study included eight healthy subjects with no history of neurological diseases or psychiatric disorders or syndromes.

The second pilot study tracked changes observed within the conventional EEG spectrum – another area of investigation that has been relatively neglected to date in the evaluation of ILF NF. This study describes changes of symptoms and EEG parameters in three depressed but unmedicated individuals after 20 sessions of ILF NF training. The clinical symptoms in each subject were rated pre- and post-treatment with three Depression Rating Scales: Montgomery-Asberg Depression Rating Scale (MADRS); Hamilton Depression Rating Scale (HAMD); and Beck Depression Inventory (BDI). The QEEG parameters were assessed in Eyes-open and Eyes-closed resting states, as well as during a visual GO/NOGO challenge.

12.4 ILF Neurofeedback in Healthy Subjects

The five men and three women (age 21–50 years) who participated in this study considered themselves to be healthy people. Despite the absence of a history of psychiatric or neurological conditions, or any medical diagnosis, they still reported physical or mental complaints of a mild to moderate degree. Among the disturbing symptoms they mentioned, for example, were fatigue, recurrent headaches, increased sensitivity to stress factors, anxiety, period-ically depressed state, mood swings, and sleep disturbances. Most of them wanted to improve their performance at work or study, and to boost memory and concentration.

We started NF training sessions with the right parietal-temporal montage (P4-T4), with the purpose of releasing physical tension in our participants – tension that was present to a greater or lesser degree in all of them. Then we used sequen-tially T4-Fp2, T3-T4 and T3-Fp1. The duration of the training in each montage was 10–15 minutes, and the total duration of the session was 40–60 minutes. The course consisted of 17–22 sessions, held 2–3 times a week for 6–8 weeks.

Before and after the course of training for each participant we recorded the 19-channel electroencephalogram (EEG) during performance of a continuous per-formance test – a visually cued GO/NOGO task. This sustained, mildly challenging test condition is likely to maintain a reasonably stable state of vigilance in the sub-ject for the duration of the test and for the EEG data acquisition.

The baseline QEEG investigation took place within seven days prior to the beginning of the training, and then again after the completion of the course of train-ing. We compared the average spectral density in the 0.01–0.5 Hz frequency band in the post-treatment QEEG with the pre-treatment baseline. Two-way repeated measures ANOVA with factors condition (before–after) and location (19 elec-trode positions) was used to estimate the statistical significance of the training effect on the slow EEG oscillations.

After the course of EEG neurofeedback all participants indicated persistent positive changes in their state: their emotional state improved, with greater sta-bility of mood; their internal stress and anxiety levels decreased; and their stress tolerance and work capacity increased. They reported improved attention, mem-ory, cognitive performance, organization, and relationships with others. Decreased frequency and intensity of headaches was reported in those who noted this symptom before the training. Those individuals who had episodes of a depressed state before the training indicated stable, positive mood and an increase of energy level after completion of the training.

According to the QEEG data, in all subjects the spectral power of ILF band increased in the range of 0.01–0.5 Hz; in some of them mainly in the frontal-central region (Figures 12.1a and b), and in the others in the parietal-occipital and posterior-temporal regions. Significant increase in the average power of ILF activity in the range of 0.01–0.5 Hz in eight subjects after the course of NF is shown in Figure 12.1c. The fact that there is considerable spread in the observed increases should not be surprising. On the contrary, the surprise is the observation of substantial systematic power increase across all participants.

In surveying Figure 12.1b, one can discern a trend toward a power-law distribution, which is the expectation for a healthy and functional EEG and SCP.[16] The best estimate for a power-law coefficient in Figure 12.1b is −1.15, which is on the high end of the expected range for this parameter. On the basis of these initial data, one may venture the expectation that changes induced in the power-law coefficient could become a useful outcome measure for ILF and other neurofeedback. It is possible that the particular contribution of ILF training is the preferential impact on state organization, as reflected within the ILF regime.

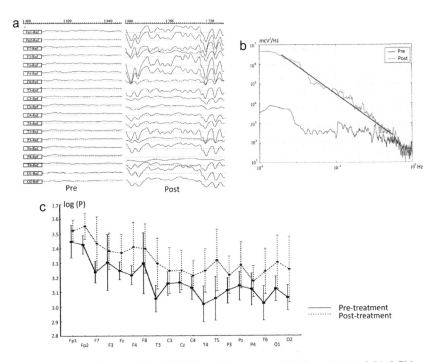

Figure 12.1 Influence of the ILF NF on the power of EEG activity in 0.01-0.5Hz frequency band

12.5 Clinical Case Studies

Case 1. Andrew, a 43-year-old psychologist, suffered from anxiety and depression from a young age. He came to us being extremely exhausted from his work and everyday troubles, and reported chronic fatigue, concentration and memory problems, chronic headache, difficulty falling asleep, and joint and eye pain. He was concerned about poor awareness of hunger and appetite as well. He has a history of early childhood psychological trauma and had several head injuries. At school, he had severe issues with social communications with peers, and was dramatically stressed because of his inability to understand their jokes and taunts. This could be a case of high-functioning autism but he was never examined to establish that diagnosis. Over time, he learned to understand the hidden subtexts and innuendo in conversations with others – studying at university in psychology helped him to acquire this skill. He never sought medical help for his psychological symptoms, nor had he ever taken any psychotropic meds. The Depression Rating Scales indicated moderate degree of depression in him: BDI rating – 16; MADRS rating – 26; HAMD rating – 21, as shown in Figure 12.2a.

QEEG investigation revealed elevated theta activity over frontal-central area in Eyes-open state and during GO/NOGO task performance; alpha power was increased over posterior regions, and beta 2 power – over frontal and posterior cortex in passive (Eyes-open and Eyes-closed) states, and during GO/NOGO task. In the course of GO/NOGO task, slow alpha rhythm spread over anterior cortical areas in his EEG. Such a sign as increased level of theta and slow alpha activity over the frontal area might correlate with poor concentration and with depressive symptoms. Elevated high-beta power over the frontal-central region could also be a sign of anxiety and ruminating thoughts.

The ILF NF course for Andrew consisted of 20 sessions. We started with the right parietal location, taking into account his physical tension, joint pain, restlessness, and difficulties falling asleep. We also intended to help him to improve his awareness of hunger, appetite, and sense of taste. Right-frontal training was added, given his childhood traumatic experience. This location should also alleviate his emotional tension and high irritability. Bilateral temporal training was done to manage his instability and symptoms of endocrine imbalance: headache, and profuse sweating. The left-frontal training was introduced to improve concentration and working memory, to suppress obsessive, ruminating thoughts, to promote positive emotions and optimism, and to alleviate the chronic joint pain.

After the first few sessions, he noticed some improvement of his mood and general tone. Session by session his energy level increased, anxiety diminished, and cheerfulness was observed. The muscle tension gradually subsided, and awareness of his body and of surrounding space improved. At around the 15th session, all positive changes stabilized.

After completion of the training course, the depressive symptoms were no longer apparent in Andrew; he reported a stable, positive mood. The Depression profile score during the second testing indicated no signs of depression: BDI rating – 1; MADRS rating – 2; and HAMD rating – 2, as shown in Figure 12.2a. Andrew also indicated that his headaches and joint pain became less intense and arose more infrequently, and his concentration had improved.

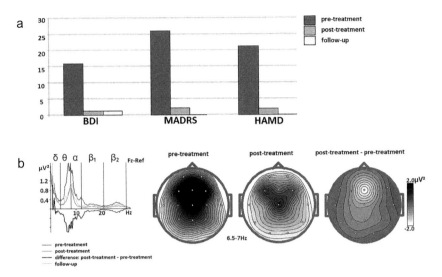

Figure 12.2 Depression scales ratings and EEG spectra after ILF NF course in Andrew (see color version in plate section)

The control QEEG assessment showed significant decrease of theta, alpha and beta 2 activity over the frontal and central cortical areas (Figure 12.2b), which could reflect increase of cortical activation in the anterior region, correlating with improved mood and cognitive functioning. In the Eyes-closed state, alpha power increased in parietal cortical areas, which might relate to a better ability to relax.

The post-training EEG pattern revealed significant enhancement of spectral power of infra-slow activity in 0.03–0.05 Hz range over the frontal region, compared to the pre-training recording.

In the follow-up investigation one year after the start of the ILF NF course, Andrew reported that all positive changes in his state had been retained, despite the fact that last year he had been busier with work than before, in addition to regularly attending educational seminars and conferences. He said that in his daily life he had been able to perceive mindfully and manage his thoughts, emotions, and moods. The headaches arose very seldom, and his improved concentration maintained. His Depression profile scores even improved as compared to the post-treatment assessment and indicated no signs of depression: BDI rating – 1; MADRS rating – 0; and HAMD rating – 0 (Figure 12.2a).

Decrease of theta activity at frontal and central sites observed after treatment remained in the third QEEG at one-year follow-up in Eyes-open and Eyes-closed states (Figure 12.2b). However, during GO/NOGO task performance theta power at anterior sites returned to the pre-treatment level. Alpha power decreased at central and parietal sites in all states, and increased at occipital sites in the last EEG, which corresponds to the normal alpha rhythm distribution.

Case 2. Paul, a 50-year-old engineer, suffered from depression and chronic fatigue for decades. Several years ago, his business crashed, his wife left him, and after the divorce he had to move from his own apartment to a communal flat. He sank into apathy and lost interest and motivation to engage in any activity. During recent years he constantly felt anxious, thinking about the war in Donbass (where he had lived as a child and where his relatives remained), about a mad neighbor in a communal flat, and his unsatisfactory income. He also experienced unreasonable fears that developed in him a tendency toward hyper-controlling behavior. In recent times, he had experienced concentration and memory problems, and learning difficulties. During the day, he felt unexplained mood swings and constant leaps from thought to thought. He had suffered from alcohol and smoking addiction, and from sleep problems for many years. He has a history of prenatal stress due to his father having behaved cruelly to his mother during pregnancy, and he experienced childhood psychological trauma. He was raised without his father, and his mother often sent him to live with grandmothers. Three times he nearly drowned as a child. At work from 28 years up to the recent time period, he felt stress and hardly survived the death of his best friend at age 31. He had not been medicated in the past and used alcohol to relieve stress.

Pre-treatment assessment using Depression Rating Scales and inventory in sum indicated moderate degree of depression in him: BDI rating – 26; MADRS rating – 20; and HAMD rating – 16. QEEG assessment revealed elevated levels of alpha activity over frontal, central, and parietal areas, as well as episodes of alpha and theta waves at temporal sites of both left and right hemispheres. These phenomena could be a marker of chronic stress, depression, fatigue, and poor concentration.

The ILF NF protocols targeting Paul's symptoms included P4-T4 to resolve physical tension and improve sleep, Fp2-T4 to calm despair and controlling behavior, as well as to decrease high emotional reactivity to stressful factors and events. T3-T4 placement was added based on his erratic shifts in mood, and T3-Fp1 took into account his obsessive worries, apathy, depressive mood, poor concentration, and working memory.

From the beginning of the training course Paul noticed becoming more relaxed, and his emotional reaction to the stressful events got smoother. He was happy to discover that during these stressful situations he managed to maintain the position of the observer. His inner tension gradually disappeared and he felt more energetic.

After completion of 20 NF sessions, Paul reported a dramatic decrease of inner tension and reactivity to stressful situations as compared to his pre-treatment state. His emotional stability increased and the level of anxiety diminished. Relationships with other people improved; he learned to understand them better. Aggressive attacks by his neighbor no longer upset his state of mental balance; consequently, she provoked him less frequently into conflict. He has significantly reduced the use of alcohol and reported that confidence, calmness, and a sense of personal efficacy has returned. The depressive mood disappeared, and he felt clarity in his mind and had constructive ideas on the organization of his future life. The Depression Rating Scale values diminished significantly and indicated no symptoms of depression: BDI rating – 2; MADRS rating – 6; and HAMD rating – 5.

His post-treatment QEEG showed a significant decrease in power of both alpha and theta activity over frontal area in Eyes-open state, and a decrease of theta power over frontal, central, and parietal area during GO/NOGO task performance, which would indicate improved activation of frontal cortex. In Eyes-closed state the maximum of alpha rhythm power shifted from the parietal to the occipital area, which is a normal distribution of the alpha rhythm with eyes closed. Spectral power of infra-slow activity in 0.02–0.03 Hz and in 0.10–0.12 Hz range increased significantly, with the most prominent increment over the parietal and occipital regions.

During our conversation one year after the pre-treatment meeting, Paul reported that improvement of his mood, emotional stability, and high level of energy gained after ILF NF remained steady. He did not suffer from the mood swings any more, and depressive and unsettling thoughts arose only rarely. He seldom used alcohol during the last year, he slept well, and experienced "lust for life." Due to his passion for Thai massage, he decided to start his own practice in that healing field and he went to medical school to get a license. In his 50th year it was not easy for him to master a new area of knowledge, and he was not satisfied with his concentration and memory. Still, he coped with the assimilation of educational material and managed to pass his exams.

One year later his Depression profile scores did not indicate signs of depression: BDI rating – 9; MADRS rating – 5; and HAMD rating – 3. Decrease of theta and alpha activity over the frontal area observed after ILF NF remained in his third QEEG in all three conditions, and frontal theta power during GO/NOGO task was even lower than in post-treatment EEG.

Case 3. Anna, a 35-year-old university lecturer, applied to us seeking help for her chronic fatigue over the last five years, and chronic sub-depressive state for the last six months. She also suffered from problems with volitional regulation, propensity to procrastination, and perfectionism. She had also experienced concentration and working memory problems for the last several years, as well as suffering from PMS, which strongly affected her both emotionally and somatically. She had a history of early childhood psychological trauma and difficulties with social communication in childhood. She was subjected to a strict upbringing, including many prohibitions. At the age of 24 months she had a case of pneumonia and was hospitalized alone, without her mother. This had been an extremely traumatic experience for her. An initial assessment using Depression scales and inventory indicated mild to moderate degree of depression: BDI rating – 18; MADRS rating – 17; and HAMD rating – 15.

Increased beta 2 activity over frontal cortical areas, and high frequency basic rhythm (11 Hz) revealed in Anna's QEEG might be the correlates of high vigilance and perfectionism. Alpha activity spread over the frontal area, and elevated theta activity over frontal and parietal areas, could reflect a diminished level of cortical activation and be associated with poor concentration, volitional regulation, and working memory, as well as with depressive complaints.

ILF NF training was started with the right parietal-temporal electrode placement (T4-P4) to reduce physical tension and hyperactivity, and the somatic manifestations of PMS. Right frontal-temporal training was added, taking into account her hyper-vigilance, perfectionism, and emotional overwhelm – probable consequences of her childhood traumatic stress. Bilateral temporal training was aimed at relieving symptoms of PMS. Left frontal was added to help her to cope with procrastination, to improve volitional regulation, concentration, and working memory.

During the first session, she experienced deep relaxation, and this pleasant state returned to her during the following days. Her worries about unfinished businesses decreased, while her performance at work gradually improved. She noticed a more positive attitude to the events in her life, including unplanned and stressful situations. She became more confident and aware of her feelings, needs, and desires. After the 15th session, she felt the need for physical activity and started cycling every day. She also felt an urge to act to achieve new goals, to organize things, along with a clear understanding of which activities are relevant and valuable for her, and which are not. For the first time she experienced a combination of three components: vivid positive emotions, readiness for activity, and at the same time – a comfortable state of physical relaxation.

After 20 NF sessions she reported remarkable improvement of her mood and decrease of anxiety level. She became calmer and more able to deal with sudden unplanned and stressful events. She started to exercise regularly and her mental performance and success at work increased remarkably.

Ratings on the Depression scales after the training course decreased significantly as compared to the pre-training results, and no longer revealed signs of depression: BDI rating – 3; MADRS rating – 4; and HAMD rating – 3.

Significant decrease of spectral power of theta and alpha activity at frontal and central sites in Eyes-open state and during GO/NOGO task in her post-training QEEG likely reflect the higher cortical activation in this area. Infra-slow activity of 0.03–0.06 Hz was elevated more over the left parietal, temporal, and occipital area.

One year after the pre-treatment investigation, all of Anna's achievements remained stable. She maintained a positive mood state and did not suffer from depression or fatigue after completion of the training. Due to her success and effectiveness at work, she was thrilled when she received an offer to become a professor at a prestigious Moscow University. She sometimes still experienced episodes of procrastination and insufficient concentration. Her Depression profile score remained at about the same level as in post-treatment assessment: BDI rating – 5; MADRS rating – 4; and HAMD rating – 3. The positive changes in Anna's EEG, such as the decrease of the initially elevated alpha and theta activity at frontal and central sites, remained constant as well.

Commonalities among the trainees were as follows: After completion of the training course, all three participants reported remarkable improvement of mood and emotional stability, decreased levels of anxiety and reactivity to stressful situations, as well as major improvements in concentration and mental performance. The post-treatment Depression Rating Scales, as compared to pre-treatment ones, revealed dramatic decrease of the depression scores closer to the norm. The new ratings were essentially retained at the one-year follow-up. The QEEG parameters in Eyes-open and Eyes-closed resting states, and during the visual GO/NOGO task, showed significant decrease of theta power over frontal and central areas in all three patients in post-treatment QEEG recordings as compared to pre-treatment EEGs, as well as other tendencies toward more normal function.

There was also considerable commonality with the eight participants in the first pilot study, all of whom indicated persistent positive changes in their emotional state, with greater stability of mood and improved stress tolerance. They too reported greater functionality in the cognitive and executive function domains, and improved work capacity. Those who initially presented with episodes of depressive mood found relief as well as higher energy levels.

Significantly, a uniform finding was elevation in ILF spectral amplitudes in the 0.01 to 0.2 Hz domain across both pilot studies. In the EEG range, the subsidence of focal elevations in band amplitudes with the training was observed even at sites that were not directly targeted in the training.

12.6 Summary and Conclusion

Our two pilot studies have shown that the ILF Neurofeedback not only has a positive effect on the psycho-emotional state and cognitive functions of healthy people and depressed individuals, but also produces changes in the physiological state of the brain, according to measurements of the power spectra in the conventional EEG bands, as well as the power of infra-low oscillations of brain potentials. Significant decrease of theta power over frontal and central areas found in depressed subjects after the neurofeedback course, and can be related to recovery of frontal cortical activation. Increase in the amplitude of the ILF oscillations of brain potentials in the second range, according to numerous studies of N.A. Aladjalova,[17, 18, 19] V.A. Ilyukhina,[20, 21] and I.V. Zabolotskikh,[22] appear to reflect the restoration of healthy dynamics in metabolic processes in brain tissue, and the re-activation of the mechanisms of adaptation in the stress regulation systems. Another interesting finding was that all participants from both studies experienced significant reduction in symptoms that were not the focus of the NF training originally. This points to a long-lived aspirational hypothesis that training of Slow Cortical Potentials in the infra-low frequency domain may have a globalizing effect on the self-regulation of the brain, leading to improved functioning in all neuro-regulatory domains.

The potential of utilizing ILF spectral amplitude distributions as a progress and quality control measure in ILF NF is indicated.

Notes

1 Aladjalova N.A. (1956). Infra-slow rhythmic changes of the brain electrical potential. *Biophysica* 1: 127–136.

2 Aladjalova N.A., Arnold O.P., Sharov V.N. (1977). Multi-minute rhythmic fluctuations of brain potentials in man and vigilance. *Hum Physiol* 3: 259–265.

3 Aladjalova N.A. (1979). *Psychophysiological aspects of brain infra-slow rhythmical activity.* Moscow: Nauka (in Russian).

4 Birbaumer N., Elbert T., Rockstroh B., Lutzenberger W. (1981). Biofeedback of event-related potentials of the brain. *Int J Psychol* 16: 389–415.

5 Rockstroh B., Birbaumer N., Elbert T., Lutzenberger W. (1984). Operant control of EEG and event-related potentials and slow brain potentials. *Biofeedback Self Regul* 9: 139–160.

6 Schneider F., Elbert T., Heimann H., Welker A., Stetter F., Mattes R., Birbaumer N., Mann K. (1993). Self-regulation of slow cortical potentials in psychiatric patients: Alcohol dependency. *Biofeedback Self Regul* 18: 23–32.

7 Kotchoubey B., Schneider D., Schleichert H., Strehl U., Uhlmann C., Blankenhorn V., Fröscher W., Birbaumer N. (1996). Self-regulation of slow cortical potentials in epilepsy: A retrial with analysis of influencing factors. *Epilepsy Res* 25: 269–276. doi: 10.1016/S0920-1211(96)00082-4.

8 Othmer S., Othmer S.F. (2009). Post-traumatic stress disorder – the neurofeedback remedy. *Biofeedback* 37(1): 24–31.

9 Othmer S., Othmer S.F., Legarda S. (2011). Clinical neurofeedback: Training brain behavior: Treatment strategies. *Pediatr Neurol Psychiatry* 2(1): 67–73.

10 Othmer S., Othmer S.F. (2016). Infra-low frequency neurofeedback for optimum performance. *Biofeedback* 44(2): 81–89.

11 Legarda S.B., McMahon D., Othmer S., Othmer S. (2011). Clinical neurofeedback: Case studies, proposed mechanism, and implications for pediatric neurology practice. *J Child Neurol* 26(8): 1045–1051. doi:10.1177/0883073811405052.

12 Grin-Yatsenko V.A., Othmer S., Ponomarev V.A., Evdokimov S.A., Konoplev Y.Y., Kropotov J.D. (2018). Infra-low frequency neurofeedback in depression: Three case studies. *NeuroRegulation* 5: 30–42.

13 Hammond D.C. (2005). Neurofeedback treatment of depression and anxiety. *J Adult Dev* 12: 131–138.

14 Pfurtscheller G., Schwerdtfeger A., Brunner C., Aigner C., Fink D., Brito J., Carmo M.P., Andrade A. (2017). Distinction between neural and vascular BOLD oscillations and intertwined heart rate oscillations at 0.1 Hz in the resting sate and during movement. *PLoS One* 4: e0168097. doi: 10.1371/journal.pone.0168097.

15 Sitaram R., Ros T., Stoeckel L., Haller S., Scharnowski F., Lewis-Peacock J., Weiskopf N., Blefari M.L., Rana M., Oblak E., Birbaumer N., Sulzer J. (2017). Closed-loop brain training: The science of neurofeedback. *Nat Rev Neurosci* 18(86): 86–100.

16 He B.J., Zempel J.M., Snyder A.Z., Raichle M.E. (2010). The temporal structures and functional significance of scale-free brain activity. *Neuron* 66(3): 353–369. doi:10.1016/j.neuron.2010.04.020.

17 Aladjalova N.A. (1979). *Psychophysiological aspects of brain infra-slow rhythmical activity*. Moscow: Nauka (in Russian).

18 Aladjalova N.A. (1957). Infra-slow rhythmic oscillations of the steady potential of the cerebral cortex. *Nature* 179(4567): 957–959.

19 Aladjalova N.A. (1962). *Slow electrical processes in the brain*. Moscow: USSR Academy of Sciences (in Russian).

20 Ilyukhina V.A., Zabolotskikh I.B. (1993). *Energodefitsitnye sostoyaniya zdorovogo i bol'nogo cheloveka (Energy-deficient states of healthy and sick individuals)*. Saint Petersburg: Russian Academy of Science, Institute of the Human Brain (in Russian).

21 Ilyukhina V.A. (2004). *Human brain in the mechanisms of information and control of interactions of the organism and the environment.* Saint Petersburg: Russian Academy of Science, Institute of the Human Brain.
22 Zabolotskikh I.B. (1993). Physiological basis of differences in the functional states in healthy and sick individuals with different tolerance of hypercapnia and hypoxia. Abstract of doctoral dissertation. Saint Petersburg (in Russian).

Acknowledgments

The authors thank Valery Ponomarev, Chief Scientist at the Laboratory of Neurobiology of Actions Programming of the Institute of the Human Brain of the Russian Academy of Sciences, Saint Petersburg, Russia, for analysis and interpretation of the EEG data, and Mark Gregory, Chief Technology Officer (CTO) of BEE Medic (GmbH. Stuttgart, Germany) for analysis of EEG data.

Chapter 13

Neurofeedback with PTSD and Traumatic Brain Injury (TBI)

Monica Geers Dahl

13.1 Introduction

> They have me on prazosin, trazodone, and sertraline. I can't take them every day, they give me cravings; ice cream, sugar and salt. When I take the meds the way they are prescribed, I gain weight, so I take them every other day, and I have nightmares 3x a week.
>
> (Jackie O, 2018 Nov)

Jackie O,[1] a DoD medic (two tours: Desert Storm and Iraq), is uniquely qualified to assess the impact of pharmaceutical interventions on her own mental, physical, and emotional well-being. In July of 2013, we initiated a 20-session protocol targeting her PTSD symptoms. After five sessions she said, "I don't need my meds to fall asleep." From 2014 until 2018, she was without neurofeedback (NF). An accident brought her back. Jackie O's experience with neurofeedback is related at the end of this chapter.

13.2 The Post-War Impact on a Warrior's Life

The warrior ideal is a state of self-control that is focused and calm under adverse conditions.[2] The enduring experience of war changes human biochemical and neurological baseline activity, possibly disrupting cerebral, visceral, interpersonal, spiritual, and environmental functions.[3] "Part of the grace of the nervous system is that it is constantly self-regulating."[4] Post-traumatic stress disorder (PTSD) disrupts the homeodynamic brain processes of rest and restoration, with deficits in the self-regulation of emotional and executive functions.[5] The debilitating, chronic symptoms of PTSD create high personal and societal costs.[6]

13.3 Standard PTSD Care in the Military

A RAND Corporation study in 2006 estimated a cost of $4–6.2 billion in the first two years post-deployment for veteran depression and PTSD care. For mild Traumatic Brain Injury (mTBI), the study estimated $591–910 million the first year

(2007 dollars);[7] the costs then appear to rise in the third and fourth years.[8] The number of veterans diagnosed with PTSD is growing; in 2004 there were 8633, in 2012 there were 65,076.[9] The prevailing Veteran's Administration (VA) model for PTSD care includes prevention, pre-treatment, acute stabilizing, post-acute, initial treatment/recovery, rehabilitation, and maintenance.[10]

The existing system of categories for diagnosing psychopathology and defining evidence-based care uses biochemical and cognitive behavioral frames of reference.[11] Concurrent treatments for comorbidity are still being explored.[12] Pharmaceutical treatment rests on a variety of medications in the search for the right combination to help active duty service members, veterans, and sometimes their family members, to adjust to post-war life. Cognitive behavioral learning strategies require communication skills and a willingness to revisit unpleasant memories and to talk about things. "(L)arge gaps in the evidence base still exist,"[13] in that both psychotherapy and pharmaceutical interventions are useful with only about 60% of the veterans who seek care through the VA.

13.4 The Trauma Memory

"All trauma is pre-verbal."[14] When the sympathetic nervous system is hyper-aroused, the ability to speak and describe what is being experienced may be impaired.[15, 16] Trauma stories tend to be non-linear (i.e., non-consecutive), fragmented, and unprocessed; the story comes out in bits of disjointed sensory experience. The declarative or explicit memory is distinct from the implicit, non-verbal, physiological, and state memory.[17] The difficulty of articulating a trauma experience is only one aspect of the larger issue of being unable to give words to experiences and feelings that in its full-blown clinical manifestation is labeled *alexithymia*.[18, 19] However, a more primary reason PTSD is resistant to talk therapy is the unitary quality of PTSD memories. Centered in the limbic structures and the autonomic nervous system, these are whole-body memories, making them relatively inaccessible to processing and resolution via cognitive faculties.

The cumulative effect of multiple threatening situations and actions creates more difficulty in articulating a coherent narrative. The emotional threads binding events together in memories can be overwhelming, triggering the avoidance aspect of PTSD.[20] Self-regulation of the physiology is needed to restore proper parasympathetic nervous system activity and re-engage the Broca's area.[21] In contrast to cognitive behavioral treatment, neurofeedback is a minimally verbal, unitary, comprehensive treatment for PTSD, as well as for co-occurring issues. In contrast to the exposure therapies, the goal of neurofeedback is systemic restoration of a calm, relaxed, and well-controlled state under benign conditions – without dwelling on images of trauma. The bioelectrically-grounded therapy addresses foundational processes of neuronal function in their spatio-temporal organization, as opposed to targeting biochemical ambients and cognitive behavioral symptoms directly. Neurofeedback training is a holistic, non-invasive approach to body–mind–spirit reintegration of the body's healing responses. Treatment effectiveness is observable in the falling away of symptoms in multiple functional domains.

13.5 Comorbidity

Whether PTSD aggravates vulnerability to addiction, or existing neurophysiological vulnerabilities to addiction promote the development and maintenance of PTSD is unclear, but there is certainly an interplay. Comorbidity creates complications in conventional treatment.[22] For veterans of Operations Enduring Freedom (OEF)/ Iraqi Freedom (OIF)/New Dawn (OND), 63% of substance or alcohol use disorders (SUD/AUD) were co-occurring with PTSD. For those who are poly-substance disordered (alcohol and other substances), the comorbidity with PTSD is 76%. A 1980s review of poly-substance disordered Vietnam vets identified 74% PTSD comorbid.[23]

Dual diagnosis PTSD and AUD may be indicative of childhood abuse and adversity.[24] Complex developmental trauma may extend into adult life from childhood neglect or abuse.[25] Bessel van der Kolk[26] has questioned the efficacy of established treatments for trauma, such as prolonged exposure therapy (PET), with individuals experiencing complex trauma, particularly those with pre-verbal experiences. Depression, concussion (mTBI), attention deficits, and PTSD have overlapping symptoms, creating complex comorbidity.[27, 28] Headaches can be indicators of mTBI (i.e. childhood falls, sports injuries, vehicular accidents, training accidents, concussive impacts from grenades, missiles, mortar, IEDs, and firing weapons).[29, 30]

In 2008, The VA handbook[31] required PTSD services and programs to serve co- occurring treatment needs of veterans with comorbid PTSD and SUD. In 2010, the VA Consensus Conference recommended that improvements be made in monitoring and collecting treatment outcomes for individuals with co-occurring pain, mTBI, and PTSD. The VA position was that clinical practice guidelines were to be followed for these issues until "[research suggesting] other approaches, or demonstrations that current clinical practice guidelines are ineffective or inappropriate for this complex population" become available.[32] In 2017, Cpt. Mike Colston[33] gave a prepared statement to the Senate Armed Services Committee regarding TBI, stating that emerging technology and novel treatments – including neurofeedback – were being studied intensively in outpatient settings. He testified that there was a "need to reduce fractured health care delivery. ... Comorbidities such as PTSD, acute stress, and sleep disruption, complicate TBI recovery and create a need for a complementary suite of mental health and rehabilitative services for effective mTBI treatment."

13.5.1 Addiction Treatment with Neurofeedback

In a matched group (N = 121) drug rehab study, the largest and most extensive controlled study ever done in neurofeedback, 40 to 50 neurofeedback sessions were integrated into existing client services.[34] Using NF protocols prevalent in the mid-nineties time frame, the experimental group demonstrated a 77% abstinence rate one-year post-neurofeedback training (36/47). The control group that received standard care demonstrated 44% abstinence at one year (12/27). The difference was significant. Further, if the outcome is referenced to the beginning of the program, where the groups were matched at ~60 each (as well as in terms of Addiction

Severity Index), the difference in outcomes was a factor of three (12/36). This is explained by the differential attrition rate during the program. 45 days into the treatment there were far fewer dropouts from the experimental group (6%) than from the control group (30%).

Follow-up after three years found that the experimental group had maintained sobriety/abstention status, whereas the control group had continued to attrition. That sustained success was highly correlated with participation in group, a key aspect of the 12-step program. One may assume that full recovery from the appeal of alcohol or drugs had not been systematically achieved in this study. Contemporary ILF neurofeedback protocols are more promising in that regard.

13.6 Pharmaceutical Care

A national sample of PTSD-diagnosed veterans between 2003 and 2004 revealed that 80% were prescribed psychotropic drugs.[35] Reliance on pharmaceutical care for PTSD is generally open-ended, possibly a lifelong commitment, the same as a 12-step program. Unfortunately, discontinuing some medications can produce nasty withdrawal symptoms or cause relapse. Weaning veterans off drugs as soon as possible appears not to be a primary concern in the existing Veteran's Administration standard care (VA SC) implementation. Some veterans say that they don't use all the drugs that get shipped in by mail. They just keep accepting them, sticking them in the closet. The explicit requests for freedom from meds appear to be driven by the striving for a restored internal locus of control, a client-driven reason for veterans to seek clinical care outside the VA.

13.7 Evidence Base for Neurofeedback Treatment of PTSD

Five studies of neurofeedback with PTSD have been analyzed with "optimistic results presented."[36] All the studies had positive outcomes. Three reported statistically significant outcomes, which "qualify neurofeedback as probably efficacious for PTSD treatment." Therapists in clinical settings tend to use behavioral change measures to assess efficacy of treatment and competence of clinical practice. A review of ten studies with interest in behavioral outcomes included three studies with randomized controls (RCTs).[37] The review acknowledged the paucity of RCTs for neurofeedback studies, and proposed that more RCTs, larger samples, and more longitudinal data are needed. "The results from all ten studies reviewed in this article demonstrated salubrious changes in at least one outcome measure of PTSD symptomology of the majority of participants in the samples." Limitations were noted in the sample size, only one was N>30,[38] as well as in the variety of NF training designs, lack of variation in ethnic background, and pre-experimental designs with no control for extraneous variables.

> In the largest published study of CBT for PTSD, more than one-third of the patients dropped out; the rest had a significant number of adverse reactions. Most of the

women in the study still suffered from full-blown PTSD after three months in the study, and only 15 percent no longer had major PTSD symptoms.[39]

Despite the reports of ineffectiveness, the governments of Canada and the United States still consider cognitive behavioral and pharmaceutical options as the only evidence-based treatments effective for veteran's with PTSD. There is also a lack of evidence as to the efficacy of these two approaches for simultaneous treatment of comorbidity.[40, 41] At the time of this writing there are no approved pharmacological treatments available for methamphetamine or cocaine addiction.[42]

[C]urrent evidence-based treatments for PTSD are not always appropriate, well-tolerated, accessible, adequate, or congruent with the patient preferences.[43]
It is critical to remember that even the most effective interventions are often ineffective with a specific case. For an individual case, the true documentation of "evidence-based" is produced only after the intervention is implemented and outcome data is produced that documents a change in the target behavior in a desired manner.[44]

13.8 Ongoing Issues with Treatment of Veterans

Veterans with PTSD risk being canalized into pharmaceutical strategies due to chronic shortages of behavioral health specialists in the VA, even when other approaches are preferred by the veteran.[45, 46, 47, 48] "Their mental health difficulties profoundly touch the lives of the U.S. general public."[49] In 2014, the Veterans Choice Act (VCA) was established to support pain management in the VA, "Veterans actively advocate for providers to communicate with them about alternatives to medication."[50] The focus on drug interventions for treating the symptoms of PTSD runs counter to the inherent military model of peak physical performance training, whereas neurofeedback training fits the peak performance training model in being entirely function-focused. It is empowering for veterans to report drug-free improvements in sleep hygiene, mood, and family and social relations. The findings of clinical effectiveness and temporal parsimony in using neurofeedback training for PTSD symptom reduction also promise a reduction in the lifelong taxpayer costs of pharmaceutical treatment.

Stress and alcoholism both involve hypothalamic pituitary adrenal (HPA) axis dysfunction.[51] It has been more than a quarter of a century since neurofeedback research in a VA setting was found effective in reducing the adverse symptoms of PTSD and its common comorbidity, alcoholism. Most veterans, mental health workers, and VA staff are unaware that neurofeedback is useful not only for reducing the symptoms of the human suffering known as PTSD; it also yields systemic benefits that exceed the expectations of simply reducing/eliminating target symptoms. Although the VA failed to continue this line of inquiry, ongoing research by private clinicians continue to replicate good findings in PTSD symptom reduction using neurofeedback training.[52, 53, 54, 55, 56, 57]

The limitations imposed by evidence-based medicine (EBM), which have only been in place since the 1990s,[58] marginalizes soft-science self-report and symptom tracking. The biochemical and cognitive behavioral perspectives skew the discussion of comorbidity by failing to address the common bioelectrical core of neuronal dysregulation underlying seemingly diverse symptoms. The relative paucity of formal research with neurofeedback for PTSD may be evidence of 1 – the difficulty in getting unambiguous data from RCT studies with people suffering from complex conditions, with varied etiologies and disparate comorbidities, using methods that are multi-fold, individualized, and adaptive; and 2 – the biases inherent in EBM regarding what data are most relevant for these types of issues and participants.

13.9 Why Neurofeedback?

Biofeedback helps "individuals become more aware of their own role in influencing health and disease; it can be quite empowering to patients."[59] Neurofeedback, aka EEG Biofeedback, is a bioelectric, non-invasive, behavioral training for restoring the brain's endogenous neuromodulation, meaning that recovery relies on the brain receiving relevant information about its own functional state.[60] Neuronal dysregulations can be refractory to talk therapy because cognitive interventions fail to stabilize and re-normalize a dysregulated nervous system efficiently.[61] From a bioelectrical network perspective, the quirks of multiple diagnoses are reframed as core regulatory issues of physiological arousal, brain instability, behavioral disinhibition, localized dysregulation, and learned fears/habits.[62] These principal failure modes are then targeted sequentially with a parsimonious set of protocols tailored to the individual and adapted continuously throughout the training process.

Neurofeedback trains the neuronal networks into optimal self-regulation, thereby ameliorating symptoms of PTSD while simultaneously reducing comorbidities, such as the sequelae of TBI, attention and learning disorders, depression, emotional reactivity, and addictions. It immediately targets the hyper-arousal that interferes with deep, drug-free sleep, and is free from the side effects service members report with pharmaceuticals. The use of medications can interfere with the ability to deploy, and with combat readiness.[63, 64, 65, 66, 67]

Neurofeedback tends to improve retention in existing programs, reduces recidivism, promotes abstinence in PTSD/substance abuse comorbid veterans, and is free from side effects and withdrawal issues of pharmaceuticals. A 20-session neurofeedback training plan that lasts from two to ten weeks can often resolve complex comorbidities. Improvements in sleep architecture generally occur after an initial session, as is reflected in the case of Jackie O described in this chapter.

Neurofeedback has demonstrated utility in both PTSD and addiction treatment. As stated in Chapters 2 and 5, High Definition Infra-Low Frequency (HD ILF) Neurofeedback training demonstrates a positive influence in restoring dynamic functional connectivity in the principal resting state network, the Default Mode Network (DMN).[68] Alpha-Theta Neurofeedback training then opens a window into traumatic memories without emotional abreaction, freeing those unresolved memories to be released and processed with less risk of client re-traumatization, or the abreaction common to cathartic release in talk and exposure therapies.[69, 70] Neurofeedback has proven to be comparable or superior to evidence-based PTSD treatment.[71] A collateral benefit is the reduced risk of secondary trauma for the clinician.

13.10 Experimental Military Treatment Programs for PTSD

No single intervention is right for every person or clinical presentation; personalized, client-driven care creates a better fit in health care for each individual.[72] With this principle in mind, Complementary and Alternative Medicine (CAM) integration was introduced at a few military bases. At Camp Lejeune, NC, Dr. Carmen Russoniello, with the Wounded Warrior Battalion East, integrated neurofeedback and heart rate variability training in 2008.[73] There was also a holistic component in the Warrior Transition Battalion at Ft. Bliss, TX.[74]

At Ft. Hood, TX, Dr. Jerry Wesch organized a team seeking to improve on the Ft. Bliss program. A year of pre-planning went into creation of the Warrior Combat Stress Reset Program (WCSRP: 2008–15, N = 850).[75, 76, 77] It applied a multi-modal approach in an 11-week process. The first three weeks were an intensive jump-start outpatient program, with two optional four-week individualized programs of follow up. Dr. Wesch states with regard to PTSD: "This is not a disease. It is a learned problem, and you can get over it."[78] The wait list was long, up to a year. Priority was given to service members intending to remain on active duty. 80% had headaches; 40% were post-concussion; 100% had pain.[79] "Wait lists are one measure of unmet demand."[80]

"(I)nterventions need to be studied to establish their evidence base and to ensure that their use does not deter patients from receiving first-line, evidence-based treatments."[81] Program evaluation was built into the Reset design. A paper file with data was collected for every participant. With funding for program evaluation available in 2012, a retrospective data base was created for analysis of multiple measures (2008–13: N = 632). The database facilitated a follow-up tracking system, and report creation. In the first six months, WCSRP used standard evidence-based care. After six months, CAM was integrated including neurofeedback. Every year, modifications were made to content and program delivery to build upon what was working.[82] For Wesch, the changes in participant outcomes on multiple standardized measures were "jaw dropping." [83]

The PCL-M[84] is a traditional measure for PTSD in military members. A five-point change is considered clinically significant. In the six months prior to CAM integration, the Reset program PTSD score change mean was −2.83 (2008). After integration of CAM, the PTSD scores showed greater participant improvement: −6.42 (2009), −9.3 (2010), −11.3 (2011), −14.6 (2012), −13.7 (2013). There were significant post-treatment reductions in PTSD symptoms (PTSD Checklist–Military version; $p < .0001$), pain (Oswestry Pain Index; $p < .0001$), anxiety (Beck Anxiety Inventory; $p < .0001$) and depression (Beck Depression Inventory II; $p < .0001$).[85]

The evaluation of WCSRP concluded:

> From the initial results, the Reset program appears very successful in meeting its stated goals and objectives. The program implementation matches the program's intent. The improvements in health outcomes are both statistically and clinically significant for reducing PTSD, anxiety and depression symptoms. Major health outcomes have improved significantly year over year. Satisfaction with the program is very high with patients, family members, program providers and staff, referring providers and leaderships.[86]

Despite its resounding success, the program was terminated in 2015. The PTSD portion was renamed and reverted to previously used "evidence-based" treatments, although CAM was still available in the mTBI and pain programs.[87]

13.10.1 Combat Operational Stress Conference (COSC)

At the 2011 COSC, San Diego, CA, preliminary clinical findings from Ft. Hood and Camp Pendleton were presented by three members of the Camp Pendleton Department of Deployment Health.[88] One of the co-presenters was Maj. Michael Villaneuva, who had just transplanted ILF NF from Camp Pendleton to Fort Hood. He summarized the results crisply: "Nobody got worse; a lot of people got a lot better. There is a return of humanity here that is not captured by our assessments." He deployed immediately after the conference, taking neurofeedback to a forward operating base in Kandahar, Afghanistan, where he became known as "the wizard" with the "magic sleep box."[89, 90] The command staff and the medical personnel came for training along with everyone else. Another co-presenter, Dr. Anna Benson, noted that the often unrecognized mTBI was treated along with the targeted PTSD symptoms. ILF neurofeedback yielded systemic enhancement in cognitive functions and overall improved regulation.[91, 92]

Symptom tracking at Camp Pendleton, with the initial cohort of over 300 being trained in the 2009–10 timeframe, documented an unusually high compliance rate of 85% (building to 95% over time). Some 65 symptom categories were tracked. Success in symptom abatement to beneath clinical significance was typically achieved in 75–80% of cases for most of the symptom categories. The highest success rate was documented for migraine, at 92% (49 cases), and the lowest was for tinnitus, at 49% response (55 cases). Success rate for depression was at 81%; for anxiety, 77% (n > 100 for both). Suicidality became a non-issue for everyone who had listed it as a concern. Some 25% of the trainees completed their recovery within 20 sessions (median just over 10 sessions), and an additional 40% achieved success by 40 sessions. The program is ongoing in 2019.

13.10.2 Torture Victims and Refugees: Red Cross Study

In 2014, a quasi-experimental pilot study with a non-equivalent control group was initiated in Malmö, Sweden, to examine the suitability of ILF neurofeedback training for "traumatized refugees who have been exposed to war and/or torture."[93] Symptom tracking was added to standardized tests used by the Red Cross for client assessment.[94] However, out of respect for patient tolerance, the full symptom tracking list was pared down substantially.[95]

In the experimental group (N = 12), the pre-post measures revealed "noticeable difference." Neurofeedback was correlated with decreases in symptoms of trauma in all measures except sleep. Improvements in the treatment group were significant. Ten sessions were a good start, but more sessions would be needed for resolution. The conclusion drawn by the researchers was that neurofeedback is an intervention tolerable for victims of war-related torture and refugees seeking to rebuild their lives and identities.

The Swedish Red Cross then conducted a follow-on study in Stockholm in 2016, one in which the training was extended from ten to twenty sessions in mid-course. Indeed, major progress in symptom abatement revealed itself in the second ten sessions. More than a 50% reduction in mean symptom severity was achieved, with progress noted at every session and with no sign of plateauing.[96]

13.10.3 Torture Victims and Refugees: Sydney, Australia

In 2017, a case study (N = 2) with neurofeedback for refugees reported, "A high proportion of these people respond poorly to current best practice treatment and remain disabled by high levels of symptomology. Thus, new evidence-based interventions are required." The published report stated that clients achieved "significant reduction in symptoms of PTSD and improvement in daily functioning post neurofeedback training."[97] It went on to say, "As these clients become better regulated and less aroused, they also become more receptive to other forms of treatment." These individuals required 50 sessions or more of intensive, personalized neurofeedback application.

13.10.4 Alpha-Theta Neurofeedback

As multiple deployments have become routine for our volunteer military, cumulative injury is an increasing concern. Research has shown that increased time in combat is linked with progressive reductions in alpha activity at the back of the brain.[98] This is consistent with a state of heightened vigilance, which is sustained by movement toward tonic over-arousal. Hyper-arousal is a tool of protection, and as such is likely refractory to talk therapy. Moreover, with veterans, there are often trust issues. Neurofeedback slips "under the radar" of hyper-vigilance, modifying the excessive arousal issue physiologically, without much talk.[99, 100]

Between 1989 and 1993, researchers in the VA tested Alpha-Theta (α-θ) brainwave neurotherapy after observing alpha was absent in the brainwaves of alcoholics.[101, 102] Alpha-theta was integrated into VA standard care for experimental treatment examining the impact of neurotherapy on alcoholism, PTSD nightmares and flashbacks, the use of psychotropic pharmaceuticals, and established measures of personality. Their replicated findings demonstrated that the veterans who received neurofeedback treatment decreased their medications more than the SC control groups, had higher rates of abstinence and relapse prevention in the 18 months following treatment than controls, and exhibited substantial reductions in severity on different personality scales, versus none among the controls.[103, 104, 105]

The goal of the initial neurofeedback training sessions described in this chapter is to stabilize the brain and to enhance its self-regulatory competence. As symptoms abate in severity or fall away entirely, Alpha-Theta training can be added to resolve deep-seated trauma. Alpha-Theta training was found to be an effective intervention for cocaine abuse, bulimia nervosa, alcoholism, and stress disorders, as well as for Vietnam combat veterans with chronic PTSD.[106] The results suggest that integration of Alpha-Theta neurofeedback into VA SC is useful in "long-term prevention of PTSD relapse," and maintenance of sobriety.[107]

13.11 The Positive Impact of Neurofeedback

It is estimated that about 40% of the veterans who develop PTSD fail to recover with traditional treatment strategies.[108, 109] If recovery is taken to mean a full restoration of what was lost, post-traumatic health may be structured on rehabilitation, adaptation, and accommodation with ongoing care.[110] The staff at Deployment Health at Camp Pendleton estimated that the full exploitation of neurofeedback, in the context of an integrative treatment program, might lead to a mere 5% residual of treatment-refractory cases.

But matters don't stop with symptom abatement. Service members and veterans start complaining about the symptom tracking when they would rather talk about what is going well in their lives. Neurofeedback aids in recovery in the fullest sense of the word. After all, neurofeedback can only build on what already works. It is inherently training toward better function. That does not stop with recovery from symptoms.

Some people who have been through trauma say those traumatic experiences ground them down, while others say those experiences revealed a healing crisis that polished them into a different form of competence and creative expression. It is a creative human capacity to transcend difficulties and achieve positive breakthroughs in personal growth and development. The peak performance and fitness benefits of neurofeedback training are observable in the emergence of positive post-traumatic growth.

13.12 A Perspective on Neurofeedback for Post-Combat Re-entry

The existing literature and history of programs integrating neurofeedback show strong evidence of clinical effectiveness in care. The findings from Ft. Hood's Reset program evaluation were statistically and clinically significant.[111] The video[112] from Ft. Hood, and presentation of excellent clinical outcomes from Camp Pendleton,[113] document a viable training strategy able to restore active duty service members and veterans to improved human functioning. The wizard and his magic sleep box passed its test by fire at a forward operating base in Afghanistan. Indeed, taking neurofeedback to front-line soldiers can reduce combat stress in the field, while at the same time increasing combat effectiveness.

The paucity of formal research into the latest methods of self-recovery is more than compensated for by the insertion of neurofeedback broadly into clinical practice. Early adopters, such as the ongoing program at the Salvation Army Bell Shelter in Los Angeles, continue to bring the demonstrated benefits of neurofeedback to our veterans. All who are being successfully recovered in these programs are testimony to the abiding inadequacy of standard care to elicit and exploit the latent recovery capacity of the brain.

The in-processing for military service is called boot camp; it is a transitional training program transforming civilians into combat-ready fighters. Thus far, there has been no similar kind of focused training to transform the combat soldiers back into civilians. When they return from their deployment many persist in warrior mode, and we need optimal stage transition training for their reintegration with their families and social lives.

Applying Reset-type training to smooth transitions for service members between missions and when separating from service could provide immediate self-care for all service members. It would avoid putting a spotlight on the individuals more adversely impacted by their service than other members of their teams, catching them before they can fall through the cracks in care. PTSD is a progressive condition among those who do not self-recover. Performance training such as that offered by the clinicians at Ft. Hood[114] and Camp Pendleton[115] could serve as a viable, cost-effective, post-deployment, and out-processing experience for service members. Integrating neurofeedback into all post-combat deployment transitional training would also remove the stigma associated with the word "treatment."

Achieving patient driven care is contingent on three variables: receptivity and responsiveness from the professionals, a supportive health care environment, and the involvement of an informed patient.[116] Clinical pilot programs continue to bring the benefits of neurofeedback for the relief from suffering of our service members and veterans. Given the lingering effects of combat trauma and related mTBI issues, combined with the relatively poor performance of evidence-based treatment modalities in current use, there is a compelling case for drawing on alternative methods in general, and on neurofeedback specifically, to address those issues.

13.13 The Case of Jackie O: Combat Medic

This section covers a case study of neurofeedback training with the female veteran quoted at the beginning of this chapter. Data were collected between 2012 and 2014, and resumed in 2018 (see Appendix B: Trend Lines). The initial 20-session training occurred in 2013 (B1: measure #5), implementing the then-existing ILF NF PTSD protocol.[117] Five booster sessions occurred in 2014 (B2: measure #10). Five more booster sessions occurred in 2018 (B3: measure #13). The findings illustrate the quality and speed of positive changes common with neurofeedback training.

History (Hx): Jackie O, a Special Ops combat medic, naturalized Hispanic American, served two decades of combined active duty and reserves.

Diagnosis (Dx): 100% disability; 70% PTSD, 30% combined mTBI and surgical reconstruction of her knee and foot, with a corpse heel, corpse navicular, and part of her own calf for the instep.

Treatment (Tx): Contemporaneous Neurofeedback Protocol Guides.

Jackie O agreed to use the established symptom tracking report (Appendix A), pay attention to and describe any perceived beneficial or detrimental effect, any progressive or regressive impact, and any surprise outcomes or unintended consequences. We discovered that she didn't like the symptom tracking questions; it was too much like interrogation with the same questions over and over ("Worst part of this whole process.")

A unique aspect of Jackie O's data set is the 3-point comparison of self-reported symptoms providing six-year trend lines of Jackie O's response to VA standard care (SC), both without and with neurofeedback. The baseline measure (2012: #1) was taken just prior to her entering VA SC specifically targeted toward PTSD, during evaluation for disability. When she arrived to initiate her first series of neurofeedback sessions (2013: A1–B1, measures #2–5) she said, "I've been attending PTSD groups for almost a year."

Jackie O was at Ft. Bragg when she separated from service on 18 prescribed meds. (The average veteran with PTSD is on ten meds.) In her Florida retirement, she researched the meds she was on and became concerned about the synergistic effects of all the pills. Some of the studies showed long-term, adverse health impacts for women. The VA SC available to her helped eliminate eight meds. She was still on ten meds when she initiated neurofeedback (A1: Measure #2). Within five sessions, she was down to two pills: blood pressure and a calcium supplement.

The full self-report on 150+ symptoms is ideally collected every five sessions to steer the lead placement decisions, using a Likert-like scale from 0 (no problem) to 10 (the worst), along with anything else that the individual perceives to be personally bothersome. Many veterans would rather track only a few symptoms (the ones most bothersome to that person), and will rarely report pain if not directly asked about it.

An online database[118] was used for entering the symptom data, creating easy to read trend lines. We targeted the symptoms with the highest reported severity, starting with sleep. A veteran struggling to express feelings and experiences may say there have been no changes in five or ten sessions. The symptoms of greatest interest to the individual may show a slower response to training than other symptoms. This is why the repetitive, self-reported symptom tracking, and visual presentation of that information over time in the form of trend lines is an important part of the process. The falling away of, or increase in, symptoms seemingly unrelated to the target symptoms are additional indicators of brain training effects, and they help to direct prospective protocol choices.

The baseline was collected on August 13, 2012, with each category of symptoms for Jackie O summarized in separate trend lines (Appendix B).

#1. August 13, 2012 – baseline measure of 62 symptoms (Sx) (ranging from 1–9 in severity).

The second measure (A1) was taken after almost a year of "evidence-based" VA SC for PTSD, and prior to neurofeedback.

#2. (A1) July 5, 2013 – 113 Sx (1–10 in severity).

The increased number of symptoms and symptom severity were a surprise.

Does this represent only the effects of evidence-based VA SC for PTSD on Jackie O's quality of life?

The reports of increased post-concussion impacts over time[119, 120] may be reflected in the emergence of Jackie O's increased number and severity of symptoms. It is obvious that the available evidence-based treatment was unable to reduce Jackie O's adverse symptom reporting. Instead, VA SC was correlated with a greater number of adverse symptoms and increased severity over time.

Jackie O trained with one-channel, ILF difference training for the first ten sessions. She optimized at 0.45 mHz on the right and 0.9 mHz on the left, meeting the expectation for a factor of two difference between left and right hemisphere training. After the first session, Jackie O was surprised by her immediate need to sleep, and then spontaneously falling asleep as soon as her head hit the pillow. Without the aid of medications, she slept deeply and awakened rested. By the fifth session, she reported that she did not need to take all her medications every day to stay calm.

With her medical training, Jackie O is uniquely qualified to assess the impact of pharmaceutical interventions. Nonetheless, a local civilian physician was recruited to evaluate this aspect of Jackie O's rehabilitative strategy. He supervised and supported Jackie O's reduction of medications. After Jackie O built up sufficient stamina for a more intensive training schedule, there were days when she trained three sessions a day with an hour off in between. Unfortunately, Jackie O's aversion to repetitive data collection meant that the first in-training data collection took place after eight neurofeedback sessions rather than five.

#3. July 10, 2013 – 41 Sx (1–8 in severity).
We took two days off after ten sessions, before three A/T (at PZ) sessions (11–13). Symptom tracking was gathered July 14, after the fourteenth neurofeedback session.

#4. July 14, 2013 – 28 Sx (2–8 in severity).
Jackie O completed the remaining sessions with the single-channel difference training at her optimized reward frequency. She was unwilling to sit through another iteration of symptom tracking. She provided data (B1) six days later, July 22, before her re-entry into VA SC.

#5. (B1) July 22, 2013 – 40 Sx (1–5 in severity).
Of the symptoms reported in measure #1, all had reduced severity. The 16 new symptoms surprised me. Did neurofeedback elicit new symptoms or adverse responses? Jackie O interpreted the change to be an increased comfort with, and awareness of, herself. She suggested that the symptoms may have been present but were not noticeable to her before because they were not as severe as the other symptoms. She agreed to stay in touch for post-training data collection, and to pay attention to any re-occurrence of symptoms, new symptoms, odd phenomena, unexpected emergent issues, indicators of distress, and surprises.

An uptick in symptoms the first week following an intensive training schedule is not uncommon. It is often followed by reports of cumulative, residual, progressive benefits in which remaining symptoms continue to melt away without additional neurofeedback. A slower pace of training twice a week over ten weeks provides a more gradual deconstruction of hyperarousal and reconstruction of a relaxed state, rarely eliciting rebound symptoms in the first week post-training. Jackie O provided symptom tracking data over the phone on August 8, three weeks post-training, after re-integrating into VA SC. It revealed the expected falling away of additional symptoms and severity.

#6. August 8, 2013 – 18 Sx (1–2 in severity).
While driving one day, Jackie O smelled smoke, visually located a dark plume, and flashed back to war-zone driving dangers. She applied cognitive behavioral strategies, reminding herself of the current civilian setting, and that the fire was

far enough away to be of no immediate threat. She thought she had calmed herself with the cognitive behavioral strategies. That night she had her first nightmare since neurofeedback training. November 29, four and a half months post training with only VA SC, Jackie O provided symptom tracking data by phone.

#7. November 29, 2013 – 80 Sx (1–10 in severity).

Research into the impact of neurofeedback training with mTBI found that 20 sessions may be insufficient, particularly if physical disruptions of neural circuits are involved. Patients with mTBI may need anywhere from 50 to 75 sessions.[121, 122] In Jackie O's case, 20 sessions were sufficient to restore, but insufficient to maintain her endogenous relaxation capacity. It is possible that her mTBI may be creating difficulty sustaining the progress of PTSD symptom reduction, implying the need for more sessions to restore and sustain her endogenous relaxation response. It appears that the VA SC without neurofeedback is limited in what it can offer Jackie O in furtherance of her rehabilitative goals and quality of life.

Surprise findings reported by Jackie O included: 1) nightmares were gone during the time of neurofeedback training and for almost a month post-training, 2) a reduction in pain, 3) her family interactions were less tense, and 4) she was able to socialize and go fishing with friends. The VA, however, was non-responsive to reports of positive outcomes with neurofeedback. None of the VA staff showed interest in the positive gains neurofeedback had elicited in her ongoing rehabilitative goals. Indeed, the VA refused to provide Jackie O with support and assistance integrating an existing, replicable treatment that she found helpful.

While attending a 2013 Veterans' Day event, Jackie O heard a helicopter in the distance and automatically jumped out of her seat to get her medic bag. Re-embedded in VA SC without neurofeedback booster sessions, she experienced olfactory and auditory triggered flashbacks, and an increase in adverse symptoms and symptom severity. During a phone interview on April 5, 2014, Jackie O reported a resumption of alcohol as a coping strategy. The number of symptoms and severity had both decreased – likely a result of the self-medication with alcohol.

#8. April 5, 2014 – 65 Sx (1–5 severity).

I was surprised by the alcohol coping strategy. How long can it mask the underlying problems before it becomes detrimental? We arranged for a field visit to bring neurofeedback sessions to Jackie O at her home; August 1st (A2) to 4th (B2).

#9. (A2) August 1, 2014 –118 Sx (1–8 in severity).

#10. (B2) August 4, 2014 – 124 Sx (1–5 in severity).

Opportunity for yet another appraisal of symptom status after five neurofeedback booster sessions was lost on the last day of training. Jackie O injured her shoulder while out walking when a dog pulled her down. Although this led to an increase in the number of symptoms, there was still an overall reduction in reported severity of the symptoms that pre-existed the dog-related injury. Symptom tracking data entry created an A1–B1–A2–B2 data set comparing VA SC without and with neurofeedback training over two years. We discussed her data, the VA's unwillingness to provide this intervention, and agreed that a home training system would be ideal for her long term self-care.

To get a home training system, Jackie O would have to fund the treatment she has found most effective for her rehabilitation goals from her disability budget. She decided that beer therapy fit her budget; it was less expensive than a neuro-feedback system. Over time, she resumed pharmaceuticals to address re-emergent sleep issues. More than four years passed in VA SC without integrative neurofeed-back training. In September of 2018, she had a near-fatal home accident. Alcohol was involved and she started to question her use of alcohol as a coping strategy. Octo-ber 28, a month after her accident, Jackie O provided symptom tracking by phone.

#11. October 28, 2018 – 85 Sx (1–10 in severity).

After she was medically cleared to drive, Jackie O drove a full day to initiate a series of neurofeedback booster sessions. November 13, she provided another data set (A3).

#12. (A3) November 13, 2018 – 78 Sx (1–8 in severity).

The original plan was two booster sessions a day, completing another accel-erated 20 sessions in two weeks. Travel for this training was delayed first by slow healing from the gruesome accident, then a back injury while walking a dog. The curtailed timeline resulted in only five sessions with the upgraded high definition (HD) software and amplifier.

We started with 20 minutes of passive infrared training (pIRx3)[123] for frontal lobe activation prior to using 2 Channel HD ILF. Jackie O optimized at 0.05 mHz. Our clinical experience was similar to the 2013 training (B1); we could only do one session a day for the first few days due to the fatigue it evoked. On the fourth day, November 16, we were able to complete two sessions. The effects of VA SC with-out (A) and with (B) neurofeedback are presented in six-year trend lines (Appendix B: A1–B1–A2–B2–A3–B3).

#13. (B3) November 16, 2018 – 42 Sx (1–8 in severity).

Jackie O attributed her new pains and increased severity to be "dog-related," plus the length of time driving for access to neurofeedback training while she still had open wounds. After five booster sessions in four days, Jackie O agreed to accept the loan of a neurofeedback system for doing supervised home training. The first morning back in her own home, she reported, "I slept like a baby. No meds, no alcohol." Two days after completing five HD ILF booster sessions, without any addi-tional sessions, she reported that her wounds were completely closed, her sleep quality was restored, and she could fall asleep without alcohol or medications, with her sleep free of nightmares.

As this book goes to press, Jackie O has integrated home training with neu-rofeedback. On January 1, 2019, she reported: "I feel great." She wants to explore her capacity to achieve long-lasting symptom amelioration, and agreed to provide symptom tracking every five sessions. Phone consultations will allow adjustment of training protocols based on her symptom reporting.

13.14 Conclusion

Infra-low frequency neurofeedback has been in continuous, intensive use at Camp Pendleton since 2009 in application to brain injury and emotional trauma. It was successfully integrated to VA SC in the multi-modal Reset training of U.S. active duty service members in 2011. In two successive studies, it has been found helpful for reducing the radical mal-adaptations elicited by war-related torture. All participants had previously failed to respond to conventional therapies. It is helpful for veterans being cared for through the Salvation Army's Bell Shelter, a program that has been underway for over a decade, and mainly serves Vietnam era veterans who had become homeless.[124] Jackie O is one of the many veterans currently being served by private practice neurofeedback clinicians working outside the existing VA SC. Many volunteer with *Homecoming for Veterans* (HC4V.org), through which neurofeedback services are provided to veterans *pro bono*.[125] The author has provided *pro bono* services as part of this program for ten years.

Ethical, client-driven clinical research needs flexibility in design. The RCT model is inappropriate to assess neurofeedback for PTSD symptom amelioration or resolution. The lack of evidence-based guidelines for PTSD care at the federal level is a strong indication that a nomothetic treatment model is a poor fit to clinical realities. An idiographic approach is called for to provide adequate care for service members who are not responding positively to VA SC.

Dr. Wesch considered the synergy of the multi-modal approach to be the most important factor in the results his team reported with their well-documented Reset program. Integrating neurofeedback into standard care has been shown to improve outcomes for combat veterans; it has been found to be better than standard care alone. Neurofeedback has the potential for improving the quality of life for those suffering from the cluster of symptoms known clinically as PTSD.

> We broke the loop. I don't go back into that loop ... I still have those memories, but they aren't forced on me ... It's liberating ... I felt like I just got a pardon from the governor from a life sentence.[126]

Notes

1 The pseudonym, Jackie O, was selected by the client for publication of her clinical outcomes, and she signed a release to that effect. www.youtube.com/watch?v=75z6AqwTRpA

2 Nash, W. P. (2007). Combat/operational stress adaptations and injuries. In C. R. Figley & W. P. Nash (Eds.), *Combat stress injury: Theory, research, and management* (pp. 33–63). New York: Routledge.

3 Tick, E. (2005). *War and the soul*. Wheaton, IL: Quest Books.

4 Levine, P. A. & Frederick, A. (1997). *Waking the tiger: Healing trauma*. Berkley, CA: North Atlantic Books. p.79.

5 Zweerings, J., Pflieger, E. M., Mathiak, K. A., Zvyagintsev, M., Kacela, A., Flatten, G., & Mathiak, K. (2018, May 30). Impaired voluntary control in PTSD: Probing

self-regulation of the ACC with real-time fMRI. *Frontiers in Psychiatry*, 9, 219. doi:10.3389/fpsyt.2018.00219. Downloaded September 22, 2018.

6   Zotev, V. A., Phillips, R., Misaki, M., Wong, C. K., Wurfel, B. E., Krueger, F., Felderner, M., & Bordurka, J. (2018, April 8). Real-time fMRI neurofeedback training of the amygdala activity with simultaneous EEG in veterans with combat–related PTSD. *Neurolmage: Clinical*, 19, 106–121. https://doi.org/10/1016/j.nicl.2018.04.010. Downloaded September 22, 2018.

7   Tanielian, T. & Jaycox, L. H. (Eds). (2008). *Invisible wounds of war: Psychological and cognitive injuries, their consequences and services to assist recovery.* Santa Monica, California: RAND Corporation MG 720- CCF (or Rand Center for Military Health Policy Research).

8   Congressional Budget Office. (2012, February 9). *The Veterans Health Administration's treatment of PTSD and traumatic brain injury among recent combat veterans.* www.cbo.gov/publication/42969. Downloaded October 1, 2018.

9   Institute of Medicine. (2014). *Treatment for post traumatic stress disorder in military and veteran populations: Final assessment.* Washington, DC: The National Academies Press. https://doi.org/10.17226/18724. p. 92. These are DoD costs, the VA spent over 3 billion on PTSD care for active duty and veterans. 2004 = 8633, cost per millions $29.6, per member, $3425, inpatient $14,172, outpatient, $2048, drugs $491. 2012 = 65,706, cost per millions $294.1, per member, $4520, inpatient $19,341, outpatient, $2095, drugs $500.

10 Hammer, P. S. (2012, Nov 27). *Defense Centers for Excellence for Psychological Health and Traumatic Brain Injury Update.* Dir. Defense Health Board. Powerpoint presentation. Downloaded Dec. 2018 online from file:///C:/Users/Admin/Downloads/122712DCOE%20Update%20(1).pdf.

11 U.S. Department of Veterans Affairs. (2017). *VA/DOD clinical practice guideline for the management of posttraumatic stress disorder and acute stress disorder: Patient education material.* (Version 3.0). Department of Veterans Affairs, Department of Defense: Author. www.healthquality.va.gov/guidelines/MH/ptsd/VADoDPTSDCPGClinicianSummaryFinal.pdf Downloaded October 22, 2018.

12 U.S. Department of Veterans Affairs. (n.d.). Treatment of co-occurring PTSD and substance use disorder in VA. *PTSD: National Center for PTSD.* Author. www.ptsd.va.gov/professional/treat/cooccurring/tx_sud_va.asp. Downloaded October 27, 2018.

13 Reiters, K., Andersen, S. B., & Carlsson, J. (2016, February 1). Neurofeedback treatment and posttraumatic stress disorder: Effectiveness of neurofeedback of posttraumatic stress disorder and optimal choice of protocol. *The Journal of Nervous and Mental Disease*, 204(2), 69–77. Wolters Kluwer, downloaded from Ovid online doi: 10.1097/NMD.0000000000000418, PMID: 26825263 p. 2.

14 Van der Kolk, B. (2014). *The body keeps the score: Brain, mind, and body in the healing of trauma.* New York, NY: Penguin Books. p. 43.

15 Gentry, J. E. (Educator, 2006, March). *Models of clinical supervision.* Sarasota: Argosy University.

16 Kano, M. & Fukudo, S. (2013). The Alexithymic brain: The neural pathways linking alexithymia to physical disorders. *Biopsychosocial Medicine*, 7, 1. www.bpsmedicine.com/content/7/1/1.

17 Busuttil, W. (2004). Presentations and management of post traumatic stress disorder and the elderly: A need for investigation. *International Journal of Geriatric Psychiatry*, 19, 429–439.

18 Imperatori, C., Marca, G. D., Brunetti, R., Carbone, G. A., Massulo, C., Valenti, E. M., Amoroso, N., Maestoso, G., Contardi, A., & Farina, B. (2016). Default Mode Network alterations in alexithymia: An EEG power spectra and connectivity study. www.nature.com/scientificreports. doi: 10.1038/srep36653.

19 Samur, D., Tops, M., Schlinkert, C., Quirin, M., Cuijpers, P., & Koole, S. L. (2013, November 19). Four decades of research on alexithymia: Moving toward clinical applications. *Frontiers in Psychology.* https://doi.org/10/3389/fpsyg.2013.00861

20 Benson, A. & LaDou, T. W. (2016). The use of neurofeedback for combat veterans with posttraumatic stress. In H. Kirk (Ed.), *Restoring the brain: Neurofeedback as an integrative approach to health* (pp. 181–200). Boca Raton, FL: CRC Press/ Taylor Francis Group.

21 Castro, C. A. (2014). The US framework for understanding, preventing, and caring for the mental health needs of service members who served in combat in Afghanistan and Iraq: A brief review of the issues and research. *European Journal of Psychotraumatology*, 5, 24731. http:/dx.doi.org/103401/ejpt.v6.24713. Downloaded October 1, 2018.

22 U.S.Veterans Association. (n.d.). *Treatment of co-occurring PTSD and substance use disorder in VA.* Author: PTSD: National Center for PTSD. www.ptsd.va.gov/ professional/treat/coocurring/tx_sud_va.asp. Downloaded October 22, 2018.

23 Castro, C. A. (2014).

24 Gilpin, N.W. & Weiner, J. L. (2017, January). Neurobiology of comorbid post-traumatic stress disorder and alcohol-use disorder. *Genes Brain Behav*, 16(1), 15–43. Downloaded October 22, 2018.

25 Fisher, S. (2014). *Neurofeedback in the treatment of development disorders: Calming the fear-driven brain.* New York, NY: W. W. Norton. & Co.

26 Van der Kolk, B. (2014).

27 Tanielian, T. & Jaycox, L. H. (Eds). (2008).

28 Gray, S. (2017). An overview of the use of neurofeedback biofeedback for the treatment of symptoms of traumatic brain injury in military and civilian populations. *Medical Acupuncture*, 29(4), 215–219.

29 Esty, M. L. & Shifflett, C. M. (2014). *Conquering concussion: Healing TBI symptoms wih neurofeedback and without drugs.* Sewickley, PA: Round Earth Publishing.

30 Colston, M. (2017, December 13). Prepared Statement regarding *The Current State and Future Aims in Traumatic Brain Injury-Research, Diagnostic Testing and Evaluations, and Treatment.* Before the Senate Armed Services Committee, Subcommittee on Personnel. Office of the Assistant Secretary of Defense-Health Affairs: Director of Mental Health Programs.

31 VA Handbook 1160.01 Uniform Mental Health Services in VA Medical Centers and Clinicals. Amended November 16, 2015. Downloaded January 2, 2019.

32 Institute of Medicine. (2012). *Treatment of posttraumatic stress disorder in military and veteran populations: Initial assessment.* Washington, DC: The National Academies Press. p. 304

33 Colston, M. (2017, December 13).

34 Scott, W.C., Kaiser, D.A., Othmer, S. Sideroff, S.I.(2005). Effects of an EEG Biofeedback Protocol on a Mixed Substance Abusing Population, *Am. J. of Drug and Alcohol Abuse*, 31(1), 455–469.

35 Institute of Medicine. (2012).

36 Van der Kolk, B. (2014).

37 Panisch, L. S. & Hai, A. H. (2018, June 11). The effectiveness of using neurofeedback in the treatment of post-traumatic stress disorder: A systematic review. *Trauma, Violence, & Abuse*, 1–10. Downloaded from Sage Journals online p.3

38 Van der Kolk. B. A., Hodgdon, H., Gapen, M., Musicaro, R., Suvak, M. K., Hamlin, E., & Spinazzola, J. (2016). A randomized controlled study of neurofeedback for chronic PTSD. *PLoS One*. 11(12). e0166752. doi:10.1371/journal.pone.0166752

39 Van der Kolk. (2014). p.221.

40 Committee on Treatment of Posttraumatic Stress Disorder, Institute of Medicine. (2003). *Treatment of posttraumatic stress disorder, an assessment of the evidence*. Washington, DC: The National Academies Press.

41 Lancaster, C. L., Teeters, J. B., Gros, D. F., & Back, S. E. (2016). Posttraumatic stress disorder: Overview of evidence-based assessment and treatment. *Journal of Clinical Medicine*, 5(105). Downloaded October 22, 2018. doi:10.3390/jcm5110105.

42 Sokhadze, T. M., Stewart, C. M., & Hollifield, M. (2007). Integrating cognitive neuroscience research and cognitive behavioral treatment with neurofeedback therapy in drug addiction comorbid with posttraumatic stress disorder: A conceptual review. *Journal of Neurotherapy*, 11(2), 13–44.

43 Strauss, J. L., Coeytaux, R., McDuffie, J., Williams, J. W., & Nagi, A. (2011, August). *Efficacy of complementary and alternative medicine therapies for posttraumatic stress disorder. VA-ESP Project #09-010*. www.ncbi.nlm.nih.gov/books/NBK82774/p.7. Downloaded December 25, 2018.

44 Curators of University of Missouri. School of Psychology. (2011). *What are evidence based interventions (EBI)?* Missoula, Missouri: Author. http://ebi.missouri.edu/?page_id=52. Downloaded January 6, 2019.

45 Tanielian, T. & Jaycox, L. H. (Eds). (2008).

46 Institute of Medicine. (2014).

47 Hester, R. D. (2017, August 18). Lack of access to mental health services contributing to the high suicide rates among veterans. *International Journal of Mental Health Systems*, 11, 47. https://ijmhs.biomedcentral.com/track/pdf/10.1186/s13033-017-0154-2. Downloaded December 24, 2018.

48 National Academies of Sciences, Engineering, and Medicine; Health and Medicine Division; Board of Health Care Services; Committee to Evaluate the Department of Veterans Affairs Mental Health Services. (2018, January 31). *Evaluation of the Department of Veterans Affairs Mental Health Services*. Washington, DC: National Academies Press (US); 16, Findings, Conclusions, and Recommendations. Available from: www.ncbi.nlm.nih.gov/books/NBK499500/.

49 Hester, R. D. (2017, August 18). Lack of access to mental health services contributing to the high suicide rates among veterans. *International Journal of Mental Health Systems*, 11, 47. https://ijmhs.biomedcentral.com/track/pdf/10.1186/s13033-017-0154-2. Downloaded December 24, 2018.

50 Giannitrapani, K., McCaa, M., Haverfield, M., Kerns, R. D., Timko, C., Dobscha, S., & Lorenz, K. (2018 November/December). Veteran experiences

seeking non-pharmacologic approaches for pain. *Military Medicine*, 183, 628–634. https://academic.oup.com/milmed/article/183/11-12/e628/4954091. Downloaded December 25, 2018.

51 Blaine, S. K., Dongju, S., & Sinha, R. (2017, March 1). Peripheral and prefrontal stress system markers and risk of relapse in alcoholism. *Addict Biol*, 22(2), 468–478.

52 Van der Kolk, B., et al. (2016).

53 Mr. Franklin Paine, Vietnam Veteran, was on 15–20 pills a day prior to starting neurofeedback. "I don't take no pain pills. I don't take no psych meds, ... I don't take none of that stuff no more." Salvation Army Bell Shelter. www.youtube.com/watch?v=oe370IjZbVI.

54 Dahl, M. G. (2010). *Dissertation: Neurofeedback for PTSD symptom reduction*. Argosy/Sarasota: Author.

55 Kelson, C. Y. (2013, October 29). *The Impact of EEG Biofeedback on Veterans' Symptoms of Posttraumatic Stress Disorder (PTSD)*. Unpublished Dissertation, Chicago School of Psychology. PQDT Open https://pqdtopen.proquest.com/doc/1492137060.html?FMT=AI. Downloaded October 27, 2018.

56 Gapen, M., van der Kolk, B. A., Hamlin, Ed., Hirshberg, L., Suvak, M., & Spinazzola, J. (2016, January 19). A pilot study of neurofeedback for chronic PTSD. *Appl. Psychophysiol Biofeedback*. Downloaded October 27, 2018. doi 10.1007/s10484-015-9326-5.

57 McReynolds, C. J., Bell, J., & Lincourt, T. M. (2017). Neurofeedback: A noninvasive treatment for symptoms of post traumatic stress disorder in veterans. *Neuroregulation*, 4(3–4), 114–124. www.neuroregulation.org. doi:10.14440/nr.4.3-4.114

58 Sur, R. L. & Dahm, P. (2011, October–December). History of evidence-based medicine. *Indian Journal of Urology*, 27(4), 487–489. www.ncbi.nlm.nih.gov/pmc/articles/PMC3263217/. Downloaded January 6, 2019.

59 Mirgain, S. A. & Singles, J. (n.d.). *Whole health: Change the conversation. Advancing skills in the delivery of personalized, proactive, patient-driven care. Educational overview: Power of the mind educational overview*. Integrative Medicine Program, Department of Family Medicine, University of Wisconsin-Madison School of Medicine and Public Health and the Pacific Institute for Research and Evaluation: VHA Office of Patient Centered Care and Cultural Transformation. http://projects.hsl.wisc.edu/SERVICE/modules/12/M12_EO_Power_of_the_Mind.pdf p.20. Downloaded December 25, 2018.

60 Othmer, S., Othmer, S., Kaiser, D. A., & Putman, J. (2012). Endogenous neuromodulation at infralow frequencies. *Seminars in Pediatric Neurology*, 20(4), 246–257.

61 Othmer, S. (2008, September 11–14). (Educator). *Four day clinical course in neurofeedback*. Woodland Hills, CA: EEGInfo.

62 Othmer, S. (2008). *Protocol guide: For neurofeedback clinicians* (2nd ed.). Woodland Hills, CA: EEGInfo.

63 Tanielian, T. & Jaycox, L. H. (Eds). (2008).

64 Sokhadze, T. M., et al. (2007).

65 Esty, M. L. & Shifflett, C. M. (2014).

66 Committee on Treatment of Posttraumatic Stress Disorder, Institute of Medicine. (2003).

67 Gray, S. (2017). An overview of the use of neurofeedback biofeedback for the treatment of symptoms of traumatic brain injury in military and civilian populations. *Medical Acupuncture*, 29(4), 215–219. doi: 10.1089/acu.2017.1220

68 Smith, M. L., Collura, T. F., Ferrera, J., & de Vries, J. (2014). Infra-slow fluctuation training in clinical prctice: A technical history. *NeuroRegulation*, 1(2), 187–207. doi:10.15540/nr.1.2.187. www.neuroregulation.org.

69 Larsen, S. (2006). Life hurts: Post-traumatic stress disorder, pain, and bereavement. In S. Larsen (Ed.), *The healing power of neurofeedback: The revolutionary LENS technique for restoring optimal brain function*. Rochester, VT: Healing Art Press. pp. 244–258.

70 Sokhadze, T. M., et al. (2007).

71 Van der Kolk, B. et al. (2016).

72 Mirgain, S. A. & Singles, J. (n.d.).

73 Ruppert, B. (2012, February 28). *Controlling post-traumatic stress could be as close as a game on a cell phone*. U.S. Army Medical Research and Material Command. www.army.mil/article/74187/controlling_post_traumatic_stress_could_be_as_close_as_game_on_cell_phone. Downloaded December 30, 2018.

74 Mattson, J. (May 30, 2012). *Holistic treatments help soldiers battle PTSD*. www.army.mil/article/80772/holistic_treatments_help_soldiers_battle_ptsd. Downloaded January 20, 2019.

75 Libretto, S., Hilton, L., Gordon, S., Zhang, W., & Wesch, J. (2015, November). Effects of integrative PTSD treatment in the military health setting. *Energy Psychology*, 7(2), 33–44. Downloaded December 25, 2018.

76 The American Institute of Stress. (2013, July). Combat Stress. Bringing you all the way home. Heros & Hope. Warrior Combat Stress Reset Program (WCSRP). Carl R. Darnall Army Medical Center. Ft Hood, TX: author. 2(3).

77 Institute of Medicine. (2014).

78 Marksberry, K. (2013, July 22). Interview of Dr. Jerry Wesch, by AIS executive director. www.youtube.com/watch?v=RIA7DET2q44.

79 Libretto, S., et al. (2015, November).

80 Herman, P. M., Sorbero, M. E., & Sims-Columba, A. C. (2017). *Complementary and alternative medicine in the military health system*. Santa Monica, CA: RAND Corporation. www.rand.org/pubs/research_reports/RR1380.html. p. xiii. Downloaded December 25, 2018.

81 Institute of Medicine. (2014).

82 Marksberry, K. (2013, July 22).

83 Wesch, J. (2012). *Pentagon's brain powered video-games might treat PTSD. Wired.* www.wired.com/2012/07/neurofeedback/.

84 PTSD(PCL-M) is a standard for measuring PTSD in service members and veterans. www.newriver.marines.mil/Portals/17/Documents/3%20PTSDTBIChecklists 20100819.pdf

85 Libretto, S., et al. (2015, November).

86 Samueli Institute: Exploring the Science of Healing. (2013). *Program evaluation of the Warrior Combat Stress Reset Program at Fort Hood*. www.healingourwarfighters.org/downloads/fort-hood-reset51713.pdf. Downloaded December 23, 2018.

87 Libretto, S., et al. (2015, November).

88 Villanueva, M., Benson, A., & LaDou, T. (2011). Clinical practice and observations of infralow neurofeedback as an adjunctive treatment within Camp Pendleton's Deployment Health Center. NCCOSC conference, April 2011.

89 Personal conversations with Villanueva, M.

90 Villanueva, M. as cited in Katie Drummond. (2013, April 18). *I think therefore I heal – The weird science of neurofeedback*. *The Verge*. www.theverge.com/2013/4/18/4226506/can-you-train-your-brain-to- heal-your-health.

91 Villanueva, M., et al. (2011).

92 Niv, S. (2013). Clinical efficacy and potential mechanism of neurofeedback. *Personality and Individual Differences*. http://dx.doi.org/10.1016/j.paid.2012.11.037

93 Nilsson, R. & Nilsson, V. (2014). *Neurofeedback treatment for traumatized refugees – A pilot study*. Psykologexamensuppsats Lunds Universitet, Institutionen för psykologi Psykologprogrammet. http://lup.lub.lu.se/luur/download?func=downloadFile&recordOld=4459760&fileOld=4459775. p. 23. Downloaded December 21, 2018.

94 The six assessments used were: *"the PTSD Checklist, Civilian Version (PCL-C), the Hopkins Symptom Checklist-25(HSCL-25), the Symptom Checklist (SCL-90), the Subscale Somatization, and the WHO-5 – Wellbeing Index (WHO-5)"* and the *Pittsburg Sleep Quality Index (PSQI)*. Nilsson & Nilsson. (2014).

95 The symptoms selected represent ~10% of the full symptom tracking list: difficulty falling asleep, disturbed sleep, nightmares, flashbacks, fear/worry/anxiety, rumination, feeling low, low self-esteem, difficulty concentrating, sensitivity to sounds, irritability, anger/ rage, fatigue, muscle tension, and headaches.

96 Metso, F. J. & Duberg, K. (2016). *Can neurofeedback reduce PTSD symptoms in severely traumatized refugees?* Stockholm, Sweden: RödaKorsets Center för torerade flykingar. (Red Cross Center for Tortured Refugees). https://nhahealth.com/neurofeedback/wp-content/uploads/2017/06/RodaKorset_update-graphics-corrected.pdf. Downloaded December 21, 2018.

97 Askovic, M., Watter, A. J., Aroche, J., & Harris, A. W. F. (2017). Neurofeedback as an adjunct therapy for treatment of chronic posttraumatic stress disorder related to refugee trauma and torture experiences: Two case studies. *Australasian Psychiatry*. 25(4). pp.358–363. Downloaded January 9, 2019.

98 Van der Kolk. (2014).

99 Othmer, S. & Othmer, S. (2009). Post-traumatic stress disorder – The concrete activities. *Biofeedback*, 37(1), 24–31.

100 Othmer, S. & Othmer, S. (Educators, 2009, March 4–8). *Four-day clinical course in neurofeedback*. Atlanta, GA: EEGInfo.

101 Peniston, E. G. & Kulkosky, P. J. (1989). α-θ brainwave training and ß-endorphin levels in alcoholics. *Alcoholism: Clinical and Experimental Research*. 13(2), 271–279.

102 Peniston, E. G. & Kulkosky, P. J. (1991). Alpha-theta brainwave neuro-feedback therapy for Vietnam veterans with combat-related post-traumatic stress disorder. *Medical Psychotherapy*, 4, 47–60.

103 Peniston, E. G., Marrinan, D. A., Deming, W. A., & Kulkosky, P. J. (1993). EEG alpha-theta brainwave synchronization in Vietnam theater veterans with combat-related post-traumatic stress disorder and alcohol abuse. *Advances in Medical Psychotherapy*, 6, 37–50.

104 Peniston, E. G. & Kulkosky, P. J. (1991a). Alpha-theta EEG biofeedback training in alcoholism & post-traumatic stress disorder. *ISSSEEM*, 5(2), 5–7.

105 Peniston, E. G. & Kulkosky, P. J. (1990). Alcoholic personality and alpha-theta brainwave training. *Medical Psychotherapy*, 3, 37–55.
106 Peniston, E. G. & Kulkosky, P. J. (1991a).
107 Peniston, E. G., et al. (1993).
108 Committee on Treatment of Posttraumatic Stress Disorder, Institute of Medicine. (2003).
109 Gerin, M. I., Fichetenholtz, H., Roy, A., Walsh, C. J., Krystal, J. H., Southwich, S., & Hampson, M. (2016, June). Real-time fMRI neurofeedback with war veterans with chronic PTSD: A feasibility study. *Frontiers in Psychiatry*, 7, 111.
110 McNally, R. J., Bryant, R. A., & Ehlers, A. (2003). Does early psychological intervention promote recovery from posttraumatic stress? *Psychological Science in the Public Interest*, 4(2), 45–79.
111 Libretto, S., et al. (2015, November).
112 Staff Sgt. Roberts, Ft. Hood, www.youtube.com/watch?v=Txw01NS9e-Q.
113 Villanueva, M., et al. (2011).
114 Marksberry, K. (2013, July 22).
115 Villanueva, M., et al. (2011).
116 Bokhour, B. G., Fix, G. M., Mueller, N. M., Barker, A. M., Lavela, S. L., Hill, J. N., Solomon, J. L., & Lukas, C .V. D. (2018). How can healthcare organizations implement patient-centered care? Examining a large-scale culture transformation. *BMC Health Services Research*, 18(168). https://doi.org/10.1186/s12913-018-2949-5. Downloaded January 11, 2019.
117 Othmer, S. (2007). *Protocol guide: Case study: PTSD*. Woodland Hills, CA: EEG Institute.
118 www.eegexpert.net/.
119 Tanielian, T. & Jaycox, L. H. (Eds). (2008).
120 Congressional Budget Office. (2012, February 9).
121 Bounias, M., Laibow, R. E., Stubblebine, A. N., Sandground, H., & Bonaly, A. (2002). EEG-neurobiofeedback treatment of patients with brain injury part 4: Duration of treatments as a function of both the initial load of clinical symptoms and the rate of rehabilitation. *Journal of Neurotherapy*, 6(1), 23–38.
122 Rostami, R., Salamati, P., Yarandi, K. K., Khoshnevisan, A., Saadat, S., Kamali, Z. S., Ghiasi, S., Zaryabi, A., Saeid, S. S. G. M., Arjipour, M., Rezaee-Aavareh, M. S., & Rahimi, Movaghar V. (2016, May 3). Effects of neurofeedback on the short-term memory and continuous attention of patients with moderate traumatic brain injury: A preliminary randomized controlled clinical trial. *Chinese Journal of Traumatology*. http://dx.doi.org/101016/j.cjtee.2016.11.007
123 Carmen, J. A. (2005). Passive infrared hemoencephalography: Four years and 100 migraines. *Journal of Neurotherapy, Investigations in Neuromodulation, Neurofeedback and Applied Neuroscience*. 8(3). Downloaded October 16, 2018.
124 Salvation Army Bell Shelter. www.youtube.com/watch?v=oe370IjZbVI.
125 Homecoming4veterans (HC4V). (n.d.). www.homecoming4veterans.org/.
126 Rand insisted on being known by his own name, refused to let his information be released under a pseudonym, and signed a release to that effect. Video of Rand online www.youtube.com/watch?v=5oK3afDGjEI. Rand's case presentation is in Chapter 10. PTSD symptom reduction with neurofeedback. Kirk, H. (Ed.). *Restoring the brain: Neurofeedback as an integrative approach to health*. Boca Raton, FL: CRC Press/Taylor Francis Group. pp. 210–216.

Appendix A

(2008) Othmer Symptom Tracking Report

(modified +2 Behavior category symptoms: Hypervigilance and Exaggerated Startle)

Date:_____Time: start_____,
complete_____Name:
data provided by:_____Symptom Tracking (0 = no problem, 10 = the worst)

Category 1 Sleep

- Bruxism
- Difficulty maintaining sleep
- Disregulated sleep cycles
- Night sweats
- Nightmares or vivid dreams
- Periodic leg movements
- Restless sleep
- Sleep walking
- Snoring
- Difficulty falling asleep
- Difficulty waking
- Narcolepsy
- Night terrors
- Nocturnal enuresis
- Restless leg
- Sleep apnea
- Talking during sleep

Category 2 Attention and Learning

- Difficulty completing tasks
- Difficulty making decisions
- Difficulty remembering names
- Difficulty shifting tasks
- Difficulty understanding
- Conversations
- Lack of alertness
- Messy handwriting
- Poor concentration
- Poor math
- Poor sustained attention
- Poor vocabulary
- Reading difficulty
- Unmotivated
- Difficulty following instructions
- Difficulty organizing personal time and space
- Difficulty shifting attention
- Difficulty thinking clearly
- Distractibility
- Lacking common sense
- Not listening
- Poor drawing ability
- Poor short-term memory
- Poor verbal expression
- Poor word finding
- Slow thinking

Category 3 Sensory

- Auditory hypersensitivity
- Motion sickness
- Somatosensory deficits
- Tinnitus
- Visual Deficits
- Chemical sensitivities
- Poor body awareness
- Tactile hypersensitivity
- Vertigo
- Visual hypersensitivity

Category 4 Behavioral

- Addictive behaviors
- Anorexia
- Binging and purging
- Compulsive behaviors
- Crying
- Excessive talking
- Hypervigilance
- Inflexibility
- Lack of sense of humor
- Manipulative behavior
- Nail biting
- Poor eye contact
- Poor social or emotional reciprocity
- Rages
- Stuttering
- Aggressive behavior
- Autistic stimming
- Class clown
- Compulsive eating
- Exaggerated startle response
- Hyperactivity
- Impulsivity
- Lack of appetite awareness
- Lack of social interest
- Motor or vocal tics
- Oppositional or defiant behavior
- Poor grooming
- Poor speech articulation
- Self-injurious behavior

Category 5 Emotional

- Agitation
- Anxiety
- Difficult to soothe
- Easily embarrassed
- Fears
- Flashbacks of trauma
- Irritability
- Lack of pleasure
- Low self-esteem
- Mood swings
- Obsessive worries
- Paranoia
- Anger
- Depression
- Dissociative episodes
- Emotional reactivity
- Feelings of unreality
- Impatience
- Lack of emotional awareness
- Lack of social awareness
- Mania
- Obsessive negative thoughts
- Panic attacks
- Suicidal thoughts

Category 6 Physical

- Allergies
- Chronic constipation
- Difficulty walking or moving
- Effort Fatigue
- Fatigue
- High blood pressure
- Immune deficiency
- Asthma
- Clumsiness
- Difficult working
- Encopresis
- Heart palpitations
- Hot flashes
- Irritable bowel

- Low muscle tone
- Muscle twitches
- Nausea
- Poor balance
- Poor gross motor coordination
- Rigidity
- Skin rashes
- Stress incontinence
- Sweating
- Tremor

- Muscle tension
- Muscle weakness
- PMS symptoms
- Poor fine motor coordination
- Reflux
- Seizures
- Spasticity
- Sugar craving and reactivity
- Tachycardia
- Urge incontinence

Category 7 Pain

- Abdominal pain
- Chronic nerve pain
- Jaw pain
- Muscle pain
- Sciatica
- Stomach aches

- Chronic aching pain
- Fibromyalgia pain
- Joint pain
- Muscle tension headaches
- Sinus headaches
- Trigeminal neuralgia

Other:

_____ _____

_____ _____

_____ _____

_____ _____

Appendix B

Trend Lines for Jackie O

Sleep

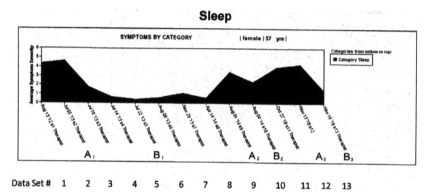

Figure 13.1 Sleep

Attention and Learning

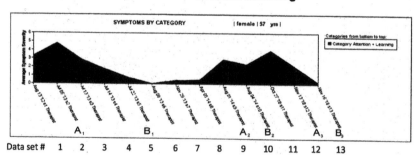

Figure 13.2 Attention and Learning

Sensory

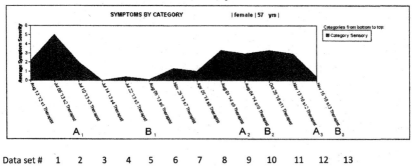

Data set #   1   2   3   4   5   6   7   8   9   10   11   12   13

Figure 13.3 Sensory

Behavior

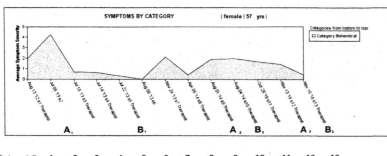

Data set #   1   2   3   4   5   6   7   8   9   10   11   12   13

Figure 13.4 Behavior

Emotions

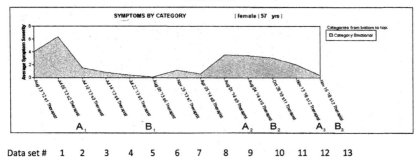

Data set #   1   2   3   4   5   6   7   8   9   10   11   12   13

Figure 13.5 Emotions

Physical

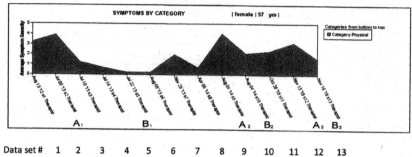

Data set #   1   2   3   4   5   6   7   8   9   10   11   12   13

Figure 13.6 Physical

Pain

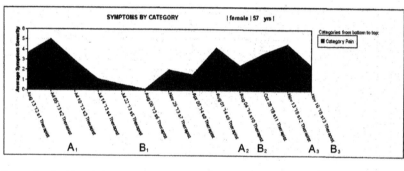

Data set #   1   2   3   4   5   6   7   8   9   10   11   12   13

Figure 13.7 Pain

Chapter 14

The Sleeping Brain
Neurofeedback and Insomnia

P. Terrence Moore

Now, blessings light on him that first invented this same sleep! It covers a man all over, thoughts and all, like a cloak; it is meat for the hungry, drink for the thirsty, heat for the cold, and cold for the hot. It is the current coin that purchases all the pleasures of the world cheap; and the balance that sets the king and the shepherd, the fool and the wise man, even. There is only one thing, which somebody once put into my head, that I dislike in sleep; it is, that it resembles death; there is very little difference between a man in his first sleep, and a man in his last sleep.

from Don Quixote, Miguel de Cervantes Saavedra

14.1 Introduction

Sleep, central to all aspects of our life and health, is highly regulated by the brain, both directly and indirectly. This chapter will discuss some basic concepts of the circadian rhythm, sleep–wake regulation (the homeostatic process) and focus on insomnia as a model for dysregulated sleep. Sleep timing and propensity results from the interplay of the circadian rhythm and the homeostatic process. While light is the primary external stimulus that "sets" the circadian clock, other factors, especially behavioral ones, can affect the circadian rhythm. There is a review of the history of biofeedback/neurofeedback in treating patients with insomnia. It concludes with two case presentations.

14.2 Aspects of Sleep

Daily I admonish my patients that there is nothing more important than good sleep. Despite having continuous real-world experience with it, few seem to regard it with the respect it is due. Every aspect of our conscious functioning depends on adequate, regular and well-organized sleep. Further, many disorders, for example epilepsy and migraine headaches, are adversely affected by poor sleep. Conversely, many illnesses can disrupt sleep resulting in familiar symptoms of excessive daytime sleepiness, maladaptive mood and impaired judgment to name a few. While having a brain is generally considered the *sine qua non* for sleep, most living organisms display a circadian rhythm that synchronizes its internal workings with the solar day and consists of alternating active and rest cycles. One of sleep's cruel ironies is that when we could get all we wanted as children, we almost always invented reasons not to go to bed. As adults we can never get enough of it!

But just what is sleep? From a medical standpoint, it may be considered the natural and regularly recurring reversible state of unconsciousness. During sleep the organism is relatively insensible to external stimuli. While specific aspects of sleep change as we age, e.g. newborns spending a third of their time in REM sleep alone, its indispensability for optimum functioning does not. Why is it important? This question is probably as much philosophical as it is scientific. Everyone has real world experience with the effects of lack of sleep, including a general feeling of malaise and lassitude, irritable mood and difficulty with mental focus and clarity. Persons without proper and adequate sleep have manifest difficulty with judgment and motor skills that may be worse than someone who is legally intoxicated. It is clearly vital to a healthy homeostasis inasmuch as persons with problematic sleep are more likely to suffer from cardiovascular disease, endocrine dysfunction and problems with immunity. Rats can be sleep-deprived to death in a straightforward manner. Mounting evidence suggests that humans can suffer the same fate, albeit over a much longer period. Exactly why these effects manifest following sleep deprivation is poorly understood.

14.3 Neurologic Control of Sleep–Wake Activity

Neuroscientists explain that sleep is the province of the brain but cannot say what it is about sleep that restores our bodies. That said, abnormal sleep often reflects a disorder of the brain and/or, conversely, results in impaired brain functioning.

The timing of sleep and wake activity is highly consistent and rigidly controlled within a given species, which strongly suggests that said timing is critical to optimum functioning. Research has suggested that sleep timing and propensity arises from the interplay of two closely related processes: the circadian rhythm, also known as process C, and the homeostatic process, AKA process S. While the timing of both REM and NREM sleep is influenced by the interaction of these processes,[1] REM sleep demonstrates a strong circadian pattern, while aspects of NREM sleep are primarily driven by homeostasis, meaning length of prior wakefulness. (See Figure 14.1)

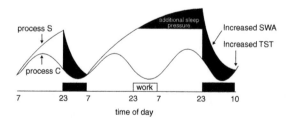

Figure 14.1 Borbely two model sleep regulation system. Process S represents the homeostatic model and process C the circadian rhythm. In this two model system, sleep propensity is directly proportional to the distance between process S and process C.
Source: Borbély A. A. and Achermann P. (1999). *Sleep homeostasis and models of sleep regulation. J. Biol. Rhythms* 14, 557–568.

Research over the last few decades has established that within the anterior hypothalamus of the brain, paired nuclei, known as the suprachiasmatic nuclei (SCN), act as the master clock that controls the circadian (from the Latin *circa* about and *diem* day) rhythm.[2] This neural pacemaker has a period of approximately 24 hours, allowing entrainment to the solar day. This internal representation of the light–dark cycle allows the organism to adapt itself to its ever-changing environment.

Incident light upon the retinae constitutes the main stimulus or time giver (*Zeitgeber*) that controls the circadian rhythm. Under normal circumstances, early morning light exposure sends impulses from the retinae via the retinohypothalamic tract (RHT)[3] to the SCN, which then resets itself – much as setting a mechanical watch daily keeps it running on time. The SCN may be viewed as something of a toggle switch that sets in motion the cyclic activity of specific wake-promoting and sleep-promoting neurons. The SCN has greater activity during the day compared to night. Targets of SCN activity are involved in modulating highly diverse activities, including autonomic and neuroendocrine function as well as sensorimotor integration and affective processes. Output of a portion of the SCN also controls the timing of melatonin release, which itself is central to bringing about sleep onset through negative feedback on the SCN.[4] Light inhibits melatonin production. (See Figure 14.2)

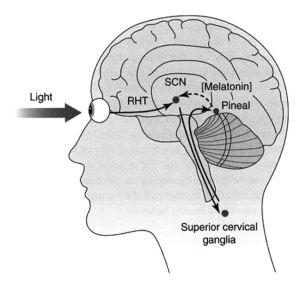

Figure 14.2 Retinal ganglion cells and Melatonin production. Retinal ganglion cells, which comprise the retinohypothalamic tract, transduce light information which is then signaled to the suprachiasmatic nucleus (SCN) of the hypothalamus. The SCN transmits these data to the pineal gland via a circuitous neural pathway passing through the superior cervical ganglion and inhibits melatonin production. In the absence of light, the inhibition is released resulting in melatonin secretion.

The oscillatory nature of circadian activity results from a transcriptional-translational molecular feedback mechanism of protein products of specific "clock genes."[5] Differences in these genes are associated with greater or lesser rates of said products, which probably account for individual predilections for being a "night owl" vs being a "lark."

While the SCN is considered the master clock, the expression of genes responsible for this molecular clock have been found in many other tissues and other regions of the brain. These peripheral oscillators, which affect things such as hormonal secretion and mental acuity, become desynchronized following damage to the SCN. For example, mental acuity is known to vary with the time of day, i.e. the phase of the circadian rhythm. Two dips in mental functioning and arousal occur approximately 12 hours apart, from about 1–3 am and again from about 1–3 pm. The latter probably accounts for the sleepiness which often occurs after lunch in persons who are already sleep-deprived to some extent. The timing of this cyclic pattern of peak mental clarity disappears following damage to the SCN.

In addition to the circadian rhythm, sleep regulation is also affected by the aforementioned homeostatic process, which may be summarized as follows: The physiologic propensity for sleep is directly proportional to the length of prior wakefulness.[6] In terms of its specific anatomic and physiologic substrate, process S is far less well understood than the circadian rhythm. Slow wave activity (SWA) power is the electroencephalographic signature of the homeostatic process. As the drive for sleep increases with extended wakefulness, the power of SWA increases with subsequent sleep, especially acutely. Adenosine and tumor necrosis factor alpha may be biochemical markers of sleepiness. Levels of adenosine and adenosine receptors in the portions of the brain correlate positively with sustained wakefulness.[7] Positron emission tomography has demonstrated increased expression of adenosine receptors during extended wakefulness. Further, both adenosine and adenosine receptor levels are reversed with recovery sleep. Caffeine, a potent wake-promoting substance, blocks adenosine receptors. While the circadian rhythm and the homeostatic process are often discussed as separate entities, one does not exist without the other in the regulation of the sleep–wake cycle. The balance between these two processes accounts for the timing, length and quality of sleep. Disruptions of signals from the circadian rhythm and/or the homeostatic process lead to complaints of insomnia or daytime sleepiness, depending on the nature of the associated perturbation. Together, the circadian rhythm and the homeostatic process have profound implications for all aspects of human behavior.

14.4 Brain Metabolic Activity during Sleep

For most animals, sleep is accompanied by physical inactivity. From a brain perspective, sleep is not a passive phenomenon. Recent research indicates that during sleep the brain undergoes active reorganization at the synaptic level, disposes of waste products that accumulate during wakefulness and consolidates new information.[8]

Many synapses that result from our daily activities and experiences are probably "pruned" when we sleep. According to the synaptic homeostasis hypothesis, salient synapses formed during the day are strengthened during sleep, allowing others to involute to save energy.[9] Further, evidence in support of synaptic reorganization and potentiation during sleep involves focal enhancement of homeostatic slow wave activity (SWA) following learning a specific motor task.[10] The enhanced focal SWA power noted in the right parietal lobe was also accompanied by improvement in performance of the task that occurred only after sleep. This enhanced performance did not occur in subjects who were re-tested after a period of wakefulness. Moreover, the degree of increased SWA power correlated with the magnitude of the reduction of directional error performing the task. Additionally, baseline SWA can be suppressed through immobilization of an extremity, further supporting the notion that SWA is the electrophysiological correlate of synaptic plasticity (at least in some instances). In contrast to the motor learning paradigm, the suppressed focal SWA correlates with impaired functioning during a motor task. Thus, SWA is thought to reflect synaptic potentiation, which arises from a cellular requirement for sleep that may result from the increased metabolic demand of learning.[11] This process of synaptic reorganization prioritizes new material, but is also necessary because the space available for the brain in the cranium allows for only so many synapses to exist. Maintaining synapses is metabolically expensive, so only those that provide the organism with optimum functioning should persist.[12]

Research into brain activity during sleep has demonstrated that the so-called glymphatic system of the brain, analogous to the systemic lymphatic system of the body, probably acts as a conduit for flushing toxins from neurons into the general circulation. Putative neurotoxins, such as beta amyloid, alpha synuclein and tau, accumulate within the interstitium (ISF) of the CNS during consciousness. The ISF is in dynamic equilibrium with the cerebrospinal fluid (CSF), resulting in convective exchange between the two fluid compartments. The channels of the ISF, referred to as the glymphatic system, envelop the neurons, glia and cerebral vasculature with CSF influxing from the arterial side and ISF into the venules. During sleep, the volume of the glymphatic system increases by approximately 60% compared to waking, which allows for enhanced clearance of the aforementioned neurotoxins.[13] The increase in clearance from this effective volume expansion is 95% compared to waking clearance. It may also be involved in neutralizing the soporific effects of adenosine that accumulates during consciousness.

Given the above, it is not surprising that the brain is metabolically very active during sleep. Despite the global reduction of cerebral blood flow and, thereby, metabolism during sleep, specific regions of the brain in both NREM and REM sleep have *increased* metabolic activity relative to wakefulness. For example, the pontine tegmentum, basal forebrain, anterior cingulate gyrus, right dorsoparietal association cortex, hypothalamus and regions of the mesial temporal lobes, become more metabolically active in NREM sleep compared to wakefulness.[14]

The mesial temporal lobe contains the amygdala and hippocampus, which are important components of emotive modulation and mnestic functioning. The increased glucose metabolism seen in the hippocampi in NREM sleep is comparable to that seen during active learning. The basal forebrain is also involved in cognition and memory. The nucleus basalis of Meynert within the basal forebrain shows profound degeneration, manifested by accumulation of beta amyloid and tau, in Alzheimer's patients.[15] Given the previously described putative clearance of neurotoxins such as beta amyloid and tau during sleep, chronic sleep deprivation may be a risk factor for dementia.[16]

PET scans obtained during REM sleep have consistently demonstrated increased activity in the pontine tegmentum and the limbic and paralimbic areas as noted in NREM.[17] The medial prefrontal cortex (MPFC) shows metabolic activity similar to that of wakefulness. The MPFC is a key component of the Default Mode Network (DMN), our principal resting state network. Additionally, the temporal and occipital cortices are active during REM, probably reflective of sensory experiences that arise with dreaming. The findings of enhanced metabolic activity in focal areas during sleep are consonant with the synaptic homeostasis model of sleep thought critical for the cerebral plasticity, which underpins a healthy homeostasis as well as learning and/or responses to novel stimuli.

The foregoing underscores the selective focal and differential character of cerebral metabolic activity during NREM and REM sleep, which in some instances is higher than during wakefulness. This is consistent with empiric evidence that sleep is an essential homeostatic process in a healthy brain. The fact that cetaceans sleep with half a brain at a time also suggests that physical inactivity may be not be essential to the function of sleep.

14.5 Insomnia

Good sleep is indispensable for normal mental functioning such as short-term memory, emotional modulation and judgment. Studies of sleep deprivation consistently show impairment in these and other areas. But what constitutes sleep deprivation? A recent study in the journal Sleep[18] demonstrated that persons getting 6 hours of sleep per night over a two-week period performed as poorly in some ways as did persons with total sleep deprivation for two days. Further, persons with 6 hours of sleep per night had far less insight into their impairment than did those with no sleep, meaning that these people made decisions thinking that their ability to perform was normal. These findings highlight the fact that even moderate chronic sleep restriction can produce serious impairment of waking functioning in otherwise healthy adults. Unfortunately, many people feel that 6 hours of sleep per night is perfectly adequate.

Insomnia in some form or another is likely the most common presenting sleep complaint at a doctor's office. It often results in symptoms of sleep deprivation. In some clinical studies, as many as 20% of adults are affected with insomnia and its consequences. According to the latest International Classification of Sleep Disorders, insomnia is defined as a persistent difficulty with sleep onset, maintenance, consolidation or quality that occurs despite adequate opportunity and circumstances for sleep and results in some form of impairment of daytime functioning.[19] To diagnose chronic insomnia, the reported sleep complaints must occur at least three nights a week for a minimum of three months. In adults, insomnia typically leads to poor performance in one's job or impairs social relationships. These persons often exhibit physical complaints such as increased muscular tension, gastrointestinal disturbances and palpitations. The Penn State Cohort study of insomnia with short sleep time in men indicates that such individuals are at increased risk of all-cause mortality.[20] Insomnia with objective short sleep is significantly associated with incident hypertension and type 2 diabetes.[21] Those affected are more likely to suffer from mental illness.[22] In children, insomnia often leads to reduced academic performance and behavioral problems.

14.6 Hyperarousal in Primary Insomnia

Insomnia has historically been approached from a behavioral perspective, but multiple lines of evidence indicate that many persons with insomnia have altered brain activity indicative of CNS hyperarousal in wakefulness and sleep compared to good sleepers. Hyperarousal, as manifested by sympathetic hyperactivity, is likely the main cause of cardiac mortality.[23]

Neuroimaging studies have demonstrated smaller differences in NREM-wake metabolism in persons with primary insomnia compared to good sleepers in multiple brain regions, including the DMN and sleep–wake neurons in the brainstem and hypothalamus.[24] These areas are strongly associated with affective modulation, cognition, self-reflection and sleep regulation. PET scans have demonstrated reduced metabolism in the DMN during waking in patients with primary insomnia.[25] Hypometabolism of the DMN may reflect psychological stress that is common among insomniacs.[26]

The concept of hyperarousal in persons with primary insomnia (PI) suggests three components of such hyperarousal, namely somatic, cognitive and neurocognitive.

Somatic arousal probably reflects hyperactivity of the sympathetic nervous system as manifested in elevated heart rate, cortisol levels, body temperature and whole-body metabolic rate described in PI.[27, 28, 29] Cognitive arousal is characterized by intrusive, repetitive and often negative thought patterns. When such patterns are induced experimentally, normal sleepers who are partially sleep-deprived demonstrate significant increases in sleep latency.[30]

EEG activity may be considered an endophenotype of what has been called neurocognitive arousal, manifested by changes in the EEG spectra of a QEEG. Beta and gamma power in QEEG are highly correlated with cognition.[31, 32, 33] Multiple QEEG studies of patients with PI have also demonstrated evidence of increased central nervous system arousal. In normal sleep, the spectral power of EEG transitions from a predominance of higher frequencies to lower frequencies.[34] In contrast, persons with PI do not demonstrate the usual reduction of high frequencies at sleep onset and during sleep maintenance.[35] Further, they exhibit increased beta power during waking,[36] increased beta and gamma power during NREM sleep,[37] and elevated beta during REM sleep.[38] They also have persistent alpha activity during sleep, despite lower levels of absolute alpha activity during wakefulness.[39, 40] Conversely, QEEG measurements have revealed significant deficits in delta power in both NREM and REM sleep.[41]

Taken together, the aforementioned data from functional neuroimaging, somatic physiology, cognitive and neurocognitive studies support a hypothesis of hyperarousal that occurs during both sleep and wakefulness in insomniacs. Thus, it may be more appropriate to view insomnia as a trait of brain dysregulation that affects individuals 24 hours a day. As we have seen, this elevated arousal is associated with endophenotypes such as elevated heart rate, blood pressure and cortisol to name a few. This may also explain the numerous co-morbidities and increased mortality associated with insomnia.

14.7 Current Treatment Recommendations for Insomnia

The most common therapy recommended in clinical practice for insomnia is pharmacotherapy. Currently, the FDA has granted approval of at least 14 different prescriptive chemical agents for the treatment of insomnia. It has been estimated that in 2013, approximately 7 million Americans received prescriptive medications for the treatment of insomnia.[42] Yet, according to the American Academy of Sleep Medicine (AASM) guidelines of 2017 using the GRADE footnote process, the evidence to recommend any of the currently available prescriptive hypnotics is "WEAK."[43] These recommendations are based on a systematic review of available randomized controlled trials of individual drugs, taking into consideration the quality of evidence, risk–benefit ratio and patient preferences. A STRONG recommendation is one that the clinician should, under most circumstances, follow. Whereas a WEAK recommendation indicates a lower degree of certainty in the outcome and appropriateness of the patient-care strategy for all patients. Downgrading the quality of evidence in this process reflects such factors as funding source for most clinical trials, the associated publication bias, and the small number of eligible trials.

It is noteworthy that the FDA has issued multiple Drug Safety Communications concerning the use of sedative-hypnotic drug products. These include warnings of next-morning impairment with zolpidem products (2013) and eszopiclone (2014), which resulted in the lowering of recommended dosing; warning of serious risk and death when combining opiates or cough medicine with benzodiazepines (2016); and warning against withholding opioid addiction medications from patients taking benzodiazepines or CNS depressants (2017).

Consonant with FDA warnings, epidemiologic evidence indicates increased all-cause mortality associated with hypnotic use. This is thought to be due to respiratory depression, especially in combination with opioids. Hypnotic usage is associated with increased serious illness and death in cancer, serious infections, disorders of mood and accidents.[44] The reported number of drug overdose deaths in 2017 was 47,055, compared to 19,854 in 2014.[45] According to *JAMA Psychiatry*, self-injury due to drug intoxication in 2013 was estimated at 68,298.[46] Multiple epidemiologic studies have demonstrated substantially elevated hazard ratios for mortality proportional to the number of doses of hypnotic per year. For example, the Geisinger Health System study showed fully-adjusted mortality ratios of 3.60 for 0.4–18 doses per year, 4.43 for 18–132 doses per year and 5.32 for more than 132 doses per year.[47] A similar study from Great Britain in 1996 revealed adjusted hazard ratios for mortality of 2.55 for 1–30 doses in a year, 3.78 for 31–60 doses in a year, 4.19 for 61–90 doses in a year and 4.51 for more than 90 doses (Figure 14.1).[48] Note that the hazard ratios for the two studies are similar. Furthermore, extrapolation of the Geisinger data to the pool of hypnotic users in the US lead to an estimated annual mortality of 300,000–500,000, more than that attributable to cigarette smoking.

Table 14.1 Adjusted mortality rates from usage of hypnotic drugs

Adjusted Mortality Ratios	Doses Per Year
3.6	.4 to 18
4.43	18 to 132
5.32	>132
Adjusted Hazard Ratios for Mortality	**Doses Per Year**
2.55	1 to 30
3.78	31 to 60
4.19	61 to 90
4.51	>90

Cognitive-behavior therapy (CBT) is founded on the premise that mental and psychological disorders are underpinned by maladaptive cognitive patterns. These patterns produce and maintain emotional distress, physiological arousal and behaviors that lead to dysfunction. Examples of maladaptive cognitions include unfounded or irrational beliefs regarding one's self, others, the world and the future – views that are particular to the patient and his circumstances. CBT utilizes tactics to counter these maladaptive cognitive patterns, resulting in a reduction of emotional distress and elimination of dysfunctional behaviors. The therapy requires active patient participation in a collaborative problem-solving dialectic, guided by the therapist, to challenge the validity of the patient's maladaptive beliefs.

A recent meta-analysis by Okajima et al.[49] reviewing 14 studies published from 1990–2009 examined the effect sizes, d, of CBT-I on sleep latency, SL, total sleep time, TST, total wake time, TWT, wake after sleep onset, WASO, early morning awakening, EMA, sleep efficiency, SE, and time in bed, TIB, from sleep diaries, polysomnograms (PSGs) or actigraphy. Subjective sleep variables from sleep diaries had medium to large effect sizes on SL (d = 0.67), TWT (d = 1.09), WASO (d = 0.07), EMA (d = 0.74), TIB (d = 0.80) and SE (d = 0.89). Medium to large d values for parameters evaluated by PSG and/or actigraphy were TWT (1.18), WASO (0.57), EMA (0.47) and SE (0.47). The authors also note that the beneficial effect of CBT-I remained in only a small number of parameters after publication bias (file drawer effect) was taken into account.

The most recent guidelines for non-pharmacologic therapy for chronic insomnia issued by the American Academy of Sleep Medicine (AASM) includes, as *Standard*, recommended therapy CBT-I, stimulus control therapy, relaxation training, and sleep restriction. A Standard recommendation is the strongest rating and refers to a generally accepted patient care strategy reflecting a high degree of clinical certainty. This recommendation is based on well-designed randomized trials with low alpha and beta errors, or on overwhelming evidence from randomized trials with high alpha and beta errors. It gives a guideline recommendation for biofeedback for treatment of chronic insomnia. Guideline evidence is a patient care strategy that reflects a moderate degree of clinical certainty based on randomized trials with high alpha and beta error or nonrandomized, concurrently controlled studies.

14.8 Behavioral Conditioning in Neurological Disease

Behavioral conditioning techniques used to treat neurological disorders have been described for more than two centuries. In 1772, Lysons[50] described a patient with focal epilepsy beginning in the feet, whose fits could be truncated by application of a tight garter at the knee. Repetition of this therapy resulted in weaker fits from the outset, until finally no treatment was needed at all. In 1881, Gowers[51] reported the arrest of Jacksonian fits by the application of a ligature just proximal to the elbow in a patient whose seizures began in the hand. After months of such treatment the seizures stopped spontaneously at the point of the previous application, even without ligature.

Multiple reports of "condition stimulating" used to produce specific physiological responses or even changes in EEG have proven that such conditioning has a direct effect on brain functioning. For example, pupillary constriction has been coupled to a sound and then to the command to "constrict."[52] Eventually, just the thought of the command was sufficient to produce the constriction. Multiple investigators have similarly conditioned alpha-blocking to nonvisual stimuli and, eventually, to the mere thought of such stimuli.[53, 54, 55] Such techniques are identical to those utilized by Pavlov to produce conditioned reflexes in dogs. These phenomena are thought to activate inhibitory neural pathways, which terminate either a normal physiological or pathological response – as in alpha-blocking or seizures, respectively.

Efron[56,57] described the fascinating case of a 41-year-old woman and professional singer with an uninterrupted 26-year history of unwaveringly rigid and stereotypic uncinate fits that were cured through a conditioned response. The seizures always began with a prolonged sense of depersonalization, followed by forced thinking, specifically, expecting a smell that never occurred. Next the patient experienced, in turn, a noxious olfactory hallucination, an auditory hallucination, and a versive head movement just before a generalized convulsive seizure. She had had from 7–18 of these spells a month with no more than a fortnight of respite from her seizures since they began at age 15. There had never been a spontaneous arrest of the seizures during this time. Further, they had been refractory to both diphenylhydantoin and phenobarbital.

Efron demonstrated that all her seizures could be successfully aborted by the application of a specific olfactory stimulus, in this case that of jasmine, provided it occurred *prior* to the appearance of the forced thinking. Further, the successful transference of seizure termination to the stimulus of viewing a silver bracelet, which had been coupled to the smell of jasmine, demonstrated a second order conditioned response. Eventually the patient could truncate the seizure by merely visualizing the bracelet in her mind. This practice was always accompanied by the olfactory hallucination of the odor of jasmine.

After the initial conditioning, the patient was exposed to I.V. metrazol to document the correlation of EEG changes with the progression of her previously well-documented semiology. It was discovered that the patient had become resistant to even high doses of this chemical.

For a six-week interval the patient was able to arrest the seizures by visualizing the bracelet. On several occasions, when she had not visualized the bracelet, she nevertheless experienced a spontaneous hallucination of the odor of jasmine, after which no further progression of the seizure occurred. For the subsequent 14 months, the patient had no episodes of depersonalization, nor did she rely on any external means to abort the seizures. Rather, she had occasional experiences of the spontaneous aroma of jasmine. She ultimately declared herself cured and was able to resume her career of singing.

14.9 Neurofeedback and Sleep

Various terms have been used to describe what is called neurofeedback. These include instrumental behavioral conditioning, instrumental SMR feedback, EEG biofeedback, neurofeedback and neurotherapy. I prefer the term neurofeedback because it is descriptive and concise. Although Margaret Ayers claimed that this therapy requires conscious awareness and effort on the part of the patient, i.e. it is operant conditioning, the evidence suggests otherwise. It is much more likely that this modality somehow appeals to the subconscious machinations of the brain that constitute a large majority of its workings.[58] Large effect sizes often seen with neurofeedback demand a reassessment of the "placebo effect." This has to be true with regard to the effect that operant conditioning had on Barry Sterman's cats, which could not have intentionally become resistant to chemically induced epilepsy, as described in Chapter 2.

In 1970, Sterman et al.[59] described the facilitation of sleep spindles (frequency approximately 12–14 Hz) in cats that had been conditioned to produce a similar pattern, known as SMR, noted over the sensorimotor cortex during quiet wakefulness. The presence of this specific EEG signature had previously been associated with inhibition of conditioned motor responses.[60] Cats so conditioned also experienced longer periods of consolidated quiet sleep, i.e. with fewer periods of phasic motor activity that typically fragment the quiet sleep of cats. These findings were strongly suggestive of a general alteration in brain functioning across waking and sleep from the operant conditioning of the SMR band.

Research has indicated that sleep spindles, which represent bursting activity of thalamocortical relay neurons, are associated with decreased activity of gamma motor neurons in the cat.[61] Moreover, patients with spinal cord injury have elevated SMR activity, attributable to reduced afferent input to thalamus.[62] SMR amplitudes and spindle-burst activity are severely reduced in some patients with epilepsy, but increases significantly following SMR training.[63] Spindles have also been associated with increases in auditory threshold during NREM sleep.[64] Conversely, differential sound oscillations which target sub-populations of spindles during NREM sleep, 11–13.5 Hz frontally and 13.5–16 Hz more posteriorly, have been found to affect the distribution of fast and slow spindles only in parietal areas.[65] These observations suggest that spindle bursts of N2 sleep correspond to a gating mechanism of sensory input and associated motor output of the central nervous system. Depending on the stimulus or sensory data involved, whether during wakefulness or sleep, spindles may interrupt input into the thalamus and the red nucleus, which is required for motoric activity, whether physiologic, such as walking, or pathologic, as in the case of epilepsy.

The published literature describing the effect of neurofeedback on persons with insomnia refers only to those with what has generally been known as primary insomnia or psychophysiological insomnia. These individuals have no known physiologic or medical condition to which their problematic sleep could be ascribed. These are subjects similar to those described as having biochemical, physiologic and neurophysiologic evidence of elevated arousal.

In 1973, Budzynski[66] reported improvement in sleep latencies in 6 of 11 insomniacs following a combination of frontalis EMG training, Alpha training and Theta training. Exact assessment protocol of the subjects was not described. Also, the combination of interventions makes it impossible to determine which had the desired effect.

Bell[67] described the improvement in self-reported sleep indices of a 42-year-old healthy woman with no history of psychiatric illness. She complained of difficulty with sleep onset despite taking nitrazepam 5 mg nightly for 5 years. Following 11 sessions of Theta neurofeedback, the patient noted improvement in time of settling down to sleep, pre-sleep intrusive cognitions, estimated sleep latency, number of awakenings and total sleep time. Following the therapy her medication was withdrawn over two weeks before being discontinued.

Her theta density increased from 9% at baseline to 17% by the final two sessions. In addition to the improved self-reported sleep parameters, the patient also demonstrated improvement in her general sense of wellbeing, based on the short version of the General Health Questionnaire. She had maintained her gains at a three months follow-up.

In 1981, Hauri[68] reported improvement in psychophysiologic insomniacs that was specific to the type of feedback used, depending on whether the subjects demonstrated high somatic or psychological tension or not. Those with elevated tension responded to theta feedback, whereas those without tension responded only to SMR feedback.

In 1982, he replicated these findings in a small randomized trial using standard protocols for both types of neurofeedback, something that was not the case in his initial study.[69] The subjects received approximately 26 sessions of either theta or SMR training over 13 weeks. It is noteworthy that with theta training SMR activity was inhibited, the converse being true with SMR training. An unexpected finding in this study was that all patients reported improvement in subjective sleep parameters, irrespective of the type of neurofeedback, but only patients who received "appropriate" therapy for their specific insomnia showed objective improvement in polysomnography (PSG), including sleep latency and sleep efficiency. Improvements were maintained or enhanced at nine months follow-up.

Berner et al.[70] explored the effect of four 10-minute sessions of neurofeedback on sleep and on a declarative memory paradigm, specifically reinforcing 11.6–16 Hz activity three hours before lights out. While this intervention did not affect the generation of spindles per se on the subsequent night's sleep, there was a trend for increased sigma band power (12–15 Hz) during NREM sleep in subjects receiving neurofeedback compared to those receiving pseudo-neurofeedback. They also noted that performance on the paired association test correlated positively with the quantitative spindle activity during the first half of sleep. Specifically, good performers had, on average, 33% higher spindle activity compared to poor performers.

A follow-up study from the same group in 2008[71] demonstrated enhanced spindle activity (sigma power) and improved sleep latency following 10 sessions of SMR training for 24 minutes each on consecutive days. These subjects also scored better on a word pair association task compared to controls who received random frequency feedback that was otherwise identical to the active arm. The transference of EEG changes to sleep from training during wakefulness is identical to that in cats described by Sterman in 1970.

To address the mechanism of neurocognitive hyperarousal in insomniacs, Cortoos reported in 2010[72] the results of tele-neurofeedback versus tele-EMG biofeedback in 17 patients with primary insomnia. The group sought ostensibly to affect EEG activity associated with cognitive processing, specifically high beta frequencies. The rationale for inhibiting theta rested on the fact that diminished theta power is associated with better daytime performance.[73] The neurofeedback group trained SMR (12 Hz) with inhibition of theta power (4–8 Hz) and high beta power (20–30 Hz) at CZ. The biofeedback group was instructed to decrease EMG at Fpz to promote relaxation. The visual display presented to each group was identical. Each group underwent 20 sessions, each lasting 20 minutes, over a period of 8 weeks.

The results on PSG indicated increased total sleep time only in the neurofeedback group. Both groups experienced shortened sleep latency compared to baseline PSG. Furthermore, only neurofeedback subjects demonstrated an overall improvement in sleep logs done at home.

Hammer[74] reported results of Z-score SMR versus QEEG-guided training for the treatment of patients with insomnia. Z scores obtained in real time were used to adjust the training parameters. Four patients were randomized to the SMR and four to the QEEG protocol, which consisted of fifteen 20-minute sessions. The primary outcome was change in sleep efficiency, SE, as measured by the Pittsburgh Sleep Quality Index (PSQI). Additionally, patients underwent pre- and post-assessments, including mental health, quality of life and insomnia status, based on multiple validated tools, such as the Insomnia Severity Index (ISI), the Minnesota Multiphasic Personality Inventory-2-Revised Form, the Psychiatric Diagnostic Screening Questionnaire and the Quality of Life Inventory. Posttreatment changes in QEEG were also reported. The patient had to be free of mental disorders or medical conditions which could interfere with sleep. They had to be free of prescription and over-the-counter medications for insomnia. Caffeine consumption was limited to fewer than five cups of coffee or caffeinated drinks per day. Shift workers were excluded.

Both groups showed improvement in all sleep parameters including the ISI, PSQI Global score and the PSQI SE. The mean increase in sleep efficiency for both groups was 16%. All participants had normal post-treatment sleep efficiencies of greater than 85%, with a mean of 93%. 7 of 8 subjects ended with a PSQI score of 5 or less, with the eighth subject having a score of 6. Similar results were found with the ISI. These improvements in sleep indices were accompanied by similar improvements in mood, sense of well-being and overall quality of life. This study strongly suggests that the simpler and more accessible protocol of SMR training was as effective as QEEG-guided neurofeedback.

Schabus et al. reported in 2014[75] the results of a counter-balanced, within subject design using 24 subjects with primary insomnia. These persons had been screened with appropriate and validated tools to exclude medical and psychiatric illnesses.

Subjects had to be free from medications and drugs and were limited in their use of caffeine and nicotine. All met AASM criteria for primary insomnia. Subjects were randomized to initial SMR instrumental conditioning at C3 or pseudo-instrumental conditioning. 12–15 Hz activity was used as feedback in the active arm and consisted of eight 3-minute blocks of conditioning for 10 sessions. Pseudo-conditioning consisted of 5 sessions of training that was identical to the active arm except for the use of random reward frequencies. Patients were instructed to move a compass needle as far to the left as they could but were given no specifics regarding how to do this. The main outcomes were enhanced sleep and performance on declarative memory.

PSG sleep parameters post-treatment demonstrated enhancement of N3 sleep and fewer awakenings. Further, there was a substantial enhancement and generation of fast sleep spindles that may have been related to the increased N3 sleep following SMR conditioning. Subjective well-being, as indicated by PSQI scores ($M = 10.83$ pre and $M = 7.00$ post), improved significantly. The study also indicated significant overnight forgetting in these insomnia subjects at baseline. While there was no overall effect of design versus pseudo-training on overnight memory or memory performance, linear correlations indicated an association between individual training success and improved memory in the design arm. Specifically, the authors suggest that the amount of 12–15 Hz enhancement during the SMR-training sessions correlated with improvement in overnight memory consolidation. They attributed the enhanced memory performance to the increase in fast spindle numbers on PSG. It is plausible that with more training sessions, a clear effect on memory could become evident, similar to that described by Hoedlmoser.[76] Finally, the data indicated that the random frequency pseudo-training had a negative effect on sleep quality.

14.10 Abnormal Sleep and ADHD

The sleep EEG (NREM) is characterized by slower frequencies and often higher voltage than that seen during wakefulness. As the focused waking alpha rhythm begins to wane, it is often replaced by theta activity, particularly in the temporal and frontal regions, with accompanying clinical manifestations of drowsiness. As noted above, the interaction between Process C and Process S plays a critical role in the timing and quality of sleep and, thereby, the regulation of vigilance. The core symptoms of ADHD can be induced in otherwise healthy children with sleep deprivation.[77] When one considers that children probably have, on average, greater than one hour less sleep compared to 100 years ago,[78] it seems quite plausible that perturbations of sleep may underpin the semiology of many persons with ADHD.

Recent clinical and electrophysiologic assessments of persons with ADHD, in fact, indicate that these syndromes may result, at least in part, from dysregulated sleep.[79] For example, the QEEGs in some patients with ADHD demonstrate findings similar to the aforementioned changes noted in drowsy individuals.[80] Further, sleep onset insomnia, which may represent a manifestation of a circadian rhythm disorder, has been found in up to 78% of unmedicated children and adults diagnosed with ADHD.[81,82,83] This finding has also been correlated with delayed dim light melatonin onset (DLMO).[84,85] Adults with ADHD are more likely to be evening types, which is thought to be due to delayed circadian phase.[86] While genetic factors are likely important in some patients with delayed circadian phase, it is clear that environmental influences, especially light exposure after sundown, contribute to dysregulated sleep as well.[87,88,89]

In 2014, Arns[90] reported the effects of SMR and theta/beta (TBR) neurofeedback on ADHD and insomnia in an open-label pilot study of 51 patients aged 6–53 years. The adult cohort was matched with 28 healthy controls aged 21–64. Adult subjects were screened for ADHD with the MINI Plus (Dutch version 5.0.0), and children with MINI KID. Inclusion in the study was based on DSM-V criteria. Subjects also completed a PSQI to assess sleep quality, including sleep latency (SOL) and duration (DUR).

Subjects underwent 2–3 sessions of neurofeedback per week of either SMR or TBR reinforcement. Specifically, the SMR group received reinforcement of 12–15 Hz at C3, C4 or Cz. The TBR group received reinforcement of beta frequencies in the ranges of 15–20 Hz and 20–25 Hz in the midline locations of Fz, FCz or Cz. Sessions lasted 20–23 minutes each. The specific protocol used was based on assessment with QEEG, which stratified subjects based on deviation from Z-scores of a normative data base (Brain Resource International). SMR training was used for subjects with low-voltage EEG whereas TBR was used for subjects with excess fronto-central theta. Each group had approximately 30 sessions of neurofeedback.

The ADHD cohort had significant correlations between symptoms of inattention and PSQI not seen in the control subjects. Abnormal SOL scores were noted in 57% of all ADHD subjects, but only 18% of controls. Sleep duration was also reduced in the ADHD cohort. Significant correlations were also noted for symptoms of inattention and PSQI.[91]

Both protocols showed improvement on cardinal ADHD symptoms and PSQI scores. Ultimate effect on SOL was also similar, but became manifest much sooner in the SMR protocol.

14.11 Case Presentations

Patient 1: A 72-year-old retired dentist presented with complaints of severe intermittent insomnia for more than 20 years. His initial Insomnia Severity Index (ISI) score was 24, indicating severe clinical insomnia. He especially had problems with sleep onset and maintenance, which he described as very severe. Additionally, the patient had severe mental rumination/anxiety about his inability to sleep, which caused a great deal of distress. His problematic sleep significantly interfered with his daytime functioning. Sleep was often worsened by life stressors and his frequent travel.

The patient had tried numerous medications including Ambien, Sonata, Lunesta and clonazepam, with limited benefit. Still, he took some form of hypnotic agent along with the clonazepam nightly. He also had some improvement with cognitive behavior therapy (CBT), including heart rate variability training, but the effects were not sustained. Additionally, he found undertaking the CBT somewhat cumbersome to maintain. His initial symptom tracker following 12 complaints had a score of 103.

The patient was also on continuous positive airway pressure (CPAP) for obstructive sleep apnea. He has historically had good compliance with CPAP with his average usage generally in the range of 7.5 hours per night.

ILF Neurofeedback was initiated with Cygnet at 0.5 mHz at T4-P4, with the frequency being optimized to 0.001 mHz over 12 sessions. Because of a persistence of racing thoughts, T4-Fp2 was added for a time to his protocol. He has had a total of 39 sessions over approximately 18 months, including 16 of both 10 Hz and 40 Hz Synchrony training. His most recent ISI score was 0, indicating no significant insomnia. His last symptom tracker composite score was 49. He takes hypnotic medications only a few times a month, usually with travel.

Patient 2: A 49-year-old realtor who was effectively house-bound by anxiety and complaints of insomnia. Following a total hysterectomy, the patient began to have crying spells and complaints of depression. She had been placed on various mood stabilizers, including Zoloft, Paxil and citalopram, but these were associated with significant side effects. For example, with Zoloft and Paxil she had paranoid episodes as well as visual hallucinations consisting of seeing blood on people. She became quite fearful. Also, she noted a burning sensation in the back and arms with these medications as well as with citalopram. She was also taking prn Xanax 2–3 times daily for acute anxiety.

She had an initial ISI score of 28, the highest possible. Her baseline symptom tracker composite score (19 items) was 185. She complained of major problems with sleep onset, maintenance and waking early, all of which had a debilitating effect on her daytime functioning. She developed severe anxiety over not being able to sleep, in addition to symptoms of generalized anxiety. She was also on nightly zolpidem CR 12.5.

ILF Neurofeedback was initiated with Cygnet at T4-P4 at 0.5 mHz. This was optimized to 0.01 mHz over the first 8 sessions, after which the patient noted significant improvement in sleep, with ISI decreasing to 20. Her insomnia worsened with ISI rebounding to 25 for reasons that were not immediately clear. Optimization at T4-P4 continued with the addition of T4-Fp2, which was associated with further improvement in insomnia. By session 12 the patient was at 0.005 mHz, with continued improvement in symptom severity. She noted also that she was no longer needing to take Xanax daily. By session 30 her ISI had decreased to 6, consistent with no clinical insomnia. By session 42 the patient had optimized to 0.001 mHz for both T4-P4 and T4-Fp2. She had also resumed her work as a realtor. Her husband endorsed what he felt was a major improvement in his wife's overall functioning.

By session 52 she had discontinued the Xanax completely. By session 55 she had discontinued the zolpidem completely. She now has intermittent sessions once or twice a month, including ILF and Synchrony for maintenance. Her most recent symptom tracker composite score was 13, and her ISI was 0. (See Figures 14.3 and 14.4.)

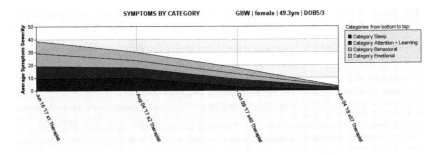

Figure 14.3 Symptom tracker for case 2 by symptom category. Note the marked reduction of all symptom categories from Jan 2017 to Jun 2018.

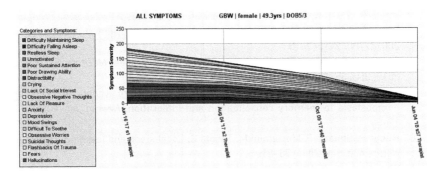

Figure 14.4 Case 2 symptom tracker by specific symptom complaints over same time interval as Figure 14.3.

14.12 Conclusions

Published reports of the benefits of neurofeedback for persons with epilepsy, insomnia and ADHD appeared in the 1970s.[92, 93, 94] This is not a new therapy. By now the collective literature is robust. Therapeutic protocols of NF are based on accepted principles of neuroanatomy and neurophysiology. Moreover, NF, through its effects on brain self-regulation, holds the promise of uncovering much of the inner workings of brain functioning. The effect size of improvements with NF compares favorably to that of pharmacotherapy, and NF avoids the potential deleterious effects of medications used to treat these conditions. Thus far there are no indications that NF produces any long-term adverse effects when it is in qualified, competent hands. Finally, the evidence indicates that effects of NF are long lasting – a clear advantage over the usual pharmacotherapy. As such, it is incumbent upon clinicians/researchers who treat persons with neuropsychological conditions to consider seriously the information contained in this chapter, and in this volume. This will require a paradigm shift among all health care professionals, but the benefits to our patients are potentially enormous.

Notes

1 Borbély AA, Daan S, Wirz-Justice A, Deboer TJ; *Sleep Res* Apr 2016; 25(2): 131–143. doi: 10.1111/jsr.12371. Epub 2016, Jan14.
2 Moore RY; The fourth C.U. Ariens Lecture. The organization of the human circadian timing system. *Prog Brain Res* 1992; 93: 101–117.
3 Dai J, Van Der Vliet J, Swaab D, Ruud M; Human Retinohypothalamic tract as revealed by in vitro postmortem tracing. *J Comp Neurol* 1998; 397: 357–370.
4 Moore RY; Suprachiasmatic nucleus. *International and Cyclic PD of Social and Behavioral Sciences* 2001; 15290–15294.
5 Von Schantz M, Archer S; Clocks, genes and sleep. *J Royal Soc Med* 2003; 96: 486–489.
6 Dai J, op. cit.
7 Elmenhorst D, Philipp T, Meyer OH, Winz AM, Ermert J, Coenen HH, Basheer R, Haas HL, Zilles K, Bauer A; Sleep deprivation increases A1 adenosine receptor binding and the human brain: A positron emission tomography study. *J Neurosci* 2007; 27(9): 2410–2415.
8 Eugene A, Masiak J; The neuroprotective aspects of sleep. *MEDtube Sci* March 2015; 3(1): 35–40.
9 Tononi G, Cirella C; Sleep and the price of plasticity: From synaptic and cellular homeostasis to memory consolidation and integration. *Neuron* Jan 2014; 81: 12–34.
10 Huber R, Ghilardi F, Massimini M, Tononi G; Local sleep and learning. *Letters to Nature* 430: July 2004; 78–81.
11 Wilhelm I, et al.; Sleep selectively enhances memory expected to be of future relevance. *J Neurosci* Feb 2011; 31(5): 1563–1569.
12 Tononi, op. cit.
13 Xie L, et al.; Sleep drives metabolic clearance from the adult brain. *Science* Oct 2013; 342(6156): 373–377.
14 Nofzinger E, Buysse D, et al.; Human regional glucose metabolism during non-rapid eye movement sleep in relation to waking. *Brain* 2002; 125: 1105–1115.
15 Whitehouse PJ, et al.; Alzheimer's disease and senile dementia: Loss of neurons in the basal forebrain. *Science* Mar 1982; 215(4537): 1237–1239.
16 Di Meco A, Joshi YB, Pratico D; Sleep deprivation impairs memory, tau metabolism, and synaptic integrity of a mouse model of Alzheimer's disease with plaques and tangles. *Neurobiol Aging* 2014; 35(8): 1813–1820.
17 Braun A, Balkin T, et al.; Dissociated pattern of activity in visual cortices and their projections during human rapid eye movement sleep. *Science* 279(5347): 91–95.
18 Van Dongen H, Maislin G, et al.; The Cumulative cost of additional wakefulness: Dose-response effects on neurobehavioral functions and sleep physiology from chronic sleep restriction and total sleep deprivation. *Sleep* 2003; 26(2): 117–126.
19 International Classification of Sleep Disorders. Third edition; Insomnia: 19–21.
20 Vgontzas AN, Liao D, Slobodanka P, et al.; Insomnia with short sleep duration and mortality: The Penn State Cohort. *Sleep* 2010; 33(9): 1159–1164.
21 Vgontzas AN, Liao D, Bixler EO, et al.; Insomnia with objective short sleep duration is associated with a high risk for hypertension. *Sleep* 2009; 32(4): 491–497.

22 Buysse DJ, Angst J, Gamma A, et al.; Pervalence, course, and comorbidity of insomnia and depression in young adults. *Sleep* 2008; 31(4): 473–480.

23 Baroldi G, Silver M; *The etiopathogenesis of coronary heart disease: A heretical theory based on morphology.* Second edition; Landes Bioscience, Austin, Texas, 2004.

24 Nofzinger E, Buysse D, et al.; Functional neuroimaging evidence for hyperarousal in insomnia. *Am J Psychiatry* 2004; 161: 2126–2129.

25 Kay D, Karim H, et al.; Sleep-wake differences in relative regional cerebral metabolic rate for glucose among patients with insomnia compared to good sleepers. *Sleep* 2016; 39: 1779–1794.

26 Hall M, Thayer J, et al.; Psychological stress is associated with heightened physiological arousal during NREM sleep in primary insomnia. *Behav Sleep Med* 5(3): 178–193.

27 Bonnet MH, Arand DL; 24-hour metabolic rate in insomniacs and matched normal sleepers. *Sleep* 1995; 18: 581–588.

28 Vgontzas AN, Bixler EO, et al.; Chronic insomnia is associated with nyctohemeral activation of the hypothalamic-pituitary-adrenal axis: Clincial implications. *J Clin Edocrinol Metab* 2001; 86: 3787–3794.

29 Rodenbeck A, Huether G, et al.; Interactions between evening and nocturnal cortisol secretion and sleep parameters in patients with severe chronic primary insomnia. *Neurosci Lett* 2002; 324: 159–163.

30 De Valck E, Cluydts R, et al.; Effect of cognitive arousal on sleep latency, somatic and cortical arousal following partial sleep deprivation. *J Sleep Res* 2004; 13: 295–304.

31 Basar-Ergolu C, Struber D, Schurmann M, et al.; Gamma-band responses in the brain: A short review of psychophysiological correlates and functional significance. *Int J Psychophysiol* 1996; 24: 101–112.

32 Jefferys JGR, Traub RD, et al.; Neuronal networks for induced "40 Hz" rhythms. *Trends Neurosci* 1996; 19: 202–208.

33 Makeig S, Jung T-P; Tonic, phasic and transient correlates of auditory awareness in drowsiness. *Cogn Brain Res* 1996; 4: 15–26.

34 De Gennaro L, Ferrara M, et al.; The boundary between wakefulness and sleep: Quantitative electroencephalographic changes during the sleep onset period. *Neurosci* 2001; 107: 1–11.

35 Staner L, Cornette F, et al.; Sleep microstructure around sleep onset differentiates major depressive insomnia from primary insomnia. *J Sleep Res* 2003; 12: 319–330.

36 Lamarche CH, Ogilvie RD; Electrophysiological changes during the sleep onset period of psychophysiological insomniacs, psychiatric insomniacs and normal sleepers. *Sleep* 1997; 20: 724–733.

37 Perlis ML, Smith MT, et al.; Beta/gamma EEG activity in patients with primary and secondary insomnia and good sleeper controls. *J Sleep Res* 2001; 24: 110–117.

38 Merica H, Blois R, et al.; Spectral characteristics of sleep EEG in chronic insomnia. *Eur J Neurosci* 1998; 10: 1826–1834.

39 Staner, op. cit.

40 Lamarche, op. cit.

41 Merica, op. cit.
42 Bertisch SM, Herzig SJ, Winkelman JW, Buettner C; National use of prescription medications for insomnia: NHANES 1999–2010. *Sleep* 2014; 37(2): 343–349.
43 Sataia M, Buysse D, et al.; Clinical practice guideline for the pharmacologic treatment of chronic insomnia in adults: An American Academy of Sleep Medicine clinical practice guideline. *J Clin Sleep Med* 2017; 13(2): 307–349.
44 Kripke D; Hypnotic drug risks of mortality, infection, depression, and cancer: But lack of benefit. *F1000Research* 2018; 5(918): 1–19.
45 Sun Y, Lin C, et al.; Association between zolpidem and suicide: A nationwide population-based case-control study. *Mayo Clin Proc* 2016; 91(3): 308–315.
46 Rockett I, Caine E; Self-injury is the eighth leading cause of death in the United States: It is time to pay attention. *JAMA Psychiatry* 2015; doi: 10.1001/jamapsychiatry.2015.1418.
47 Hartz A, Ross JJ; Cohort study of the association of hypnotic use with mortality in postmenopausal women. *BMJ Open* 2012; 2(1): pii: e001413.doi: 10.1136/bmjopen-2102-001413.
48 Kripke DF, Langer RD, Kline LE; Hypnotics' association with mortality or cancer: A matched Cohort study. *BMJ Open* 2012; 2(1): e000850.
49 Okajima I, Komada Y, Inoue Y; A meta-analysis on the treatment of effectiveness of cognitive behavioral therapy for primary insomnia. *Sleep Biol Rhythms* 2011; 9: 24–34.
50 Lysons D; *Practical Essays upon Intermitting Fevers*. Bath, 1772.
51 Gowers W; *Epilepsy and Other Chronic Convulsive Conditions*. London, 1881.
52 Hudgins CV; Conditioning and the voluntary control of the pupillary light reflex. *J General Psychol* 8: 3–51.
53 Jasper H, Shagass C; Conditioning of the occipital alpha rhythm in man. *J Exp Psychol* 1941; 28(5): 373–388.
54 Jasper H, Shagass C; Conscious time judgements related to conditioned time intervals and voluntary control of the alpha rhythm. *J Exp Psychol* 1941b; 28: 503–508.
55 Travis LE, Egan JP; Conditioning of the electrical response of the cortex. *J Exp Psychol* 1938; 22(6): 524–531.
56 Efron R; The effect of olfactory stimuli in arresting uncinate fits. *Brain* Jun 1956; 79(2): 267–281.
57 Efron R; The conditioned inhibition of uncinate fits. *Brain* Jun 1957; 80(2): 251–262.
58 van Lommel P. *Consciousness Beyond Life: The Science of the Near Death Experience*. Harper Collins, New York, 2010.
59 Sterman MB, Howe RC, Macdonald LR; Facilitation of spindle-burst sleep by conditioning of electroencephalographic activity while awake. *Science* 167(3921): 1146–1148.
60 Roth SR, Sterman MB, Clemente CD; Comparison of EEG correlates of reinforcement, internal inhibition and sleep. *Electroencephalogr Clin Neurophysiol* 1967; 23: 509–520.
61 Hongo T, Kubota K, Shimazu H; EEG spindle and depression of gamma motor activity. *J Neurophysiol* 1963; 26: 568–580.

62 Sterman MB; Effects of Sensorimotor EEG Feedback Training on Sleep and Clincal Manifestations of Epilepsy. *Biofeedback and Behavior*, 167–200. Plenum Press, New York, 1977.

63 Sterman, op. cit.

64 Bonnet MH, Moore SE; The threshold of sleep: Perception of sleep as a function of time asleep and auditory threshold. *Sleep* 1982; 5(3): 267–276.

65 Antony JW, Paller KA; Using oscillating sounds to manipulate sleep spindles. *Sleep* 2016; 40(3): 1–8.

66 Budzynski TH, Biofeedback procedures in the clinic. *Seminars in Psychiatry* 1973; 5(4): 537–547.

67 Bell SJ, The use of EEG theta biofeedback in the treatment of a patient with sleep-onset insomnia. *Biofeedback Self Regul* 1979; 4(3): 229–236.

68 Hauri P, Treating psychophysiological insomnia with biofeedback. *Arch Gen Psychiatry* 1981; 38: 752–758.

69 Hauri P, The treatment of psycholphysiologic insomnia with biofeedback: A replication study. *Biofeedback Self Regul* 1982; 7(2): 223–235.

70 Berner I, Schabus M, et al.; The significance of sigma neurofeedback training on sleep spindles and aspects of declarative memory. *Appl Psychophysiol Biofeedback* 2006; 31(2): 97–113.

71 Hoedlmoser K, Pecherstorfer MS, et al.; Instrumental conditioning of human sensorimotor rhythm (12–15 Hz) and its impact on sleep as well as declarative learning. *Sleep* 2008; 31(10): 1401–1408.

72 Cortoos A, De Valck E, Arns M; An exploratory study of the effects of tele-neurofeedback and tele-biofeedback on objective and subjective sleep in patients with primary insomnia. *Appl Psychophysiol Biofeedback* 2010; 35: 125–134.

73 Klimesch W, Sauseng P, Hanslmayer G, et al.; Event-related phase reorganization may explain evoked neural dynamics. *Neurosci Biobehav Rev* 2007; 31: 1003–1016.

74 Hammer B, Colbert A, Brown K, Ilioi E; Neurofeedback for insomnia: A pilot study of Z-Score SMR and individualized protocols. *Appl Psychophysiol Biofeedback* 2011; 36: 251–264.

75 Schabus M, Heib D, Lechinger J, et al.; Enhancing sleep quality and memory in insomnia using instrumental sensorimotor rhythm conditioning. *Biol Psychol* 2014; 95: 126–134.

76 Hoedlmoser, op. cit.

77 Golan N, Shahar E, Ravid S, Pillar G; Sleep disorders and daytime sleepiness in children with attention-deficit/hyperactive disorder. *Sleep* 2004; 27(2): 262–266.

78 Matricciani L, Olds T, Petkov J; In search of lost sleep: Secular trends in the sleep time of school-aged children and adolescents. *Sleep Med Rev* 2012; 16(3): 203–211.

79 Arns M, Kenemans JL; Neurofeedback in ADHD and insomnia: Vigilance stabilization through sleep spindles and circadian networks. *Neurosci Biobehav Rev* 2014; 44: 183–194.

80 Arns M, Conners CK, Kraemer HC; A decade of EEG theta/beta ratio research in ADHD: A meta- analysis. *J Atten Disord* 2013; 17: 374–383.

81 Van der Heijden KB, Smits MG, Van Someren EJ, Gunning WB; Idiopathic chronic sleep onset insomnia in attention-deficit/hyperactivity disorder: A circadian rhythm sleep disorder. *Chronobiol Int* 2005; 22(3): 559–570.

82 Smits MG, Nagtegaal JE, van der Heijden J, et al.; Melatonin for chronic sleep onset insomnia in children: A randomized placebo-controlled trial. *J Child Neurol* 2001; 16: 86–92.
83 Van Veen MM, Kooij JJ, Boonstra AM, et al.; Delayed circadian rhythm in adults with attention-deficit/hyperactivity disorder and chronic sleep-onset insomnia. *Biol Psychiatry* 2010; 67(11): 1091–1096.
84 Smits MG, Nagtegaal JE, van der Heijden J, et al.; Melatonin for chronic sleep onset insomnia in children: A randomized placebo-controlled trial. *J Child Neurol* 2001; 16: 86–92.
85 Van Veen MM, Kooij JJ, Boonstra AM, et al.; Delayed circadian rhythm in adults with attention-deficit/hyperactivity disorder and chronic sleep-onset insomnia. *Biol Psychiatry* 2010; 67(11): 1091–1096.
86 Rybak Y, McNeely H, Mackenzie B, et al.; Seasonality and circadian preference in adult attention-deficit/hyperactivity disorder: Clinical and neuropsychological correlates. *Comp Psych* 2007; 48: 562–571.
87 Baird AL, Coogan AN, Siddiqui A, et al.; Adult attention-deficit hyperactivity disorder is associated with alterations in circadian rhythms at the behavioural, endocrine and molecular levels. *Mol Psych* 2012; 17: 988–995.
88 Bijlenga D, van der Heijden KB, Breuk M, et al.; Associations between sleep characteristics, seasonal depressive symptoms, lifestyle and ADHD symptoms in adults. *J Atten Disord* 2013; 17(3): 261–275.
89 Arns M, van der Heijden KB, Eugene Arnold L, et al.; Reply to: Attention-deficit/hyperactivity disorder: The sunny perspective. *Biol Psychiatry* 2013; 76: e21–e32.
90 Arns M, Feddema I, Kenemans JL; Differential effects of theta/beta and SMR neurofeedback in ADHD on sleep onset latency. *Front Human Neurosci* 2014; 8: 1–10.
91 Lubar JF; Shouse MN. EEG and behavioral changes in a hyperkinetic child concurrent with training of the sensorimotor rhythm (SMR): A preliminary report. *Biofeedback Self Regul* 1976; 3: 293–306.
92 Sterman, op. cit.
93 Bell, op. cit.
94 Ayers M; Assessing and Treating Open Head Trauma, Coma and Stroke Using Real-Time digital EEG Neurofeedback. In *Introduction to Quantitative EEG and neurofeedback*, 203–222. Academic Press, 1999.

Chapter 15

Conclusion

The Future of Neurofeedback

Siegfried Othmer

The optimal subjects in whom to intervene therapeutically are those who are destined but not yet manifest.

C.R. Jack, The Living Brain and Alzheimer's Disease, 2004

15.1 Introduction

Making projections for the future of neurofeedback is a challenge because the barriers are no longer either technical or conceptual. They are sociological and political and economic. On the larger canvas, they are also cultural. Neurofeedback is representative of an emerging class of technologies that exploit latent brain plasticity to improve functionality and remediate mental dysfunction. This is quite literally a scientific revolution, and revolutions are always messy and unpredictable in their particulars. Often they don't come into focus except in retrospect. In this case, as in others, the emergent technology goes against a number of established beliefs, deeply entrenched practices, powerful economic interests, and basic cultural proclivities. Progress is going to be fitful until some kind of tipping point is reached, and the environment switches from an adversarial to a competitive one. At present, the neurofeedback pilot vessel plows forward like an icebreaker, creating the circumstances that are favorable for its continued movement as it goes. Some thick ice needs to be broken up every step of the way. Not many step in to assist its progress, as they are convinced that the cargo is nothing but fool's gold. Once it is discovered that it is indeed carrying real gold, there will be a struggle over who gets to pilot the ship and who has title to the treasure.

The full acceptance of neurofeedback is contingent on a transition in our understanding of how the brain is organized, and in this book we have tried to create that understanding. As pointed out in Chapter 1, we need to move collectively beyond an understanding mainly in terms of neurotransmitter and neuromodulator systems to an understanding in terms of neural network models and their organization. As pointed out in Chapters 2 and 3, brain behavior is organized with great spatial specificity and temporal precision. Its failures lie there as well. The operative assumption is that brain-based dysfunctions are traceable in large measure to the established behavior patterns of neural networks. These are to be regarded in three aspects: There is the realm of the core structural networks; there is the realm of functional connectivity that organizes itself on those networks around core functions; and there is the realm of brain dynamics, in which the brain maintains its homeodynamic status in real time, while exercising all of its responsibilities in terms of managing the interface with the outside world.

As shown in Part III, many, if not most, mental dysfunctions are sustained by patterns of network organization that have established themselves either through trauma or injury, or through a learning process. Hence these patterns of organization are predominantly acquired characteristics. Only in extreme cases, or only at the margins, are they grounded in flaws at the level of the core structural networks. This means that they lie in the functional domain and are largely accessible to us for remediation, which presents a substantial therapeutic opportunity. But that is not all. Genetic flaws may also be compensated for within the scope of brain plasticity.

15.2 The Ideal Future of Neurofeedback

One way to envision neurofeedback in its maturity is to imagine its application over the lifespan. The following assumes that financial barriers have been largely surmounted and a certain technological maturity has developed within the population at large. In this idyllic future, the idea of training the brain to improved functionality is broadly accepted, and there is some appreciation of the principles underlying the method.

Matters begin even before birth, as the mother-to-be takes advantage of neurofeedback to prepare herself for labor. As a result, the birth process goes much more smoothly than expected. After birth, the likelihood of post-partum depression has surely been reduced by the prior training, but in the event that it occurs, neurofeedback is used to pull the mother out of her depressed state. The infant seems fine, but in the event that it is difficult to soothe, is at times inconsolable, does not allow the parents any sleep, threatens to become a fussy eater, or has only fitful bowel function, a few sessions of neurofeedback are undertaken to let the brain find its way toward calmer and more controlled states.

Early on, if the child shows signs of not engaging with other people, perhaps withdrawing from eye contact, neurofeedback training would again be brought to bear. A few years later, it might be drawn upon to help with bedwetting. In the event of febrile convulsions or mild head injuries some sessions of neurofeedback training would be done as a matter of course, irrespective of any evidence of functional deficits. In the first days of school, neurofeedback training might help with separation anxiety.

In elementary school, if the child falls behind academically or shows any sign of struggling with mastery of the material, neurofeedback would be recruited as a matter of course. The same would hold if the child has difficulty fitting into the class because of social anxiety. The class bully would also be invited to undergo brain training. If attentional deficits manifest, then neurofeedback training would be drawn upon at once. As academic challenges mount in later years, more training may be done to shore up the child's native abilities. If any child cannot master the challenges presented in elementary school with ease, is disengaged or overwhelmed, then most likely neurofeedback can help.

During the years of insecurity in adolescence, the child may be offered Alpha-Theta training in order to get a bearing on who they really are, and to wind up their personal gyroscope to set their internal compass to carry them through those awkward years. The Alpha-Theta training enhances ego strength in the fragile adolescent, and acquaints him with his core self. This experience may well buffer him against the importuning of ostensible friends.

As the young adult enters college there may well be issues of performance anxiety that could benefit from neurofeedback. Issues of personal identity may surface that could benefit from Alpha-Theta training. Academic struggles could be eased by means of neurofeedback practice. Participation in sports may motivate additional training sessions to enhance skills.

As the fresh college graduate faces the world of work, neurofeedback may quell any concerns about poor performance in interviews and auditions. The stresses of the working world can be ameliorated as necessary with the occasional training session. Performance artists could add neurofeedback training to their preparatory routines, and professional athletes could prepare for each competition with a booster session. Individuals who do a lot of traveling could use neurofeedback to reduce the impact of time zone changes on their productivity and on their sleep cycles.

In later years, the familiar training would be utilized in order to maintain mental sharpness and good memory access, retain good sleep architecture, and aid in pain management, if necessary. And as the end of life is approached, neurofeedback could be very helpful with the mental pre-occupations involved in that transition. Alpha-Theta training can be very helpful in giving the person perspective on life and relationships, and conferring equanimity in the confrontation of death. If the person wishes to nourish spiritual impulses, the training can serve to reinforce and deepen them. It is entirely a question of what the person brings to the experience. The training will move to whatever state the person finds comforting, because inherently it moves toward the person's core self.

The broad diffusion of neurofeedback into society presupposes the emergence of a suitable technological vehicle that allows the training to be conducted with the sole guidance of the person at interest or of a parent or other family member. Infra-Low Frequency training does not fit readily into this mold because the training is so sensitively dependent on the specifics. A trained practitioner should always be in charge. On the other hand, the beginnings of a personal care model are already unfolding, with ILF training being inserted into home care for autistic children, dementia, and other conditions.

At present, home training is only being done selectively in cases where long-term training is needed, and where responsible parents or caregivers are managing the process. This option can be complemented with remotely guided training, where the clinician selects the training parameters remotely. Over time, ILF training will become more fault-tolerant through the integration of software that manages the frequency optimization procedure on the basis of a variety of independent measures of physiological function.

In this manner, neurofeedback can propel us to a future in which people increasingly take responsibility for their own well-being. This future was projected years ago by John Knowles, then President of the Rockefeller Foundation: "The next major advance in the health of the American people will result from the assumption of individual responsibility for one's own health."

15.3 Predicting Future Developments

We are already seeing trends toward making information on physiological measures available to people in real time. This is being driven first of all by the exercise market, where heart rate monitors are ubiquitous. Also on the horizon are devices for cueing drivers and pilots on their state of alertness. In these cases, the feedback is to the person in order to inform his judgment, rather than to the person's brain in order to influence its activity. But the latter may not be far behind.

The elements are all there. In the future, there will be increasing reliance placed on monitors of physiological activity that will inform feedback to the person or to his brain directly. The intelligence will be lodged in software that translates information on physiological state into the most effective kind of feedback to the brain.

The first wave of neurofeedback will involve its insertion broadly into clinical practice within psychiatry, neurology, geriatrics, pediatrics, primary care, psychology, family therapy, and the rehabilitative disciplines of osteopathy, physical therapy, occupational therapy, and educational therapy. The second wave will be the broad adoption of neurofeedback among athletes, performers in the arts, corporate executives, and cultural creatives, etc. for their personal benefit. The third wave will involve the emergence of the prevention model of neurofeedback, in which it will be applied routinely starting as early in life as the need for it is recognized, and leading ultimately to the universal adoption of neurofeedback training as an aid in child-raising.

The cost barrier with respect to instrumentation is easily surmounted in this electronic age. The electronics are not intrinsically expensive. The cost is volume-driven. The real cost driver is the clinician involvement. This is a clear requirement in the application to clinical conditions. However, even in that domain trainees can reach the point where they are sufficiently acquainted with their own response to the training that they can monitor the process on their own. And this indicates the path forward. Once people get acquainted with their brains with the help of a clinician, they can start to take responsibility for their own training and only use the clinician as an intermittent resource to move the process along as their needs change.

Perhaps even more significant than the cost barrier is the issue of time commitment. It is a well-known problem that exercise equipment bought for the home soon sits idle in the basement or garage. Exercise gyms are packed on January second, but fishing for customers by September. The answer is to incorporate neurofeedback into other activities. ILF training can be done in the background while the trainee is reading the newspaper on his computer screen or watching television. For youngsters it can be incorporated into video games. And auditory neurofeedback could even be done while taking a walk or commuting. Finally, if all else fails and time has to be set aside for the training, the trainee can always busy himself with video material that engages him. Neurofeedback does not need to be boring.

15.4 Neurofeedback in the Family

We can project a future in which caring parents not only get to know their children intimately, but they also know their neurofeedback protocols. And when spouses start to bicker, they will not blame each other but rather propose that the spouse's brain may not be in a propitious state at that moment, and for that matter, the state of their own brain may be the issue. They will both be reminded to train their brains, and they could even do that jointly in couples training. In consequence, the warring atmospheres that prevail in so many households can reach disarmament status without nicks to any egos. There are no winners and losers. Neurofeedback can play a major role in relationship repair precisely because the process is not cognitive, and is therefore not judgmental. It resolves relationship problems without getting egos tied in a knot.

This is also the pathway to the resolution of multi-generational trauma that is incubated in dysfunctional families, which is likely the single most significant mental health issue faced by our society.

15.5 Neurofeedback in Social Services and Criminal Justice

In this ideal future, neurofeedback will be broadly introduced into the foster care system. Many foster parents find themselves taking on children with Developmental Trauma that they cannot handle. This is no personal failing; these problems cannot, in fact, be handled by ordinary means available to parents. Neurofeedback is the only known remedy. The remedy is also cost-effective, if comparison is made to the absence of neurofeedback that we have presently. A study in Utah years ago found that the average cost to the State of a foster child that aged out of the system was $50,000 per year. In comparison, neurofeedback is a bargain.

Neurofeedback will also be broadly introduced into the juvenile justice system. This is yet another system of care in which we temporarily house those with unre-mediated Developmental Trauma. By the same token, neurofeedback will be broadly diffused into the prison system. This may take a while, however, as the system is not presently oriented toward rehabilitation. Neurofeedback will also be struggling uphill because the system is presently structured to bring about the destruction of personhood, particularly in its increasing reliance on solitary confinement. It is difficult to escape the impression that in today's prisons the disintegration of personhood is the explicit, if unspoken, objective. Once neurofeedback is well rec-ognized in society, the return of the prison system to a rehabilitation model will be only a matter of time.

15.6 Neurofeedback in Education

Brain training for school children will assume a place in the minds of parents analogous to gym class. If a child might benefit from neurofeedback, then it is in our society's interest to provide the opportunity. Once again, the cost–benefit ratio is substantial. Just as a solid case can be made for providing pre-school opportunities to children, an even stronger case can be made for neurofeedback. That is principally because this intervention works with even the most challenged children. School systems expend collectively 20% on special education services, with a cost factor of 1.9 with respect to regular students. The addition of neurofeedback to the special education curriculum would substantially decrease the residence time in special education settings for most of these children. This can be accomplished for less than the cost of one year of special services. The real payoff to society, though, comes from the fact that the trained individual is much more functional than would have been the case otherwise.

15.7 Summary and Conclusion

In this chapter we have assumed that the insertion of neurofeedback into our society will take two principal forms. On the one hand it will come to play a dominant role in the field of mental health, as well as a supportive role in health care in general. On the other it will come to be broadly adopted by the lay public for aid in meeting life's challenges. This transition is contingent on three major conceptual shifts: 1) The adoption of the Dysregulation Model in mental health and the incorporation of Functional Medicine into the health care field in general; 2) The recognition of self-regulation as the appropriate remedy for Disorders of Dysregulation; and 3) A shift toward the broad adoption of the Prevention Model in health care.

In the public sphere, there will be a movement to appropriate this technology for the augmentation of function on the one hand, and for self-discovery and spiritual practice on the other. The former will be driven, initially, by parents in need of help with their children, and the other by the seekers, the cultural creatives. The insertion of neurofeedback into society will lead to the adoption of new modes of thinking about our own nature and how it is constrained by physiology. This, in turn, will have profound implications for child care, for the field of education, for the criminal justice system, and for how we deal with addictions. The impact on our culture will be as substantial as the direct effect on our collective well-being.

Coming to terms with our brains will be the defining watershed of the 21st century. The belated acceptance of the concept of brain plasticity in the closing years of the 20th century opened the door to the entry of neurofeedback into the mainstream of medicine. Historian Arnold Toynbee projected that the 21st would be the century of spirituality. That will likely come true, but in a more inclusive and expansive frame than perhaps he had the means to intimate. This is the century in which the right hemisphere assumes its rightful place, one it relinquished at the dawn of the Enlightenment. Right hemisphere consciousness is breaking the boundaries on left hemisphere thinking that has constrained our sense of self and shaped our modern institutions.

Infra-Low Frequency Neurofeedback with the right hemisphere gives us access to the experiencing self, and facilitates the person's more intimate communion with self. In this manner, we build the capacity for nurturing the self and for fostering strong relationships. A future in which all may live up to their full potential is one worth striving for.

Index

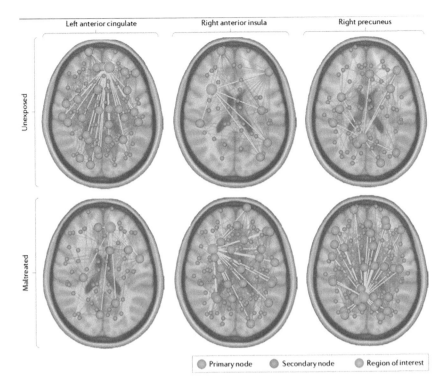

Figure 3.1

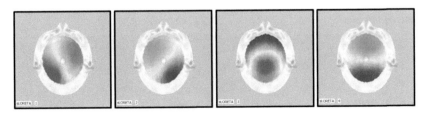

Figure 3.7

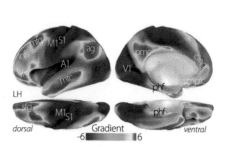

Figure 3.4

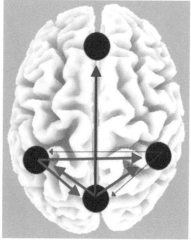

Figure 3.8

Results Summary:

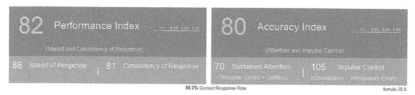

Figure 10.1

RAW DATA	Period 1 Sect. 1 Low Demand	Period 2 Sect. 1 Low Demand	Period 3 Sect. 2 High Demand	Period 4 Sect. 2 High Demand	Period 5 Sect. 3 Low Demand	Sect. 1	Sect. 2	Sect 3	Total
Omissions(#)	0	0	1	0	0	0	1	0	1
Outliers	1	0	1	14	3	1	15	3	19
Commissions(#)	0	0	2	1	1	0	3	1	4
Response time(ms)	393	440	394	444	482	417	417	482	423
Variability(ms)	61	91	90	125	83	81	110	83	90

Figure 10.2

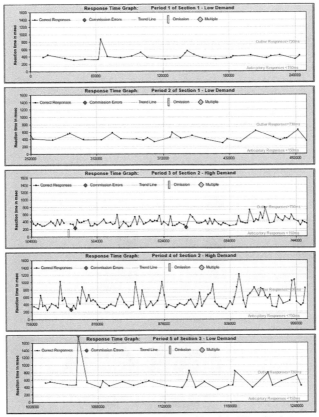

X-Axis for all charts: time into QIKtest in msec, with vertical gridlines of 1 minute

Figure 10.3

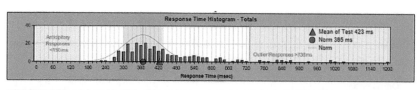

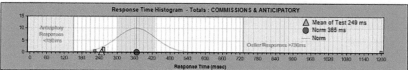

Norms: the blue line represents a normal distribution of reaction times for this age and group: compare by form and position to your data in red. The light blue area represents 68.2% (or ±1σ) of a normal distribution.

Figure 10.4

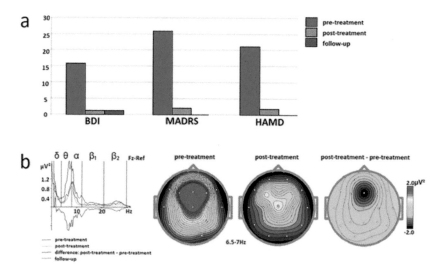

Figure 12.2